Moller's Essentials of Pediatric Cardiology

T0188758

Moller's Essentials of Pediatric Cardiology

FOURTH EDITION

Walter H. Johnson, Jr., MD
Professor of Pediatrics
Department of Pediatrics
Division of Pediatric Cardiology
University of Alabama at Birmingham
Birmingham, AL, USA

Camden L. Hebson, MD
Associate Professor of Pediatrics
Department of Pediatrics
Division of Pediatric Cardiology
University of Alabama at Birmingham
Birmingham, AL, USA

WILEY Blackwell

Contents

Preface

Since the first printing of this text 50 years ago, pediatric cardiac catheterization, echocardiography, computed tomography, and magnetic resonance imaging have developed and less emphasis has been placed on the more traditional methods of evaluating a cardiac patient. Most practitioners, however, do not have access to these refined diagnostic techniques or the training to apply them. To evaluate a patient with a finding that could suggest a cardiac issue, a practitioner therefore relies upon either the combination of physical examination, electrocardiogram, and chest X-ray, or referral to a cardiac diagnostic center.

This book formulates guidelines by which a practitioner, medical student, or house officer can approach the diagnostic problem presented by an infant or child with a cardiac finding. Through proper assessment and integration of the history, physical examination, electrocardiogram, and chest X-ray, the type of problem can be diagnosed correctly in many patients, and the severity and hemodynamics correctly estimated.

Even though a patient may ultimately require referral to a cardiac center, the practitioner will appreciate and understand better the specific type of specialized diagnostic studies performed, and the approach, timing, and results of operation or management. This book helps select patients for referral and offers guidelines for timing of referrals.

The book has 12 chapters:

Chapter 1 (Tools to diagnose cardiac conditions in children) includes sections on history, physical examination, electrocardiography, and chest radiography, and discusses functional murmurs. A brief overview of special procedures, such as echocardiography and cardiac catheterization, is included.

Chapter 2 (Environmental and genetic conditions associated with heart disease in children) presents syndromes, genetic disorders, and maternal conditions commonly associated with congenital heart disease.

Chapters 3–7 are "Classification and physiology of congenital heart disease in children," "Anomalies with a left-to-right shunt in children" (acyanotic and with increased pulmonary blood flow), "Conditions obstructing blood flow in children" (acyanotic and with normal blood flow), "Congenital heart disease with a right-to-left shunt in children" (cyanosis with increased or decreased pulmonary blood flow), and "Unusual forms of congenital heart disease in children." This set of chapters discusses specific congenital cardiac malformations. The hemodynamics of the malformations are presented as a basis for understanding the physical findings, electrocardiogram, and chest radiographs. Emphasis is placed on features that permit differential diagnosis.

Chapter 8 (Unique cardiac conditions in newborn infants) describes the cardiac malformations leading to symptoms in the neonatal period and in the transition from the fetal to the adult circulation.

Chapter 9 (The cardiac conditions acquired during childhood) includes cardiac problems, such as Kawasaki disease, rheumatic fever, and the cardiac manifestations of systemic diseases which affect children.

Chapter 10 (Abnormalities of heart rate and conduction in children) presents the practical basics of diagnosis and management of rhythm disorders in children.

Chapter 11 (Congestive heart failure in infants and children) considers the pathophysiology and management of cardiac failure in children. Medical and surgical (including circulatory support devices, and transplantation) treatments are discussed.

Chapter 12 (A healthy lifestyle and preventing heart disease in children) discusses preventive issues for children with a normal heart (the vast majority), including smoking, hypertension, lipids, exercise, and other risk factors for cardiovascular disease that become manifest in adulthood. Prevention and health maintenance issues particular to children with heart disease are also discussed.

This book is not a substitute for the many excellent and encyclopedic texts on pediatric cardiology, or for the expanding number of electronic resources. The "Additional reading" sections accompanying some chapters and the additional reading section at the end of the book include both traditional and online resources chosen to be of greatest value to readers.

Certain generalizations are made. In pediatric cardiology, as in all fields, exceptions occur. Therefore, not all instances of cardiac abnormality will be correctly diagnosed on the basis of the criteria set forth here.

Chapter 1
Tools to diagnose cardiac conditions in children

Much of the information presented in this chapter relates best to older infants and children. Diagnosis in newborn infants is more difficult, because the patient may be very ill and in need of an urgent diagnosis for prompt treatment. In this age group, echocardiography is often the initial diagnostic method. The unique challenges in newborns are discussed in Chapter 8.

The history and physical examination are the keystones for diagnosis of cardiac problems. A variety of other diagnostic techniques can be employed beyond the history and physical examination. With each technique, different aspects of the cardiovascular system are viewed, and by combining the data derived, an accurate assessment of the patient's condition can be obtained.

Moller's Essentials of Pediatric Cardiology, Fourth Edition.
Walter H. Johnson, Jr. and Camden L. Hebson.
© 2023 John Wiley & Sons Ltd. Published 2023 by John Wiley & Sons Ltd.

HISTORY

General principles of the cardiovascular history

The suspicion of a cardiovascular abnormality may be raised initially by specific symptoms, but more commonly the presenting feature is the discovery of a cardiac murmur. Many children with a cardiac abnormality are asymptomatic because the malformation does not result in major hemodynamic alterations. Even with a significant cardiac problem, the child may be asymptomatic because the myocardium is capable of responding normally to the stresses placed upon it by the altered hemodynamics. A comparable lesion in an adult might produce symptoms because of coexistent coronary arterial disease or myocardial fibrosis.

In obtaining the history of a child suspected of cardiac disease, one seeks three types of data: those suggesting a diagnosis, assessment of severity, and the etiology of the condition.

Diagnostic clues

Diagnostic clues and other more general factors include the following.

Gender. Certain cardiac malformations have a definite gender predominance. Atrial septal defect (ASD) and patent ductus arteriosus (PDA) are two to three times more likely in female than in male children. Coarctation of the aorta, aortic stenosis, and transposition of the great arteries occur more commonly in male children.

Age. The age at which a cardiac murmur or a symptom develops may give a diagnostic clue. The murmurs of congenital aortic stenosis and pulmonary stenosis are often heard on the first examination after birth. Ventricular septal defect (VSD) is usually first recognized because of symptoms and murmur at two weeks of age. The murmur of an ASD may not be discovered until the preschool examination. A functional (innocent) murmur is found in at least half of school-age children.

Severity of the cardiac condition

Information that suggests the condition's severity (e.g. dyspnea or fatigue) should be sought.

Etiology

The examiner should seek information that suggests an etiology of cardiac condition (e.g. maternal lupus).

Chief complaint and/or presenting sign

Certain presenting complaints and signs are more common in particular cardiac disorders and the "index of suspicion" aids the medical professional in organizing the data to make a differential diagnosis. For many of the signs and symptoms discussed later, *noncardiac causes are often more likely than cardiac causes* (e.g. acute dyspnea in a previously healthy four-month-old infant with no murmur is more likely a result of bronchiolitis than of congestive heart failure). Therefore, a complete history must be integrated with the physical examination and other diagnostic studies to arrive at the correct cardiac diagnosis.

The most common symptoms or signs found in an outpatient setting are murmur, chest pain, palpitations, and near-syncope (fainting).

Murmur

Murmur is the most common presenting finding because virtually all children and adults with a normal heart have an innocent (normal) murmur sometime during their lifetime. Certain features are associated with an innocent murmur; the child is asymptomatic and murmurs appearing after infancy tend to be innocent. The murmur of ASD is one important exception.

Chest pain

Chest pain is a common and benign symptom in older children and adolescents, estimated to occur at some time in 70% of school-aged children. About 1 in 200 visits to a pediatric emergency room is for chest pain.

Chest pain rarely occurs with cardiovascular disease during childhood. Myocardial ischemic syndromes (e.g. Kawasaki disease with coronary artery aneurysms; hypertrophic cardiomyopathy) may lead to true angina. Patients with connective tissue disorders (e.g. Marfan syndrome) may have chest (or back) pain from aortic dissection. Although pericarditis may cause chest pain, it is almost always associated with fever and other signs of inflammation. Occasionally, chest pain accompanies supraventricular tachycardia. Most children with congenital cardiac malformations, including those who are fully recovered from surgery, do not have chest pain, and most children and adolescents who present with chest pain as their chief complaint do not have a cardiac malformation or disease.

Most chest pain is benign. It is usually transient, appearing abruptly, lasting from 30 seconds to five minutes, and localized to the parasternal area. It is distinguished from angina by the absence of diaphoresis, nausea, emesis, and paresthesias in an ulnar distribution. Benign chest pain is typically well localized, sharp in character (not "crushing" like angina), short in duration (seconds to minutes), often aggravated by certain positions or movements, and occasionally can be induced by palpation over the area. Benign chest pain may also occur as a result of chest wall tenderness. These characteristics are strong evidence against cardiac cause for the pain. Some noncardiac conditions (e.g. asthma) may be associated with childhood chest pain. Benign pain is often described as "functional" because an organic cause cannot be found.

Palpitations

Palpitations, the sensation of irregular heartbeats, "skipped beats," or, more commonly, rapid beats, are also common in the school-aged child and adolescent. They frequently occur in patients with other symptoms, such as chest pain, but often not simultaneously with the other symptoms. Palpitations are often found to be associated with normal sinus rhythm when an electrocardiogram is monitored during the symptom. Palpitations are not usually present in patients with known premature beats. Palpitations of sudden onset (approximately the time span of a single beat) and sudden termination suggest tachyarrhythmia.

Syncope and orthostatic intolerance

Syncope is a sudden, brief loss of consciousness associated with loss of postural tone, with a spontaneous recovery. It is a common presenting symptom to the cardiology clinic, present in up to 15% of children, especially during the adolescent years. Life-threatening etiologies are rare but possible, and, when present, are often cardiac in nature. Worrisome historical features, such as lack of any prodrome, occurrence during exercise, or antecedent strong palpitations necessitate a more extensive work-up. Cardiac causes for syncope include electrical (i.e. long QT syndrome [LQTS], Brugada) and structural (hypertrophic cardiomyopathy, coronary anomalies, aortic stenosis, pulmonary hypertension) conditions. Further clues as to these diagnoses may come from the family history, which should be explored for sudden death, syncope, seizures, sudden infant death syndrome (SIDS), swimming deaths, and single-occupant motor vehicle fatalities.

Despite the concern a syncopal episode often generates, benign etiologies are often the culprit, with vasovagal syncope being the most common pediatric diagnosis (>80% of pediatric syncope). Vasovagal syncope occurs when the autonomic nervous system overreacts to a trigger, such as dehydration, pain, or emotional upset, with the result being bradycardia and/or vasodilation and thus significant cerebral hypoperfusion, leading to loss of consciousness and tone. With a fall to the ground, gravity no longer hinders restoration of cerebral perfusion and the patient quickly reawakens. Further history obtained from these patients typically includes inadequate fluid and salt intake, preceding postural change or prolonged upright body position, and, importantly, prodromal dizziness prior to syncope. Frequent postural dizziness without syncope often also is present. When persistent and sufficiently distressing to the patient, this is referred to as orthostatic intolerance. Orthostatic intolerance is quite common in teenagers due to the higher metabolic needs during adolescence, lack of adequate fluid and salt intake by the teenagers to meet these needs, and propensity for anxiety as a result of the symptoms generated. In addition to dizziness, patients with orthostatic intolerance complain of headaches, palpitations, fatigue, and difficulty concentrating. Patient and family education and counseling are vital to improve these symptoms, as a sufficient and consistent plan, to improve fluid and salt intake and deal with emotional upset, is needed. Vitamin D and iron deficiency are common in those with persistent symptoms and can be supplemented when present. Most patients improve considerably over time.

Dyspnea

Dyspnea (labored breathing) is different from tachypnea (rapid breathing). It is a symptom present in patients with pulmonary congestion from either left-sided cardiac failure or other conditions that raise pulmonary venous pressure or from marked hypoxia. Dyspnea is manifested in neonates and infants by rapid, grunting respirations associated with retractions. Older children complain of shortness of breath. The most common causes in children are asthma and bronchitis, whereas in the first year of life it is often associated with pulmonary infections or atelectasis.

Fatigue

Fatigue on exercise must be distinguished from dyspnea as it has a different physiologic basis. In neonates and infants, fatigue on exercise is indicated by difficulty while feeding. The act of sucking while feeding requires energy and is "exercise." It is manifest by infants by stopping frequently during nursing to rest, and the feeding may take an hour or more.

Exercise intolerance of cardiac origin indicates an inability of the heart to meet the increased metabolic demands for oxygen delivery to the tissues during this state. This can occur in three situations:

- *Cyanotic congenital heart disease* (arterial oxygen desaturation).
- *Congestive cardiac failure* (inadequate myocardial function).
- *Severe outflow obstructive conditions or those causing cardiac filling impairment* (inadequate cardiac output).

Fatigue on exercise or exercise intolerance is a difficult symptom to interpret because other factors, such as motivation or amount of training, influence the amount of exercise that an individual can perform. To assess exercise intolerance, compare the child's response to physical activity with that of peers and siblings or with their previous level of activity.

The remaining symptoms are found more commonly in neonates and infants.

Growth retardation

Growth retardation is common in many children who present with other cardiac symptoms within the first year of life.

Infants with cardiac failure or cyanosis. These infants show retarded growth, which is more marked if both are present. Usually, the rate of weight increase is more delayed than that of height. The cause of growth retardation is unknown, but it is probably related to inadequate caloric intake due to dyspnea and fatigue during feeding and to the excessive energy requirements of congestive cardiac failure.

Growth. Growth may also be retarded in children with a cardiac anomaly associated with a syndrome, such as Down syndrome, which in itself causes growth retardation.

Developmental milestones. Developmental milestones requiring muscle strength may be delayed, but usually mental development is normal. To assess the significance of a child's growth and development, obtaining growth and development information about siblings, parents, and grandparents is helpful.

Congestive cardiac failure

Congestive cardiac failure leads to the most frequently described symptom complex in infants and children with cardiac disease. In infants and children, 80% of instances of heart failure occur during the first year of life; these are usually associated with a cardiac malformation. The remaining 20% that occur during childhood are related more often to acquired conditions. Infants with cardiac failure are described as slow feeders who tire when feeding, this symptom indicating dyspnea on exertion (the act of sucking a bottle). The infant perspires excessively, presumably from increased catecholamine release. Rapid respiration, particularly when the infant is asleep, is an invaluable clue to cardiac failure in the absence of pulmonary disease. The ultimate diagnosis of cardiac failure rests on a compilation of information from the history, the physical examination, and laboratory studies such as chest X-ray and echocardiography. Management of congestive cardiac failure is discussed in Chapter 11.

Respiratory infections

Respiratory infections, particularly pneumonia and respiratory syncytial virus (RSV), are frequently present in infants, and, less commonly, in older children with cardiac anomalies, especially those associated with increased pulmonary blood flow (left-to-right shunt) or with a greatly enlarged heart. The factors leading to the increased incidence of pneumonia are largely unknown but may be related to compression of the major bronchi by either enlarged pulmonary arteries, an enlarged left atrium, or distended pulmonary lymphatics.

Atelectasis may also occur, particularly in the right upper or middle lobe, in children with greatly increased pulmonary blood flow, or in the left lower lobe in children with a cardiomyopathy and massively dilated left atrium and ventricle.

Cyanosis

Cyanosis is a bluish or purplish color of the skin caused by the presence of at least 5 g/dL of reduced hemoglobin in capillary beds. The desaturated blood imparts a bluish color to the appearance, particularly in areas with a rich capillary network, such as the lips or oral mucosa. The degree of cyanosis reflects the magnitude of unsaturated blood. Mild degrees of arterial desaturation may be present without cyanosis being noted. Usually, if the systemic arterial oxygen saturation is less than 88%, cyanosis can be recognized – this varies with skin pigmentation, adequacy of lighting, and experience of the observer. A minimal degree of cyanosis may appear as a mottled complexion, darkened lips, or plethoric fingertips. Clubbing develops with more significant degrees of cyanosis.

Cyanosis is classified as either peripheral or central.

Peripheral cyanosis. Peripheral cyanosis, also called *acrocyanosis*, is associated with normal cardiac and pulmonary function. Related to sluggish blood flow through capillaries, the continued oxygen extraction eventually leads to increased amounts of desaturated blood in the capillary beds. It typically involves the extremities and usually spares the trunk and mucous membranes. Exposure to cold is the most frequent cause of acrocyanosis, leading to blue hands and feet in neonates and circumoral cyanosis in older children. Peripheral cyanosis disappears upon warming. The normal polycythemia of neonates may contribute to the appearance of acrocyanosis.

Central cyanosis. Central cyanosis is related to any abnormality of the lungs, heart, or hemoglobin that interferes with oxygen transport from the atmosphere to systemic capillaries. Cyanosis of this type involves the trunk and mucous membranes in addition to the extremities. A variety of pulmonary conditions, such as atelectasis, pneumothorax, and respiratory distress syndrome, can cause cyanosis. Areas of the lungs, although not ventilated, are perfused, and blood flowing through that portion of the lung remains unoxygenated. Thus, desaturated blood returns to the left atrium and mixes with fully saturated blood from the ventilated portions of the lungs. Rarely, dysfunctional hemoglobin disorders, such as excessive levels of methemoglobin, result in cyanosis because hemoglobin is unable to bind normal quantities of oxygen.

Cardiac conditions cause central cyanosis by either of two mechanisms:

(1) *Structural abnormalities*. Structural abnormalities that divert portions of the systemic venous return (desaturated blood) away from the lungs can be caused by two categories of cardiac anomalies:
   (a) *Conditions with obstruction to pulmonary blood flow and an intracardiac septal defect* (e.g. tetralogy of Fallot).
   (b) *Conditions in which the systemic venous and pulmonary venous returns are mixed in a common chamber before being ejected* (e.g. single ventricle).
(2) *Pulmonary edema of cardiac origin*. Mitral stenosis and similar conditions raise pulmonary capillary pressure. When capillary pressure exceeds oncotic pressure, fluid crosses the capillary wall into the alveoli. The fluid accumulation interferes with oxygen transport from the alveolus to the capillary so that hemoglobin leaving the capillaries remains desaturated.

Cyanosis resulting from pulmonary edema may be strikingly improved by oxygen administration, whereas cyanosis occurring with structural cardiovascular anomalies may show little change with this maneuver.

Squatting

Squatting is a relatively specific symptom, occurring almost exclusively in patients with tetralogy of Fallot. It has virtually disappeared except in countries where children with tetralogy of Fallot do not have access to surgery. When experiencing a hypercyanotic or "tet" spell, cyanotic infants assume a knee/chest position, whereas older children squat in order to rest. In this position, the systemic arterial resistance rises, the right-to-left shunt decreases, and the patient becomes less desaturated.

Neurologic symptoms

Neurologic symptoms may occur in children with cardiac disease, particularly those with cyanosis, but are seldom the presenting symptoms. Brain abscess may accompany endocarditis in severely cyanotic children. Stroke may be seen in cyanotic patients and the rare acyanotic child with "paradoxical" embolus occurring via an ASD. Stroke may also occur intra- or postoperatively, or as a result of circulatory support devices, and in cardiomyopathy, and rarely in children with arrhythmia.

In otherwise apparently normal children, *seizures* stem from arrhythmias, such as the ventricular tachycardia seen in the LQTS, and may be the sole presenting symptom.

Prenatal history
A prenatal history may also suggest an etiology of the cardiac malformation if it yields information such as maternal rubella, drug ingestion, other teratogens, or a family history of cardiac malformation. In these instances, a fetal echocardiogram is often performed to identify possible anomalies of the heart or other organ systems.

Family history
The examiner should obtain a complete family history and pedigree to disclose the presence of congenital cardiac malformations, syndromes, or other disorders, such as hypertrophic cardiomyopathy (associated with sudden death in young persons) or LQTS (associated with a family history of seizures, syncope, and sudden death).

Other facts obtained on the history that may be diagnostically significant will be discussed in this book in relation to specific cardiac anomalies.

PHYSICAL EXAMINATION
When examining a child with suspected cardiac abnormalities, the examiner may focus too quickly on the auscultatory findings, overlooking the general physical characteristics of the child. In some patients, these findings equal the diagnostic value of the cardiovascular findings.

Cardiac abnormalities are often an integral part of generalized diseases and syndromes: recognition of the syndrome can often provide a clinician with either an answer or a clue to the nature of the associated cardiac disease. These syndromes are discussed in Chapter 2.

Vital signs

Blood pressure
In all patients suspected of cardiac disease, examiners should record accurately the blood pressure in both arms and one leg. Doing this aids in diagnosis of conditions causing aortic obstruction, such as coarctation of the aorta, recognition of conditions with "aortic runoff," such as PDA, and identification of reduced cardiac output.

Many errors can be made in obtaining the blood pressure recording. The patient should be in a quiet, resting state, and the extremity in which blood pressure is being recorded should be at the same level as the heart. A properly sized blood pressure cuff must be used because an undersized cuff causes false elevation of the blood pressure reading. A slightly oversized cuff is unlikely to affect readings greatly. Therefore, blood pressure cuffs of various sizes should be available. A guide to the appropriate size for each age group is given in Table 1.1.

Table 1.1 Recommended dimensions for blood pressure cuff bladders.

Age range	Width (cm)	Length (cm)	Maximum arm circumference (cm)[a]
Newborn	4	8	10
Infant	6	12	15
Child	9	18	22
Small adult	10	24	26
Adult	13	30	34
Large adult	16	38	44
Thigh	20	42	52

[a]Calculated so that the largest arm would still allow the bladder to encircle the arm by at least 80%.

This is a work of the US government, published in the public domain by the American Academy of Pediatrics, available online at http://pediatrics.aappublications.org/content/114/supplement_2/555 and http://www.nhlbi.nih.gov/health/prof/heart/hbp/hbp_ped.htm.

Source: Adapted from National High Blood Pressure Education Program Working Group on High Blood Pressure in Children and Adolescents. The Fourth Report on the Diagnosis, Evaluation, and Treatment of High Blood Pressure in Children and Adolescents. *Pediatrics*, 2004, **114** (2 Suppl. 4th Report), 555–576.

Generally, the width of the inflatable bladder within the cuff should be at least 40% of the circumference of the limb, and the bladder length should encompass 80–100% of the circumference of the limb at the point of measurement. In infants, placing the cuff around the forearm and leg rather than around the arm and thigh is easier.

Although a 1-inch-wide cuff is available, it should never be used because it leads uniformly to a falsely elevated pressure reading except in the tiniest premature infants. A 2-inch-wide cuff can be used for almost all infants.

Failure to pause between readings does not allow adequate time for return of venous blood trapped during the inflation and may falsely elevate the next reading.

Methods. Four methods of obtaining blood pressure can be used in infants and children – three manual methods (flush, palpatory, and auscultatory) and an automated method (oscillometric).

For manual methods, the cuff should be applied snugly and the manometer pressure quickly elevated. The pressure should then be released at a rate of 1–3 mmHg/s and allowed to fall to zero. After a pause, the cuff can be reinflated. Pressure recordings should be repeated at least once.

Flush method. A blood pressure cuff is placed on an extremity, and the hand or foot is tightly squeezed. The cuff is rapidly inflated and the infant's hand or foot is released. As the cuff is slowly deflated, the value at which the blanched hand or foot flushes reflects the mean arterial pressure. By connecting two blood pressure cuffs to a single manometer and placing one cuff on the arm and the other cuff on the leg, simultaneous blood pressure can be obtained.

Palpation. Palpation can also be used in infants. During release of the pressure from the cuff, the pressure reading at which the pulse appears distal to the cuff indicates the systolic blood pressure. A more precise but similar method uses an ultrasonic Doppler probe to register the arterial pulse in lieu of palpating it.

Auscultation. In an older child, blood pressure can be obtained by the auscultatory method: in the arm, by listening over the brachial artery in the antecubital space, or in the leg and in the thigh, by listening over the popliteal artery. The pressure at which the first Korotkoff sound (K_1) is heard represents the systolic pressure. As the cuff pressure is released, the pressure at which the sound muffles (K_4) and the pressure at which the sound disappears (K_5) should also be recorded. The diastolic blood pressure is located between these two values.

Automated methods. Automated methods have largely replaced the manual methods. They are widely used in ambulatory, hospital, and intensive care settings. These oscillometric methods use a machine that automatically inflates and deflates the cuff while monitoring pulse-related air pressure fluctuations within the cuff. Deflation is performed in a stepwise fashion, and at each step the machine pauses for two seconds or less while the cuff pressure oscillations are recorded. The amplitude of these pulsatile oscillations begins to increase as the cuff pressure falls to the level of the systolic blood pressure, reaches a maximum amplitude at a cuff pressure equal to mean blood pressure, and diminishes as cuff pressure falls to diastolic levels. Because the method depends on measurement of faint pulsatile pressure oscillations, irregular heart rhythm (e.g. atrial fibrillation), conditions with beat-to-beat variability in pulse pressure (e.g. the pulsus alternans of heart failure or mechanical ventilator-induced changes), and patient movement may lead to inaccurate or absent readings.

Normal values. The normal blood pressure values for different age groups are given in Figure 1.1 and Tables 1.2 and 1.3. The blood pressure in the leg should be the same as that in the arm. Leg blood pressure should also be taken with an appropriate-sized cuff, usually larger than the cuff used for measurement of the arm blood pressure in the same patient. Since the same-sized cuff is frequently used at both sites, the pressure values obtained may be higher in the legs than in the arms. Coarctation of the aorta is suspected when the systolic pressure is 20 mmHg lower in the legs than in the arms.

Blood pressure must be recorded properly by listing in the patient's record the systolic and diastolic pressure values, the method of obtaining the pressure, the extremity used, and whether upper- and lower-extremity blood pressures were measured simultaneously or sequentially. When using automated methods requiring nonsimultaneous measurement, recording the heart rate measured with each pressure reading may be helpful, since wide rate variations may give a clue to varying states of anxiety and may help in the interpretation of differing pressure values.

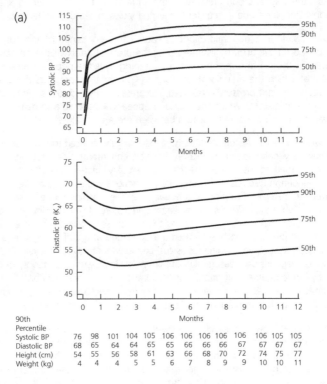

90th Percentile												
Systolic BP	76	98	101	104	105	106	106	106	106	106	106	105	105
Diastolic BP	68	65	64	64	65	65	66	66	66	67	67	67	67
Height (cm)	54	55	56	58	61	63	66	68	70	72	74	75	77
Weight (kg)	4	4	4	5	5	6	7	8	9	9	10	10	11

Figure 1.1 Upper limits of blood pressure for (a) girls and (b) boys from birth to one year of age. Source: From Report of the Second Task Force on Blood Pressure Control in Children. *Pediatrics*, 1987, **79**, 1–25. The material is a work of the US Government in the public domain; it is reprinted with acknowledgement from the American Academy of Pediatrics.

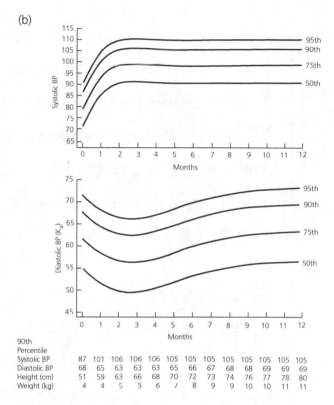

Figure 1.1 (*continued*)

Pulse pressure. Pulse pressure (the difference between the systolic and diastolic pressures) normally should be approximately one-third of the systolic pressure. A narrow pulse pressure is associated with a low cardiac output or severe aortic stenosis. Pulse pressure widens in conditions with an elevated cardiac output or with abnormal runoff of blood from the aorta during diastole. The former occurs in such conditions as anemia and anxiety, whereas the latter is found in patients with conditions such as PDA or aortic regurgitation.

Table 1.2 Blood pressure levels for boys by age (1–17 years) and height percentile.

Age (years)	BP percentile	Systolic BP (mmHg) ← Percentile of height →							Diastolic BP (mmHg) ← Percentile of height →						
		5th	10th	25th	50th	75th	90th	95th	5th	10th	25th	50th	75th	90th	95th
1	50th	80	81	83	85	87	88	89	34	35	36	37	38	39	39
	90th	94	95	97	99	100	102	103	49	50	51	52	53	53	54
	95th	98	99	101	103	104	106	106	54	54	55	56	57	58	58
	99th	105	106	108	110	112	113	114	61	62	63	64	65	66	66
2	50th	84	85	87	88	90	92	92	39	40	41	42	43	44	44
	90th	97	99	100	102	04	105	106	54	55	56	57	58	58	59
	95th	101	102	104	106	108	109	110	59	59	60	61	62	63	63
	99th	109	110	111	113	115	117	117	66	67	68	69	70	71	71
3	50th	86	87	89	91	93	94	95	44	44	45	46	47	48	48
	90th	100	101	103	105	107	108	109	59	59	60	61	62	63	63
	95th	104	105	107	109	110	112	113	63	63	64	65	66	67	67
	99th	111	112	114	116	118	119	120	71	71	72	73	74	75	75
4	50th	88	89	91	93	95	96	97	47	48	49	50	51	51	52
	90th	102	103	105	107	109	110	111	62	63	64	65	66	66	67
	95th	106	107	109	111	112	114	115	66	67	68	69	70	71	71
	99th	113	114	116	118	120	121	122	74	75	76	77	78	78	79
5	50th	90	91	93	95	96	98	98	50	51	52	53	54	55	55
	90th	104	105	106	108	110	111	112	65	66	67	68	69	69	70
	95th	108	109	110	112	114	115	116	69	70	71	72	73	74	74
	99th	115	116	118	120	121	123	123	77	78	79	80	81	81	82
6	50th	91	92	94	96	98	99	100	53	53	54	55	56	57	57
	90th	105	106	108	110	111	113	113	68	68	69	70	71	72	72
	95th	109	110	112	114	115	117	117	72	72	73	74	75	76	76
	99th	116	117	119	121	123	124	125	80	80	81	82	83	84	84

(continued)

Age (year)	BP percentile	SBP (mmHg) — percentile of height							DBP (mmHg) — percentile of height						
		5th	10th	25th	50th	75th	90th	95th	5th	10th	25th	50th	75th	90th	95th
7	50th	92	94	95	97	99	100	101	55	55	56	57	58	59	59
	90th	106	107	109	111	113	114	115	70	70	71	72	72	73	74
	95th	110	111	113	115	117	118	119	74	74	75	76	77	78	78
	99th	117	118	120	122	124	125	126	82	82	83	84	85	86	86
8	50th	94	95	97	99	100	102	102	56	57	57	59	60	60	61
	90th	107	109	110	112	114	115	116	71	72	72	73	74	75	76
	95th	111	112	114	116	118	119	120	75	76	77	78	79	79	80
	99th	119	120	122	123	125	127	127	83	84	85	86	87	87	88
9	50th	95	96	98	100	102	103	104	57	58	59	60	61	61	62
	90th	109	110	112	114	115	117	118	72	73	74	75	76	76	77
	95th	113	114	116	118	119	121	121	76	77	78	79	80	81	81
	99th	120	121	123	125	127	128	129	84	85	86	87	88	88	89
10	50th	97	98	100	102	103	105	106	58	59	60	61	61	62	63
	90th	111	112	114	115	117	119	119	73	73	74	75	76	77	78
	95th	115	116	117	119	121	122	123	77	78	79	80	81	81	82
	99th	122	123	125	127	128	130	130	85	86	86	88	88	89	90
11	50th	99	100	102	104	105	107	107	59	59	60	61	62	63	63
	90th	113	114	115	117	119	120	121	74	74	75	76	77	78	78
	95th	117	118	119	121	123	124	125	78	78	79	80	81	82	82
	99th	124	125	127	129	130	132	132	86	86	87	88	89	90	90
12	50th	101	102	104	106	108	109	110	59	60	61	62	63	63	64
	90th	115	116	118	120	121	123	123	74	75	75	76	77	78	79
	95th	119	120	122	123	125	127	127	78	79	80	81	82	82	83
	99th	126	127	129	131	133	134	135	86	87	88	89	90	90	91
13	50th	104	105	106	108	110	111	112	60	60	61	62	63	64	64
	90th	117	118	120	122	124	125	126	75	75	76	77	78	79	79
	95th	121	122	124	126	128	129	130	79	79	80	81	82	83	83
	99th	128	130	131	133	135	136	137	87	87	88	89	90	91	91
14	50th	106	107	109	111	113	114	115	60	61	62	63	64	65	65
	90th	120	121	123	125	126	128	128	75	76	77	78	79	79	80
	95th	124	125	127	128	130	132	132	80	80	81	82	83	84	84
	99th	131	132	134	136	138	139	140	87	88	89	90	91	92	92

Table 1.2 (continued)

Age (years)	BP percentile	Systolic BP (mmHg) ← Percentile of height →							Diastolic BP (mmHg) ← Percentile of height →						
		5th	10th	25th	50th	75th	90th	95th	5th	10th	25th	50th	75th	90th	95th
15	50th	107	108	109	110	111	113	113	64	64	64	65	66	67	67
	90th	120	121	122	123	125	126	127	78	78	78	79	80	81	81
	95th	124	125	126	127	129	130	131	82	82	82	83	84	85	85
	99th	131	132	133	134	136	137	138	89	89	90	91	91	92	93
16	50th	108	108	110	111	112	114	114	64	64	65	66	66	67	68
	90th	121	122	123	124	126	127	128	78	78	79	80	81	81	82
	95th	125	126	127	128	130	131	132	82	82	83	84	85	85	86
	99th	132	133	134	135	137	138	139	90	90	90	91	92	93	93
17	50th	108	109	110	111	113	114	115	64	65	65	66	67	67	68
	90th	122	122	123	125	126	127	128	78	79	79	80	81	81	82
	95th	125	126	127	129	130	131	132	82	83	83	84	85	85	86
	99th	133	133	134	136	137	138	139	90	90	91	91	92	93	93

The height percentiles are based on data available online at http://www.cdc.gov/growthcharts.

Source: Adapted from National High Blood Pressure Education Program Working Group on High Blood Pressure in Children and Adolescents. The Fourth Report on the Diagnosis, Evaluation, and Treatment of High Blood Pressure in Children and Adolescents. *Pediatrics*, 2004, **114** (2 Suppl. 4th Report), 555–576. This is a work of the US government, published in the public domain by the American Academy of Pediatrics, available online at http://pediatrics.aappublications.org/content/114/supplement_2/555 and http://www.nhlbi.nih.gov/health/prof/heart/hbp/hbp_ped.htm.

Modifications to these data to exclude children with BMI≥ 85th percentile and better reflect normal values for children of normal weight are available. Flynn JT, Kaelber DC, Baker-Smith CM, et al. Clinical Practice Guideline for Screening and Management of High Blood Pressure in Children and Adolescents [published correction appears in Pediatrics. 2018 Sep;142(3):1]. Pediatrics. 2017;140(3):e20171904. doi:10.1542/peds.2017-1904.

Table 1.3 Blood pressure levels for girls by age (1–17 years) and height percentile.

Age (years)	BP percentile	Systolic BP (mmHg) ← Percentile of height →							Diastolic BP (mmHg) ← Percentile of height →						
		5th	10th	25th	50th	75th	90th	95th	5th	10th	25th	50th	75th	90th	95th
1	50th	83	84	85	86	88	89	90	38	39	39	40	41	41	42
	90th	97	97	98	100	101	102	103	52	53	53	54	55	55	56
	99th	108	108	109	111	112	113	114	64	64	65	65	66	67	67
2	50th	85	85	87	88	89	91	91	43	44	44	45	46	46	47
	90th	98	99	100	101	103	104	105	57	58	58	59	60	61	61
	95th	102	103	104	105	107	108	109	61	62	62	63	64	65	65
	99th	109	110	111	112	114	115	116	69	69	70	70	71	72	72
3	50th	86	87	88	89	91	92	93	47	48	48	49	50	50	51
	90th	100	100	102	103	104	106	106	61	62	62	63	64	64	65
	95th	104	104	105	107	108	109	110	65	66	66	67	68	68	69
	99th	111	111	113	114	115	117	117	73	73	74	74	75	76	76
4	50th	88	88	90	91	92	94	94	50	50	51	52	52	53	54
	90th	101	102	103	104	106	107	108	64	64	65	66	67	67	68
	95th	105	106	107	108	110	111	112	68	68	69	70	71	71	72
	99th	112	113	114	115	117	118	119	76	76	76	77	78	79	79
5	50th	89	90	91	93	94	95	96	52	53	53	54	55	55	56
	90th	103	103	105	106	107	109	109	66	67	67	68	69	69	70
	95th	107	107	108	110	111	112	113	70	71	71	72	73	73	74
	99th	114	114	116	117	118	120	120	78	78	79	79	80	81	81
6	50th	91	92	93	94	96	97	98	54	54	55	56	56	57	58
	90th	104	105	106	108	109	110	111	68	68	69	70	70	71	72
	95th	108	109	110	111	113	114	115	72	72	73	74	74	75	76
	99th	115	116	117	119	120	121	122	80	80	80	81	82	83	83

(continued)

Table 1.3 (continued)

Age (years)	BP percentile	Systolic BP (mmHg) ← Percentile of height →							Diastolic BP (mmHg) ← Percentile of height →						
		5th	10th	25th	50th	75th	90th	95th	5th	10th	25th	50th	75th	90th	95th
7	50th	93	93	95	96	97	99	99	55	56	56	57	58	58	59
	90th	106	107	108	109	111	112	113	69	70	70	71	72	72	73
	95th	110	111	112	113	115	116	116	73	74	74	75	76	76	77
	99th	117	118	119	120	122	123	124	81	81	82	82	83	84	84
8	50th	95	95	96	98	99	100	101	57	57	57	58	59	60	60
	90th	108	109	110	111	113	114	114	71	71	71	72	73	74	74
	95th	112	112	114	115	116	118	118	75	75	75	76	77	78	78
	99th	119	120	121	122	123	125	125	82	82	83	83	84	85	86
9	50th	96	97	98	100	101	102	103	58	58	58	59	60	61	61
	90th	110	110	112	113	114	116	116	72	72	72	73	74	75	75
	95th	114	114	115	117	118	119	120	76	76	76	77	78	79	79
	99th	121	121	123	124	125	127	127	83	83	84	84	85	86	87
10	50th	98	99	100	102	103	104	105	59	59	59	60	61	62	62
	90th	112	112	114	115	116	118	118	73	73	73	74	75	76	76
	95th	116	116	117	119	120	121	122	77	77	77	78	79	80	80
	99th	123	123	125	126	127	129	129	84	84	85	86	86	87	88
11	50th	100	101	102	103	105	106	107	60	60	60	61	62	63	63
	90th	114	114	116	117	118	119	120	74	74	74	75	76	77	77
	95th	118	118	119	121	122	123	124	78	78	78	79	80	81	81
	99th	125	125	126	128	129	130	131	85	85	86	87	87	88	89
12	50th	102	103	104	105	107	108	109	61	61	61	62	63	64	64
	90th	116	116	117	119	120	121	122	75	75	75	76	77	78	78
	95th	119	120	121	123	124	125	126	79	79	79	80	81	82	82
	99th	127	127	128	130	131	132	133	86	86	87	88	88	89	90

Age	BP percentile	SBP (mmHg) by height percentile							DBP (mmHg) by height percentile						
13	50th	104	105	106	107	109	110	110	62	62	62	62	63	64	65
	90th	117	118	119	121	122	123	124	76	76	76	76	77	78	79
	95th	121	122	123	124	126	127	128	80	80	80	80	81	82	83
	99th	128	129	130	132	133	134	135	87	87	88	88	89	90	91
14	50th	106	106	107	109	110	111	112	63	63	63	63	64	65	66
	90th	119	120	121	122	124	125	125	77	77	77	78	79	80	80
	95th	123	123	125	126	127	129	129	81	81	81	81	82	83	84
	99th	130	131	132	133	135	136	136	88	88	88	89	90	91	92
15	50th	107	108	109	110	111	113	113	64	64	64	64	65	66	67
	90th	120	121	122	123	125	126	127	78	78	78	78	79	80	81
	95th	124	125	126	127	129	130	131	82	82	82	82	83	84	85
	99th	131	132	133	134	136	137	138	89	89	89	90	91	92	93
16	50th	108	108	110	111	112	114	114	64	64	64	65	66	67	68
	90th	121	122	123	124	126	127	123	78	78	78	79	80	81	82
	95th	125	126	127	128	130	131	132	82	82	83	83	84	85	86
	99th	132	133	134	135	137	138	139	90	90	90	91	92	93	93
17	50th	108	109	110	111	113	114	115	64	65	65	66	67	67	68
	90th	122	122	123	125	126	127	128	78	79	79	79	80	81	82
	95th	125	126	127	129	130	131	132	82	83	83	83	84	85	85
	99th	133	133	134	136	137	138	139	90	90	91	91	92	93	93

Source: Adapted from National High Blood Pressure Education Program Working Group on High Blood Pressure in Children and Adolescents. The Fourth Report on the Diagnosis, Evaluation, and Treatment of High Blood Pressure in Children and Adolescents. *Pediatrics*, 2004, **114** (2 Suppl. 4th Report), 555–576.
This is a work of the US government, published in the public domain by the American Academy of Pediatrics, available online at http://pediatrics.aappublications.org/content/114/Supplement_2/555 and http://www.nhlbi.nih.gov/health/prof/heart/hbp/hbp_ped.htm. Modifications to these data to exclude children with BMI ≥ 85th percentile and better reflect normal values for children of normal weight are available. Source: Flynn JT, Kaelber DC, Baker-Smith CM, et al. Clinical Practice Guideline for Screening and Management of High Blood Pressure in Children and Adolescents [published correction appears in *Pediatrics*. 2018 Sep;142(3):1]. *Pediatrics*. 2017;140(3):e20171904. doi:10.1542/peds.2017-1904.

Pulse

In palpating a child's pulse, not only the rate and rhythm but also the quality of the pulse should be carefully noted, as the latter reflects pulse pressure. Brisk pulses reflect a widened pulse pressure, whereas weak pulses indicate reduced cardiac output and/or narrowed pulse pressure. Coarctation of the aorta, for example, can be considered by comparing the femoral with the upper-extremity arterial pulses. Mistakes have been made, however, in interpreting the quality of femoral arterial pulses. Palpation alone is not sufficient either to diagnose or to rule out coarctation of the aorta. Blood pressures must be taken in both arms and one leg.

Respiratory rate and effort

The respiratory rate and respiratory effort should be noted. Normal values for the respiratory rate are given in Table 1.4. Although the upper limit of the normal respiratory rate for an infant is frequently given as 40 breaths per minute, observed rates can be as high as 60 breaths per minute in a normal infant; the respiratory effort in such infants is easy. Difficulty with breathing is indicated by intercostal or suprasternal retractions or by flaring of the alae nasae. Premature infants or neonates may show periodic breathing, so the rate should be counted for a full minute.

Cardiac examination

Inspection

Cardiac examination begins with inspection of the thorax. A precordial bulge may be found along the left sternal border in children with cardiomegaly. The upper sternum may bulge in children with a large left-to-right shunt and pulmonary hypertension or with elevated pulmonary venous pressure.

Table 1.4 Normal respiratory rates at different ages.

Age	Rate (breaths/min)[a]
Birth	30–60 (35)
First year	30–60 (30)
Second year	25–50 (25)
Adolescence	15–30 (15)

[a] Respiratory rates (breaths/min) vary with changes in mental state and physical activity. Sleeping rates are slower and are indicated in parentheses. Depth of respirations and effort expended by the patient are equally or more important than the rate itself.

Palpation

Several findings may be discovered by palpation; the most important is the location of the cardiac apex, an indicator of cardiac size. Obviously, if the apex is in the right hemithorax, there is dextrocardia.

Apical impulse. In infants and children under four years of age, the apex impulse, which is the most lateral place that the cardiac impulse can be palpated, should be located in the fourth intercostal space at the mid-clavicular line. In older children, it is located in the fifth intercostal space at the mid-clavicular line. Displacement laterally or inferiorly indicates cardiac enlargement.

Thrills. These are best identified by palpation of the precordium with the palmar surfaces of the metacarpophalangeal and proximal interphalangeal joints. Thrills are coarse, low-frequency vibrations occurring with a loud murmur, and are located in the same area as the maximum intensity of the murmur. In any patient suspected of congenital heart disease, the suprasternal notch also should be palpated but with a fingertip. A thrill at this site indicates a murmur originating from the base of the heart, most commonly aortic stenosis, less commonly pulmonary stenosis. In patients with PDA or aortic insufficiency, the suprasternal notch is very pulsatile.

Heaves. Forceful, outward movements of the precordium (heaves) indicate ventricular hypertrophy. Right ventricular heaves are located along the right sternal border, and left ventricular heaves are located at the cardiac apex.

Percussion

Percussion of the heart can substantiate estimation of cardiac size in addition to that obtained by inspection and palpation.

Auscultation

Auscultation of the heart provides perhaps the most useful diagnostic information and should be performed in a systematic way to obtain optimum information.

Instrumentation. A good stethoscope is a must. It should have short, thick tubing, snug-fitting earpieces, and both a bell and a diaphragm. Low-pitched sounds and murmurs are heard best with the bell and high-pitched sounds with the diaphragm. For most children, a 3/4 -inch bell and a 1-inch diaphragm are suitable for auscultation, although an adult-sized bell and diaphragm are preferable if adequate contact can be made with the chest wall. A diaphragm 1 inch in diameter can be used in children of all ages, since only part of the diaphragm need be in contact with the chest wall to transmit sound. Smaller-sized diaphragms provide poor sound transmission.

Position and technique. In infants, initially auscultate through the clothing despite the often-quoted admonition that auscultation should never be performed in such a manner. Sometimes removing the clothes disturbs the child and results in a fussy state that precludes adequate auscultation. After the initial period of listening, the clothing can be removed to listen further. Make certain that the chest pieces of the stethoscope are warm.

With children between the ages of one and three years, listening is easier if they are sitting on their parent's lap, because children of this age are often frightened by strangers. In older children, they can sit on the examination table and the examination can proceed as in adults.

When auscultating, sitting alongside the child is helpful. This position is neither fatiguing to the examiner nor threatening to the child.

Auscultation of the heart should proceed in an orderly, stepwise fashion. Both the anterior and posterior thorax is auscultated with the patient in the upright position. Then the precordium is re-examined with the patient reclining. Each of the five major areas (aorta, pulmonary, tricuspid, mitral, and back) is carefully explored. Both the bell and diaphragm should be used in auscultation of each site. High-pitched murmurs and the first and second heart sounds are heard better with the diaphragm; low-pitched murmurs and the third heart sound are most evident with the bell. The diaphragm should be applied with moderate pressure; the bell must be applied with only enough pressure for uniform contact and not enough force to stretch the underlying skin into a "diaphragm," which alters the sensitivity to low frequencies. When auscultating the heart, attention is directed not only to cardiac murmurs but also to the quality and characteristics of the heart sounds.

Physiologic basis of auscultation. The events and phases of the cardiac cycle should be reviewed. Figure 1.2 represents a modification of a diagram by Wiggers and shows the relationship between cardiac pressures, heart sounds, and electrocardiogram. In studying this diagram, relate the events both vertically and horizontally.

Systole

The onset of ventricular systole occurs following depolarization of ventricles and is indicated by the QRS complex of the electrocardiogram. As the ventricles begin to contract, the papillary muscles close the mitral and tricuspid valves. The pressure in the ventricles soon exceeds the atrial pressure and continues to rise until it reaches the diastolic pressure in the great vessel, at which point the semilunar valves open. The period of time between closure of the atrioventricular (AV) valves and the opening of the semilunar valves represents the *isovolumetric contraction period*. During this period, blood neither enters nor leaves the ventricles. During the next period, the ejection period, blood leaves the ventricles, and the ventricular pressure slightly exceeds the pressure in the corresponding great artery. As blood flow decreases, eventually the pressure in the ventricle falls below that in the great vessel, and the semilunar valve closes. This point represents the end of systole. The pressure in the ventricles continues to fall until it reaches the pressure of the corresponding atrium, at which time the AV valve opens. The period between closure of the semilunar valves and the opening of the AV valves is termed the *isovolumetric relaxation period* because blood neither enters nor leaves the ventricles.

Diastole

Diastole is divided into three consecutive phases:

- **Early**. Early diastole is defined as the portion of ventricular diastole comprising the isovolumetric relaxation period, a time when ventricular pressures are falling but the volume is not changing because all cardiac valves are closed.
- **Mid**. Mid-diastole begins with the opening of the AV valves; 80% of the cardiac output traverses the AV valves during mid-diastole. It has two distinct phases: a rapid and a slow filling phase. The rapid filling phase comprises approximately the first 20% of diastole, during which about 60% of blood flow into the ventricle occurs. When a third heart sound (S_3) is present, it occurs at the transition between the rapid and slow filling phases (Figure 1.2).
- **Late**. Late diastole begins with atrial contraction, and the remaining 20% of ventricular filling occurs.

Interpretation of cardiac sounds and murmurs

The timing and meaning of cardiac sounds and murmurs are easily understood by considering their location within the cardiac cycle and the corresponding cardiac events. Although the origin of heart sounds remains controversial, we will discuss them as originating from valvar events.

Heart sounds. The first heart sound (S_1) represents closure of the mitral and tricuspid valves (Figure 1.2) and occurs as the ventricular pressure exceeds the atrial pressure at the onset of systole. In children, the individual mitral and tricuspid components are usually indistinguishable, so the first heart sound appears single. Occasionally, two components of this sound are heard. Splitting of the first heart sound can be a normal finding.

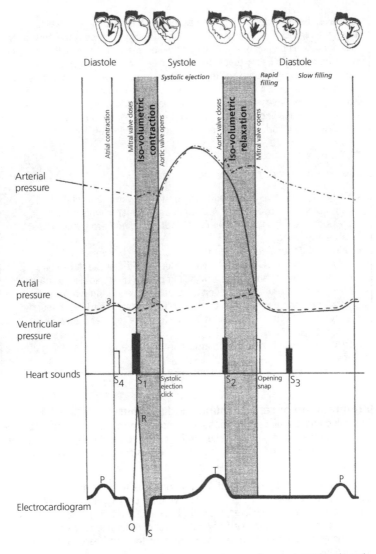

Figure 1.2 Relationship between cardiac pressures, electrocardiogram, heart sounds, and phases of the cardiac cycle. S_1, first heart sound; S_2, second heart sound, etc.

The first heart sound is soft if the impulse conduction from the atrium to the ventricle is prolonged. This delay allows the valves to drift closed after atrial contraction. The first heart may also be soft if myocardial disease is present.

The first heart sound is accentuated in conditions with increased blood flow across an AV valve (as in left-to-right shunt) or in high cardiac output. The second heart sound (S_2) is of great diagnostic significance, particularly in a child with a cardiac malformation. The normal second heart sound has two components which represent the asynchronous closure of the aortic and pulmonary valves. These sounds signal the completion of ventricular ejection. Aortic valve closure normally precedes closure of the pulmonary valve because right ventricular ejection is longer. The presence of the two components, aortic (A_2) and pulmonic (P_2), is called splitting of the second heart sound (Figure 1.3).

The time interval between the components varies with respiration. Normally, on inspiration the degree of splitting increases because a greater volume of blood returns to the right side of the heart. Since ejection of this augmented volume of blood requires a longer time, the second heart sound becomes more widely split on inspiration. On expiration, the degree of splitting is shortened.

The second heart sound can be split abnormally:

Wide Splitting

Conditions prolonging right ventricular ejection lead to wide splitting of the second heart sound because P_2 is delayed further than normal. This phenomenon is present in three hemodynamic states:

- Conditions in which the right ventricle ejects an increased volume of blood (e.g. ASD – but not VSD).
- Obstruction to right ventricular outflow (e.g. pulmonary stenosis).
- Delayed depolarization of the right ventricle (e.g. complete right bundle branch block).

Paradoxical Splitting

Paradoxical splitting of the second heart sound is probably of greater importance in understanding the physiology of heart sounds than in reaching a cardiac diagnosis in children. Conditions prolonging left ventricular ejection may delay the aortic component, causing it to follow the pulmonary component (Figure 1.3). Thus, as P_2 varies normally with respiration, the degree of splitting widens paradoxically on expiration and narrows on inspiration. Left ventricular ejection is prolonged in conditions in which the left ventricle ejects an increased volume of blood into the aorta (e.g. PDA), in left ventricular outflow obstruction (e.g. aortic stenosis), and in delayed depolarization of the left ventricle (complete left bundle branch block).

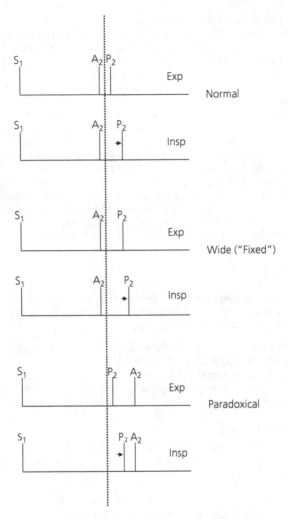

Figure 1.3 Respiratory variations in splitting of the second heart sound. In a normal individual, P_2 (pulmonary component of second heart sound) is delayed on inspiration. Wide splitting occurs in conditions prolonging right ventricular ejection. Paradoxical splitting occurs in conditions delaying A_2 (aortic component of second heart sound). P_2 changes normally with inspiration. Thus, the interval between P_2 and A_2 narrows on inspiration and widens on expiration.

Thus, wide splitting and paradoxical splitting of the second heart sound occur from similar cardiac abnormalities but on opposite sides of the heart. Paradoxical splitting is associated with severe left-sided disorders.

In assessing a child with a cardiac anomaly, particular attention also should be directed toward the intensity of the pulmonic component (P_2) of the second heart sound. The pulmonic component of the second sound is accentuated whenever the pulmonary arterial pressure is elevated, whether this elevation is related to pulmonary vascular disease or to increased pulmonary arterial blood flow. In general, as the level of pulmonary arterial pressure increases, the pulmonic component of the second heart sound becomes louder and closer to the aortic component.

The finding of a single second heart sound usually indicates that one of the semilunar valves is atretic or severely stenotic because the valve involved does not contribute its component to the second sound. The second heart sound also is single in patients with persistent truncus arteriosus (common arterial trunk) because there is only a single semilunar valve or whenever pulmonary arterial pressure is at systemic levels, and the aortic and pulmonary artery pressure curves are superimposed.

Third heart sound (S_3) may be present in a child without a cardiac anomaly but may be accentuated in pathologic states. This sound occurs early in diastole and represents the transition from rapid to slow filling phases. In conditions with increased blood flow across either the mitral valve (as in mitral regurgitation) or the tricuspid valve (as in ASD), the third heart sound may be accentuated. A gallop rhythm found in congestive cardiac failure often represents exaggeration of the third heart sound in the presence of tachycardia.

Fourth heart sounds (S_4) are abnormal. Located in the cardiac cycle late in diastole, they occur with the P wave of the electrocardiogram and exist synchronous to the atrial "a" wave. They are found in conditions in which either the atrium forcefully contracts against a ventricle with decreased compliance, as from fibrosis or marked hypertrophy, or when the flow from the atrium to the ventricle is greatly increased. The fourth heart sound may be audible as a presystolic gallop, particularly if tachycardia is present.

Systolic ejection clicks are abnormal and occur at the time the semilunar valves open. Therefore, they mark the transition from the isovolumetric contraction period to the onset of ventricular ejection. Ordinarily this event is not heard, but in specific cardiac conditions, a sound (systolic ejection click) may be present at this point in the cardiac cycle and because of its timing may be confused with a split first heart sound.

Systolic ejection clicks indicate the presence of a dilated great vessel, most frequently from poststenotic dilation. These sharp, high-pitched sounds have a clicky quality. Ejection clicks of aortic origin are heard best at the cardiac apex or over the left lower thorax when the patient is in a supine position; they vary little with respiration. Aortic ejection clicks are common in patients with valvar aortic stenosis or a bicuspid aortic valve with concomitant poststenotic dilation. Ejection clicks may also originate from a dilated pulmonary artery, as present in pulmonary valvar stenosis or significant pulmonary arterial hypertension. Pulmonic ejection clicks are best heard in the pulmonary area when the patient is sitting and vary in intensity with respiration. Ejection clicks in patients with a stenotic semilunar valve occur more commonly in mild or moderate cases; they may be absent in patients with severe stenosis.

Clicks are not associated with subvalvar stenosis since there is no poststenotic dilation.

Opening snaps are abnormal and occur when an AV valve opens. At this point, the ventricular pressure is falling below the atrial pressure, the isovolumetric relaxation period is ending, and ventricular filling is beginning. Ordinarily, no sound is heard at this time, but if the AV valve is thickened or fibrotic, a low-pitched noise may be heard when it opens. Opening snaps, rare in children, are almost always associated with rheumatic mitral valvar stenosis.

Murmurs. Cardiac murmurs are generated by turbulence in the normal laminar blood flow through the heart. Turbulence results from narrowing the pathway of blood flow, abnormal communications, or increased blood flow.

> Five aspects of a cardiac murmur provide knowledge of the underlying cause of turbulence: location in cardiac cycle (timing), location on thorax, radiation of murmur, loudness, and pitch and character.

Murmurs may be classified by their location within the cardiac cycle (Figure 1.4). A murmur is heard only during that portion of the cardiac cycle in which turbulent blood flow occurs.

Two types of systolic murmurs exist: holosystolic and systolic ejection. Holosystolic murmurs (synonyms are pansystolic or systolic regurgitant) start with the first heart sound and continue into systole, often extending to the second heart sound. Therefore, these murmurs involve the isovolumetric contraction period.

> Only two conditions permit blood flow during isovolumetric contraction:
>
> - VSD.
> - AV valve regurgitation (mitral, tricuspid, or the "common" valve in AV septal defect).

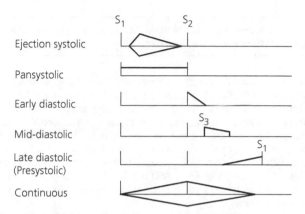

Figure 1.4 Classification of murmurs, showing location within the cardiac cycle and usual contour. S_1, first heart sound; S_2, second heart sound; S_3, third heart sound.

In VSD, flow occurs between the left and right ventricles from the onset of systole, whereas in AV valve regurgitation the high-pressure ventricle is in communication with the lower-pressure atrium from the time of the first heart sound.

Because holosystolic murmurs begin so close to the first heart sound, that sound may be masked at the location of maximum murmur intensity. This masking can be a clue to a holosystolic murmur, particularly in patients with rapid heart rate.

Systolic ejection murmur (SEM) results from turbulent forward blood flow across a semilunar valve (aortic, pulmonary, or truncal valve), a great vessel, or ventricular outflow tract. Since turbulent flow in these locations cannot begin until the semilunar valves open, an interval (the isovolumetric contraction period) exists between the first heart sound and the onset of the murmur. Although often diamond shaped (crescendo/decrescendo), SEMs are distinguished by the delayed onset of the murmur until after the isovolumetric contraction period.

Ejection murmurs are found in conditions such as ASD, aortic stenosis, and pulmonary stenosis. In contrast to holosystolic murmurs, the first heart sound is distinctly audible at the site where the SEM is best heard.

Diastolic murmurs can also be classified according to their timing in the cardiac cycle. Early diastolic murmurs occur immediately following the second heart sound and include the isovolumetric relaxation period. During this time, blood can only flow from a higher-pressure great vessel into a lower-pressure ventricle.

> Early diastolic murmurs indicate regurgitation across a semilunar valve (aortic, pulmonary, or truncal valve regurgitation).

Usually decrescendo, their pitch depends on the level of diastolic pressure within the great vessel: high pitched in aortic or truncal regurgitation and lower pitched with pulmonary regurgitation (unless pulmonary hypertension is present).

Mid-diastolic murmurs (sometimes called inflow murmurs) occur at the time of maximum passive ventricular filling and usually result from increased forward blood flow across a normal AV valve. In children, they occur most commonly in conditions with increased pulmonary blood flow and, therefore, with increased blood flow into the ventricles (as in ASD or VSD). These low-pitched rumbles are usually heard only with the bell of the stethoscope and are easily overlooked by an inexperienced examiner.

Late diastolic murmurs represent organic obstruction of an AV valve. These murmurs crescendo with a low pitch. Rheumatic mitral stenosis is a typical example.

A continuous murmur indicates turbulence beginning in systole and extending into diastole. It may last throughout the cardiac cycle. Usually it occurs when communication exists between the aorta and the pulmonary artery or other portions of the venous side of the heart or circulation. PDA is the classic example, but continuous murmurs are heard with other types of systemic arteriovenous fistulae.

The similarities and differences between regurgitant murmurs and those due to forward blood flow, whether in systole or diastole, are summarized in Table 1.5.

Table 1.5 Characteristics of murmurs.

Location in cardiac cycle	Type of murmur	
	Regurgitant	Forward flow

Systolic	Holosystolic
	  Begins with S_1
	  Includes isovolumetric
	    contraction period
		Ejection
		  Follows S_1
		  Occurs after isovolumetric
		    contraction period

Diastolic	Early diastolic
	  Begins with S_2
	  Includes isovolumetric
	    relaxation period
		Mid- or late diastolic
		  Follows S_2
		  Occurs after isovolumetric
		    relaxation period

Continuous	Systole and diastole Continues through S_2	

S_1, first heart sound; S_2, second heart sound.

Regurgitant murmurs begin with either the first or second heart sound and include the isovolumetric periods, whereas those related to abnormalities of forward flow begin after an isovolumetric period and may be associated with an abnormal cardiac sound (systolic ejection click or opening snap). A notable exception to these rules is the murmur associated with mitral valve prolapse. Table 1.6 presents differential diagnosis of murmurs by timing.

The location of the maximum intensity of murmurs on the thorax (Figure 1.5) provides information about the anatomic origin of the murmur:

(1) *Aortic area*: from the mid-left sternal border to beneath the right clavicle.
(2) *Pulmonary area*: the upper left sternal border and beneath the left clavicle.
(3) *Tricuspid area*: along the lower left and right sternal border.
(4) *Mitral area*: the cardiac apex.

In these areas, the murmurs of aortic stenosis, pulmonary stenosis, tricuspid insufficiency, and mitral insufficiency, respectively, are found. In infants and children, listening over both sides of the back is essential. For example, the murmur of coarctation of the aorta is heard best in the left paraspinal area, directly over the anatomic site of the aortic narrowing. The murmur of peripheral pulmonary artery stenosis is heard over both sides of the back and axillae.

Radiation, the direction of transmission of the murmur, is also helpful, as it reflects the direction of turbulent flow, which often is along major blood vessels. Murmurs originating from the aortic outflow area (e.g. aortic valvar stenosis) radiate toward the neck and into the carotid arteries. Murmurs from the pulmonary outflow area are transmitted to the left upper back. Mitral murmurs are transmitted toward the cardiac apex and left axilla; occasionally, mitral regurgitation is heard in the middle back.

Loudness of a cardiac murmur is graded on a scale in which grade 6 represents the loudest murmur. Conventionally, loudness is indicated by a fraction in which the numerator indicates the loudness of the patient's murmur and the denominator indicates the maximum grade possible. Although somewhat arbitrary, the classification is based on sound intensity and chest wall vibration (thrills).

1/6 is very soft – heard only with careful attention.
2/6 is not loud but is easily heard.
3/6 is loud but no thrill can be palpated.
4/6 is loud and associated with a thrill.
5/6 is very loud.
6/6 is very loud – heard even with the stethoscope held just off the chest wall.

Table 1.6 Differential diagnosis of murmurs by location in the cardiac cycle.

Location in cardiac cycle	Timing	Physiology	Possible conditions
Systolic	Holosystolic	Flow, ventricle to ventricle	VSD
		Regurgitation, ventricle to atrium	AV valve regurgitation (MR, TR, common AV valve regurgitation)
	Ejection	Flow, ventricle to artery	Semilunar valve, outflow tract, or branch pulmonary artery flow (normal)
			Increased pulmonary valve flow (e.g. ASD, AVM – abnormal)
		Stenosis, ventricle to artery	Semilunar valve stenosis (e.g. AS, PS, truncal valve stenosis), subvalvar stenosis, or supravalvar stenosis
	Mid- to late systolic	Regurgitation, ventricle to atrium, only with AV valve prolapse	Mitral valve prolapse with regurgitation
Diastolic	Early diastolic	Regurgitation, artery to ventricle	Semilunar valve regurgitation (AI, PI, truncal valve regurgitation)
	Mid- or late diastolic	Flow, atrium to ventricle	Increased flow via AV valve (e.g. mitral mid-diastolic murmur in VSD, PDA, or severe MR; tricuspid valve mid-diastolic murmur in ASD, AVM)
		Stenosis, atrium to ventricle	AV valve stenosis (e.g. MS, TS)
Continuous	Systolic accentuation	Flow, artery to artery	PDA
			Surgical systemic artery to pulmonary artery shunt
		Flow, artery to vein	AVM
		Flow, within artery	Arterial bruit
	Respiratory accentuation	Flow, within vein	Venous hum

AI, aortic insufficiency (regurgitation); AS, aortic stenosis; ASD, atrial septal defect; AV, atrioventricular; AVM, arteriovenous malformation; MR, mitral regurgitation; MS, mitral stenosis; PDA, patent ductus arteriosus; PI, pulmonary insufficiency (or regurgitation); PS, pulmonary stenosis; TR, tricuspid regurgitation; TS, tricuspid stenosis; VSD, ventricular septal defect.

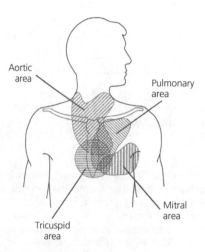

Figure 1.5 Primary areas of auscultation. Source: Reprinted from Pelech, A.N. The cardiac murmur: when to refer? *Pediatr. Clin. North Am.*, **45**, 107–122. Copyright 1998, with permission from Elsevier.

Pitch can be described as high, medium, or low. High-pitched murmurs (heard with a diaphragm) occur when a large pressure difference in the turbulent flow exists, such as in aortic or mitral insufficiency. Low-pitched murmurs (heard with a bell) occur when there is a small pressure difference, as in the mid-diastolic mitral inflow murmur accompanying a VSD.

The character of the murmur can be helpful in distinguishing certain causes. Soft murmurs tend to be from laminar flow and are often normal murmurs. Harsh murmurs are typical of severe outflow stenosis as in aortic valvar stenosis when a large pressure difference is present, are associated with turbulence and multispectral frequencies, and are often abnormal.

Normal murmurs. Distinction between a normal or functional (innocent) and a significant (organic) murmur can be difficult in some children. Although this text describes the characteristics of the commonly heard functional murmurs, only by experience and careful auscultation can one become proficient in distinguishing a functional murmur from a significant murmur.

> Functional murmurs have four features that help to distinguish them from significant murmurs: (i) normal heart sounds, (ii) normal heart size, (iii) lack of significant cardiac signs and symptoms, and (iv) loudness of grade 3/6 or less.

Some mild forms of cardiac abnormalities may have these features. Thus, the ability to categorize the murmur as a specific type of functional murmur is helpful.

Six types of normal or functional murmurs follow:

(1) *Still's murmur*. Often called "musical" or "twangy string," this soft (grade 1/6–3/6) low-pitched vibratory SEM is heard between the lower left sternal border and apex. Because of this location on the thorax, it may be misinterpreted as a VSD. It can be distinguished because it begins after, not with, the first heart sound (as in VSD) and lacks the harsh quality of a VSD murmur.

(2) *Pulmonary flow murmur*. This soft (grade 1/6–3/6) low-pitched SEM is heard in the pulmonary area. The murmur itself may be indistinguishable from ASD. With this functional murmur, however, the characteristics of the second heart sound remain normal, whereas in ASD the components of the second heart sound show wide, fixed splitting.

(3) *Normal neonatal pulmonary artery branch flow murmur*. This soft SEM is heard in many premature neonates, often at the time their physiologic anemia reaches its nadir, and in many term infants. It is characterized by a soft systolic flow murmur best heard in the axillae and back, and poorly heard, if at all, over the precordium. To avoid confusion with true pulmonary artery pathology, the synonym peripheral pulmonic stenosis, or PPS, should not be used.

(4) *Venous hum*. This murmur might be confused with a PDA because it is continuous. It is heard best, however, in the right infraclavicular area. Venous hum originates from turbulent flow in the jugular venous system. Several characteristics distinguish it from PDA: it can be louder in diastole and varies with respiration; it is best heard with the patient sitting; it diminishes and usually disappears when the patient reclines; and it changes in intensity with movements of the head or with pressure over the jugular vein.

(5) *Cervical bruit*. In children, a soft systolic arterial bruit may be heard over the carotid arteries. They are believed to originate at the bifurcation of the carotid arteries. The bruit should not be confused with the transmission of cardiac murmurs to the neck, as in aortic stenosis. Aortic stenosis is associated with a suprasternal notch thrill.

(6) *Cardiopulmonary murmur*. This sound (more along the mid left sternal border than right) originates from compression of the lung between the heart and the anterior chest wall. This murmur or sound occurs during systole, becomes louder in mid-inspiration and mid-expiration, and sounds close to the ear.

In most children with a functional cardiac murmur, a chest X-ray, electrocardiogram, or echocardiogram is unnecessary, as the diagnosis can be made with certainty from the physical examination alone. In a few patients, these studies may be indicated to distinguish a significant and a functional murmur. If it is a normal (innocent) murmur, the parents and the patient should be reassured of its benign nature. No special care is indicated for these children, and the child can be monitored at intervals dictated by routine pediatric care by their own medical provider. Many (not all) functional murmurs disappear in adolescence, and the murmurs may be accentuated during times of increased cardiac output, such as during fever and anemia.

Abdominal examination

The abdomen should be carefully examined for the location and size of the liver and spleen. The examiner should be alert to the presence of situs inversus. The hepatic edge should be palpated and its distance below the costal margin measured. If the edge is lower than normal, the upper margin of the liver should be percussed to determine the span of the liver. In patients with a depressed diaphragm (e.g. from asthma), the liver edge is also depressed downward; in this instance, the upper extent of the liver is also depressed. The liver edge normally is palpable until four years of age. Pulsatile motion may be palpated over the liver in severe tricuspid regurgitation or transmitted through soft tissues from a hyperdynamic heart in the absence of AV valve regurgitation.

The spleen ordinarily should not be palpable. It may be enlarged in patients with chronic congestive cardiac failure or infective endocarditis.

LABORATORY EXAMINATION

Electrocardiography

Electrocardiography plays an integral part in the evaluation of a child with cardiac disease. It is most useful in reaching a diagnosis when combined with other patient data. The electrocardiogram permits the assessment of the severity of many cardiac conditions by reflecting the anatomic changes of cardiac chambers resulting from abnormal hemodynamics imposed by the cardiac anomaly.

For example, left ventricular hypertrophy (LVH) develops in patients with aortic stenosis. The electrocardiogram reflects the anatomic change; and the extent of electrocardiographic change roughly parallels the degree of hypertrophy, yielding information about the severity of the obstruction. However, a pattern of LVH is not diagnostic of aortic stenosis because other conditions, such as systemic hypertension or coarctation of the aorta, also cause anatomic LVH and the associated electrocardiographic changes. Occasionally, electrocardiographic patterns are specific enough for diagnosis of a particular cardiac anomaly (e.g. anomalous left coronary artery, tricuspid atresia, or AV septal defect).

The electrocardiogram is used to assess cardiac rhythm disturbances (see Chapter 10) and electrolyte abnormalities. Ambulatory electrocardiography (24-hour electrocardiogram or "Holter monitor") is used for surveillance of subclinical arrhythmias, to access the range and variability of heart rate, and to document the rhythm during symptoms. When symptoms suspected of originating from arrhythmia occur less frequently than daily, an *event monitor* allows recording of brief (one to two minutes) electrocardiograms *during symptoms* for transmission via cellphone.

Developmental changes

The electrocardiogram of children normally changes with age; the greatest changes occur during the first year of life, reflecting developmental changes in the circulation. At birth, the right ventricle weighs more than the left ventricle because during fetal life it supplied blood to the aorta by way of the ductus arteriosus and had a greater stroke volume than the left ventricle. As the child grows, the left ventricular wall thickens as systemic arterial pressure rises slowly; meanwhile, the right ventricular wall thins as pulmonary arterial pressure falls. These anatomic changes primarily affect those portions of the electrocardiogram reflecting ventricular depolarization (QRS complex) and repolarization (T waves).

Therefore, in infancy, the thicker than normal right ventricular wall directs the QRS axis more toward the right with tall R waves in lead V_1 and relatively deep S waves in lead V_6. With age, the QRS axis shifts toward the left, and leads V_1 and V_6 assume a pattern similar to that seen in adults (Figure 1.6).

In interpreting the electrocardiogram of a child, these changes and others that occur with age must be considered. Table 1.7 shows the range of normal values for several electrocardiographic intervals and wave forms.

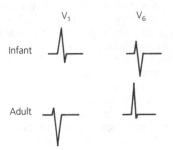

Figure 1.6 Comparison of the contour of QRS complex in leads V_1 and V_6 of infants and adults.

Table 1.7 Normal values of important electrocardiographic parameters.

Age	QRS Axis (°)	R wave in V_1 (mm)	S wave in V_1 (mm)	R wave in V_6 (mm)	S wave in V_6 (mm)
0–24 hours	137 (70–205)	16 (6–27)	10 (0–25)	4 (0–8)	4 (0–12)
1–7 days	125 (75–185)	17 (4–30)	10 (0–20)	6 (0–16)	3 (0–12)
8–30 days	108 (30–190)	13 (3–24)	7 (0–18)	8 (0–20)	2 (0–9)
1–3 months	75 (25–125)	10 (2–20)	7 (0–18)	9 (2–16)	2 (0–6)
3–6 months	65 (30–96)	10 (2–20)	7 (2–12)	10 (2–16)	1 (0–5)
6–12 months	65 (10–115)	10 (2–20)	8 (2–15)	12 (3–20)	1 (0–3)
1–3 years	55 (6–108)	9 (2–18)	10 (2–25)	12 (3–21)	1 (0–3)
3–5 years	62 (20–105)	7 (1–16)	13 (2–25)	13 (4–21)	1 (0–3)
5–8 years	65 (16–112)	7 (1–16)	14 (2–25)	14 (6–24)	1 (0–3)
8–12 years	62 (15–112)	6 (1–16)	14 (2–25)	14 (8–21)	1 (0–3)
12–16 years	65 (20–116)	5 (0–16)	15 (2–25)	13 (8–20)	1 (0–3)

Technical factors

Analysis of an electrocardiogram should proceed in an orderly sequence to gain maximum information from the tracing. The speed and sensitivity of the recording should be noted, and variation from the "standard" speed of 25 mm/s and amplitude of 10 mm/mV must be considered with comparison with normal values.

Rate and rhythm. The initial step should be to recognize any cardiac arrhythmias or major conduction abnormalities. These can usually be detected by answering the following three questions:

- Are there P waves?
- Is each P wave followed by a QRS complex?
- Is each QRS complex preceded by a P wave?

If the answer to any of these questions is no, the type of rhythm disturbance should be further investigated by following the instructions given in Chapter 10.

Components of the electrocardiogram. The next step is the analysis of each component of the electrocardiographic tracing. This is accomplished not by looking at each lead from left to right, as in reading a newspaper, but by reading up and down. In each lead, first assess the P waves, then the QRS complexes, and finally the T waves.

For each wave form, four features are analyzed: axis, amplitude, duration, and any characteristic pattern (such as the delta wave of Wolff–Parkinson–White syndrome). Using groups of leads, axis is analyzed: the limb leads are used to derive frontal–plane axes, and the chest or precordial leads are used for horizontal plane axes.

Sometimes confusion exists about the word axis. Commonly the term "the axis" is used to describe the QRS in the standard leads. But, just as the direction of the QRS can be described indicating the axis, so can the direction of P and T waves; the principle is the same.

P wave. The P wave is formed during depolarization of the atria. Depolarization is initiated from the sinoatrial node located at the junction of the superior vena cava and right atrium. It generally proceeds inferiorly and leftward toward the AV node located at the junction of the atrium and ventricle, low in the right atrium and adjacent to the coronary sinus. The direction of atrial depolarization also proceeds slightly anteriorly. Since atrial depolarization begins in the right atrium, the initial portion of the P wave is formed primarily from right atrial depolarization, whereas the terminal portion is formed principally from left atrial depolarization.

The following three characteristics of the P wave should be studied:

(1) *P-wave axis.* The P-wave axis indicates the net direction of atrial depolarization (Figure 1.7). Normally, the P-wave axis in the frontal plane is +60° (+15° to +75°), reflecting the direction of atrial depolarization from the sinoatrial to the AV nodes.

> Therefore, the largest P waves are usually in lead II; the P waves are normally positive in leads I, II, and aVF, always negative in lead aVR, and positive, negative, or diphasic in leads aVL and III.
>
> In the horizontal plane, the P-wave axis is directed toward the left (approximately lead V_5). Therefore, the P wave in lead V_1 may be positive, negative, or diphasic.

The P-wave axis changes when the pacemaker initiating atrial depolarization is abnormally located. One example is mirror-image dextrocardia associated with situs inversus, in which the anatomic right atrium and the sinoatrial node are located on the left side, so atrial depolarization occurs from left to right. This leads to a P-wave axis of +120° with the largest P waves in lead III. Another example is junctional rhythm, in which atrial depolarization proceeds from the AV node in a superior-rightward direction.

(2) *P-wave amplitude.* The P wave should not exceed 3 mm in height. Because most of the right atrium is depolarized before the left atrium, the early portion of the P wave is accentuated in right atrial enlargement.

> P waves taller than 3 mm indicate right atrial enlargement. This condition causes tall, peaked, and pointed P waves, usually found in the right precordial leads or in leads II, III, or aVF.

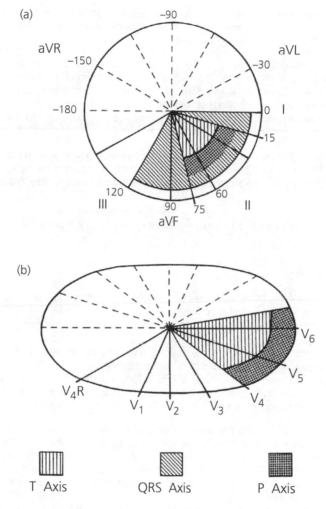

Figure 1.7 Electrocardiogram normal axes. Relationship of limb leads in frontal plane (a) and precordial leads in horizontal plane (b). The normal ranges for the P-wave, QRS-complex, and T-wave axes in the frontal plane and the P- and T-wave axes in the horizontal plane are shown.

(3) *P-wave duration*. The P wave should be less than 100 ms in duration. When longer, left atrial enlargement or intra-atrial block (much rarer) is present.

In left atrial enlargement, the P wave is broad and notched, particularly in leads I, aVL, and/or V_5 and V_6; a wide negative component of the P wave may also exist in lead V_1 because the latter part of the P wave principally represents left atrial depolarization and because the left atrium faces the left precordial leads so the terminal P-wave forces are accentuated and directed leftward.

PR interval. The PR interval is the time from the onset of the P wave to the onset of the QRS complex. It represents the transmission of the impulse from the sinoatrial node through the atria and then through the AV node and the Purkinje system.

The normal values of PR interval measured in leads I, II, or III are as follows:

- 100–120 ms in infancy,
- 120–150 ms in childhood, and
- 140–220 ms in adulthood.

However, the PR interval varies with heart rate in addition to age, becoming shorter with faster rates.

A PR interval longer than these values is caused by prolongation of AV nodal conduction, such as that caused by acute febrile illness or digoxin. The PR interval may also be shorter than normal if an ectopic focus for atrial depolarization exists, as in low atrial rhythm, or if an accessory conducting pathway into the ventricle with pre-excitation is present, as in Wolff–Parkinson–White syndrome.

QRS complex. The QRS complex represents ventricular depolarization. Ventricular depolarization starts on the left side of the interventricular septum near the base and proceeds across the septum from left to right. Depolarization of the free walls of both ventricles follows. The posterior basilar part of the left ventricle and the infundibulum of the right ventricle are the last portions of ventricular myocardium to be depolarized.

The QRS complex should be analyzed for the following features:

(1) *QRS axis*. The QRS axis represents the net direction of ventricular depolarization. In children, the axis varies because of the hemodynamic and anatomic

changes that occur with age. The value of the QRS axis in the frontal plane for various ages is shown in Table 1.7.

In neonates, the QRS axis range is +70° to +215°, but with age the axis comes into the range 0° to +120°. Most of the change occurs by three months of age (Figure 1.7).

Right-axis deviation is diagnosed when the calculated value for the QRS axis is greater than the upper range of normal, which for older children is more than +120°. Right-axis deviation is almost always associated with right ventricular hypertrophy (RVH) or enlargement (RVE).

Left-axis deviation is indicated when the calculated QRS axis is less than the smaller value of the normal range. Left-axis deviation is associated with myocardial disease or ventricular conduction abnormalities, such as those that occur in AV septal defect, but uncommonly with isolated LVH.

When the QRS axis lies between −90° and −150° (+210° and +270°), deciding if this represents marked right-axis deviation or marked left-axis deviation is difficult. In such patients, the practitioner should interpret the location of the axis in light of the patient's cardiac anomaly.

Calculation of the direction of the mean QRS vector in the horizontal plane is more difficult, but the vector can be generally described as anterior, posterior, leftward, or rightward. Determination of the horizontal QRS axis can be combined with information about QRS amplitude to determine ventricular hypertrophy.

(2) *QRS amplitude.* In infants and children, little diagnostic information is obtained from the QRS amplitude of the six standard leads except when low voltage is present in these leads. Normally, the QRS complex in leads I, II, and III exceeds 5 mm in height, but if smaller it suggests conditions such as pericardial effusion.

In the precordial leads, QRS amplitude is used to determine ventricular hypertrophy. Leads V_1 and V_6 should each exceed 8 mm; if smaller, pericardial effusion or similar conditions may be present.

Ventricular hypertrophy is manifested by alterations in ventricular depolarization and amplitudes of the QRS complex. The term ventricular hypertrophy is partly a misnomer, as it applies to electrocardiographic patterns in which the primary anatomic change is ventricular chamber enlargement and to patterns associated with cardiac conditions in which the ventricular walls are thicker than normal.

> Generally, hypertrophy is the response to pressure loads upon the ventricle (e.g. aortic stenosis), whereas enlargement reflects augmented ventricular volume (e.g. aortic regurgitation).

Interpretation of an electrocardiogram for ventricular hypertrophy must be made relative to the normal evolution of the QRS complex, particularly to the amplitude of the R and S waves in leads V_1 and V_6 (Table 1.7).

Right ventricular hypertrophy. In RVH, the major QRS forces are directed anteriorly and rightward. This usually leads to right-axis deviation, a taller than normal R wave in lead V_1, and a deeper than normal S wave in lead V_6.

RVH can be diagnosed by either of the following criteria: (i) the R wave in lead V_1 is greater than normal for age or (ii) the S wave in lead V_6 is greater than normal for age.

A positive T wave in lead V_1 in patients between the ages of 7 days and 10 years supports the diagnosis of RVH.

RVH/RVE Criteria

R in V_1 > normal for age.
S in V_6 > normal for age.
RSR′ in V_1 with R′ > R and R′ > 5 mm.
Upright T wave in V_1 between age 1 week and 12 years.
RAD (right-axis deviation of QRS frontal plane axis).

Differentiating RVH and RVE

Patterns reflecting increases in right ventricular muscle mass ("hypertrophy") usually show a tall R wave in lead V_1, whereas patterns showing RVE usually show an RSR′ pattern in lead V_1 and a QRS complex in lead V_6 with a large broad S wave. Usually, the R′ exceeds 10 mm. This distinction is not absolute; variations occur.

Left ventricular hypertrophy. The major QRS forces are directed leftward and, at times, posteriorly. LVH can be diagnosed by this "rule of thumb:" (i) an R wave in lead V_6 >25 mm (or >20 mm in children less than six months of age) and/or (ii) an S wave in lead V_1 >25 mm (or >20 mm in children less than six months of age) (Figure 1.8).

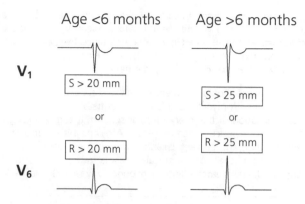

Figure 1.8 Electrocardiographic criteria for LVH/LVE by "rule of thumb."

Combined with ST-segment changes and inversion of the T wave in lead V_6, this is referred to as a pattern of "strain" and may be seen in severe left ventricular outflow obstruction.

Differentiating LVH and LVE

Distinction between LVH and LVE is difficult. LVH may show a deep S wave in lead V_1 and a normal amplitude R wave in lead V_6, whereas LVE shows a tall R wave in lead V_6 associated with a deep Q wave and a tall T wave.

Biventricular hypertrophy. This condition is diagnosed by criteria for both RVH and LVH or by the presence of large equiphasic R and S waves in the mid-precordial leads with a combined amplitude ≥70 mm (Katz–Wachtel phenomenon).

The electrocardiographic standards presented are merely guidelines for interpretation. The electrocardiograms of a few normal patients may be interpreted as ventricular hypertrophy, and indeed, with utilization of these standards only, the electrocardiograms of some patients with heart disease and anatomic hypertrophy may not be considered abnormal.

(3) *QRS duration.* The width of the QRS complex should be measured in lead V_1. The normal range is from 60 to 100 ms; however, infants show shorter QRS intervals. If the duration of the QRS complex exceeds 100 ms, a conduction abnormality of ventricular depolarization, such as right or left bundle branch

block, is most likely present. In complete right bundle branch block, an RSR' pattern appears in lead V_1 and the R' is wide. In lead V_6, the S wave is frequently broad and deep. Right bundle branch block frequently results from operative repair of tetralogy of Fallot. Another example of prolonged QRS duration is Wolff–Parkinson–White syndrome.

Q wave. The Q waves should be carefully analyzed; abnormal Q waves may be present in patients with myocardial infarction. Normally, the Q wave represents primarily depolarization of the interventricular septum. It can be exaggerated if infarction of the left ventricular free wall exists. After the initial 20 ms of the ventricular depolarization, the left ventricular free wall begins to depolarize. With left ventricular infarction, the right ventricular depolarization is unopposed and directed rightward. This creates a larger and longer Q wave in the left-side leads.

---

(1) *Q-wave amplitude.* Except in leads aVR and aVL, the Q-wave amplitude should not exceed 25% of the combined amplitude of the QRS complex. If it is larger, the initial QRS forces are accentuated, usually a result of either left ventricular myocardial damage or abnormal septal hypertrophy.
(2) *Q-wave duration.* The Q-wave duration in leads I, II, and V_6 should be less than 30 ms. If it is longer, myocardial infarction is suspected.

ST segment. The QRS complex returns to the baseline before forming the T wave. The segment (ST) between the QRS complex and the T wave should be isoelectric; but in normal children, particularly adolescents, it may be elevated 1 mm in the limb leads and 2 mm in the mid-precordial leads. It should not be depressed more than 1 mm.

Alterations in the ST segment beyond these limits occur because of myocardial ischemia (depression), pericarditis (elevation), or digoxin (coving depression). The ST segment and T wave are often considered as a unit but should be analyzed separately. ST–T abnormalities are not specific as they can occur in many conditions (e.g. electrolyte disturbances) or in normal children (so-called early depolarization).

T wave. The T wave represents repolarization of the ventricles. Whereas ventricular depolarization takes place from the endocardium to the epicardium, repolarization is considered to occur in the opposite direction. Thus, the direction of the T-wave axis is generally that of the QRS axis.

(1) *T-wave axis.* The T-wave axis in the frontal plane is normally between +15° and +75°; in the horizontal plane it is between −15° and +75° (Figure 1.7). In neonates, it begins closer to −15° and moves gradually toward +75° during

childhood. Thus, in the horizontal plane, the T wave should always be positive in lead V_6. In V_1, the T wave is upright in the first three days of life and then becomes inverted until 10–12 years of age, when it again changes to positive.

When both the T wave and the QRS complex are abnormal, showing either hypertrophy or conduction abnormalities, the T-wave abnormalities are most likely secondary to the QRS changes.

If, however, the T wave is abnormal whereas the QRS complex is normal, the T-wave changes represent primary repolarization abnormalities. These may be caused by a variety of factors, such as electrolyte abnormality, metabolic abnormality, pericardial changes, or medication effect.

(2) *T-wave amplitude*. There are no rigid criteria for the amplitude of T waves, although the general rule is the greater the amplitude of the QRS, the greater is that of the T wave. The average T-wave amplitude is approximately 20% of the average QRS amplitude. T waves normally range from 1 to 5 mm in standard leads and from 2 to 8 mm in precordial leads.

T-wave amplitude is affected by the serum potassium concentration. Hypokalemia is associated with low-voltage T waves and hyperkalemia with tall, peaked, and symmetrical T waves. A variety of T-wave patterns have been associated with other electrolyte abnormalities.

(3) *T-wave duration*. This is best measured by the QT interval, defined as the time from onset of the Q wave to termination of the T wave, and it varies naturally with heart rate. Therefore, it needs to be corrected for heart rate by measuring the interval between R waves (R–R). The equation representing this is

$$QT_c = \frac{QT}{\sqrt{R-R}}$$

where QT_c is the corrected QT interval (seconds), QT is the measured QT interval (seconds), and R–R is the measured interval between R waves (seconds).

Males:
   normal QT_c ≤ 440 ms
Females:
   normal QT_c ≤ 450 ms

The QT_c normally does not exceed 440 ms for males and 450 ms for females. Hypercalcemia and digitalis shorten the QT_c; hypocalcemia lengthens it. Medications may variably affect the QT_c.

LQTS is a familial condition associated with syncope, seizures, ventricular tachycardia, and sudden death. In this condition, the QT_c often exceeds 480 ms.

U wave. In some patients, a small deflection of unknown origin, the U wave, follows the T wave. It can be prominent in patients with hypokalemia or hypothermia.

Chest X-ray

Chest X-rays should be considered for every patient suspected of cardiac disease. Study of the X-ray films reveals information about cardiac size, the size of specific cardiac chambers, the status of the pulmonary vasculature, and the variations of cardiac contour, vessel position, and organ situs. Two views of the heart are usually obtained: posteroanterior and lateral.

Cardiac size

Size can be evaluated best on a posteroanterior projection.

> Cardiac enlargement indicates an augmented volume of blood in the heart. Any condition that places a volume load upon the heart (e.g. a regurgitant valve or a left-to-right shunt) leads to cardiac enlargement proportional to the amount of volume overload.
>
> In contrast, ventricular hypertrophy, meaning increased thickness of the myocardium, does not show cardiac enlargement on the chest X-ray, although it might change the contour of the heart.

Care must be taken in interpreting X-rays of neonates, particularly those obtained in intensive care units with portable equipment. Three factors in this situation can result in an image that falsely appears as cardiomegaly: the films are usually obtained in anteroposterior rather than posteroanterior projection; the X-ray source-to-film distance is short (40 inches rather than the standard 72 inches); and the infant is supine (in all supine individuals, cardiac volume is greater).

The anatomic position of the cardiac chambers on chest X-ray views is shown in Figure 1.9. Several important anatomic features are illustrated. The atria and ventricles, rather than being positioned in a true right-to-left relationship, have a more anteroposterior orientation. The right atrium and right ventricle are anterior and to the right of the respective left-sided chambers. The interatrial and interventricular septae are not positioned perpendicular to the anterior chest wall but at a 45° angle to the left and tilted away 35% from the midline of the body.

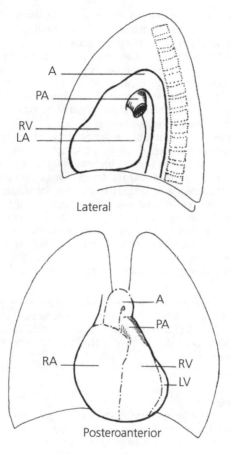

Figure 1.9 Relationship of cardiac chambers observed in posteroanterior and lateral chest X-rays. A, aorta; LA, left atrium; LV, left ventricle; PA, pulmonary artery; RA, right atrium; RV, right ventricle.

In the posteroanterior projection, the right cardiac border is formed by the right atrium. Prominence of this cardiac border may suggest right atrial enlargement, but this diagnosis is difficult to make from the roentgenogram.

The left cardiac border is composed of three segments: the aortic knob, pulmonary trunk, and broad sweep of the left ventricle. The right ventricle does not contribute to the left cardiac border in this projection.

Prominence of the aorta or the pulmonary trunk may be found in this view. Enlargement of either of these vessels occurs in three hemodynamic situations: increased blood flow through the great vessel, poststenotic dilation, or increased pressure beyond the valve, as in pulmonary hypertension. A concave pulmonary arterial segment suggests pulmonary artery atresia or hypoplasia and diminished volume of pulmonary blood flow.

On the lateral film, the margins of the cardiac silhouette are formed anteriorly by the right ventricle and posteriorly by the left atrium. This view is preferred for showing left atrial enlargement because the left atrium is the only cardiac chamber that normally touches the esophagus. An esophageal contrast swallow study can be used to delineate the esophagus. In a normal individual, the left atrium may indent the anterior esophageal wall, but the posterior wall is not displaced. If both anterior and posterior walls are displaced, left atrial enlargement is present.

Normally, the lower part of the right ventricle abuts the sternum and the air-filled lung extends down between the sternum and the right ventricle and pulmonary artery. When the retrosternal space is obliterated by cardiac density, RVE is present. In infants, however, this space may also be obliterated by the thymus.

> Both the electrocardiogram and the chest X-ray may be used to assess cardiac chamber size. Left atrial enlargement is best detected by chest X-ray, whereas ventricular or right atrial enlargement is detected better by an electrocardiogram.

Cardiac contour
In addition to the search for information about cardiac size on the posteroanterior view of the heart, the practitioner should direct attention to distinctive cardiac contours, such as the boot-shaped heart of tetralogy of Fallot. In conditions with RVH, the cardiac apex may be turned upward, whereas conditions with LVH or dilation lead to displacement of the cardiac apex outward and downward toward the diaphragm.

Situs
Note situs of the heart, stomach, and especially the aortic arch. In infants with a prominent thymus, the aortic knob is usually obscured, and normal aortic arch position is inferred from the rightward displacement of the trachea in a properly

positioned posteroanterior chest film. A right aortic arch is common in tetralogy of Fallot and truncus arteriosus and can be diagnosed by leftward displacement of the trachea.

Pulmonary vasculature

The status of the pulmonary vasculature is the most important diagnostic information derived from the chest X-ray; this function has not been replaced by the echocardiogram. The radiographic appearance of the blood vessels in the lungs reflects the degree of pulmonary blood flow. Because many cardiac anomalies alter pulmonary blood flow, proper interpretation of pulmonary vascular markings is diagnostically helpful. It is one of the two major features discussed in this book for initiating the differential diagnosis.

The lung fields are assessed to determine if the vascularity is increased, normal, or diminished, reflecting augmented, normal, or decreased pulmonary blood flow, respectively. As a check of the logic of interpretation, the vascular markings should be compared with cardiac size. If a large-volume left-to-right shunt exists, the heart size has to be larger than normal.

Pulmonary vascular markings may be more difficult to analyze from portable films obtained in a neonatal care unit because the X-ray exposure time is longer, resulting in blurred images from rapid respirations, and from the redistributed pulmonary blood volume in the supine patient.

With experience obtained from viewing a number of chest X-rays, the status of pulmonary vasculature can be judged. With increased vascularity, the lung fields show increased pulmonary arterial markings, the hilae are plump, and vascular shadows radiate toward the periphery. With decreased vascularity, the lungs appear dark or lucent; the hilum is small; and the pulmonary arterial vessels are stringy.

Summary of Chest X-ray Parameters

Situs (heart, stomach, and aortic arch)
Cardiac size
Cardiothymic silhouette, shape, and contour
Pulmonary artery silhouette
Pulmonary vascular markings (normal, increased, or decreased; symmetric versus asymmetric)

Pulse oximetry

Because oxyhemoglobin and deoxyhemoglobin absorb light differently, spectro-photometry can be used to measure the percentage of hemoglobin bound to oxygen.

Pulse oximeters utilize a light source and light sensor applied to the surface of a patient's skin to compare noninvasively the light absorption of moving blood (during arterial flow) with the light absorption of nonmoving blood and tissue during arterial diastole (analogous to a reference sample).

Functional arterial oxygen saturation (SaO_2) in percent is calculated automatically and displayed along with pulse rate.

Pulse oximeters do not detect dysfunctional hemoglobin (e.g. methemoglobin and carboxyhemoglobin), so patients with important concentrations of these types of abnormal hemoglobin have a factitiously high SaO_2 compared with their true fractional saturation as measured from a blood sample using a standard laboratory co-oximeter.

Other factors that affect pulse oximeter results include skin pigmentation, poor skin perfusion, tachycardia, ambient light, and shifts in the oxyhemoglobin absorption spectrum that can accompany chronic cyanosis.

Neonates with cyanotic heart malformations (e.g. transposition of the great vessels) or obstructive lesions (e.g. coarctation of the aorta) may have differential cyanosis, a measurable inequality in the pulse oximetry readings from preductal (right-hand) compared with postductal (foot) sites, even though the difference is not apparent by physical examination (discussed more fully in Chapter 8).

Blood counts

In infants and children with cyanotic forms of congenital cardiac disease, hypoxemia stimulates the bone marrow to produce more red blood cells (polycythemia), thus improving oxygen-carrying capacity. As a result, both the total number of erythrocytes and the hematocrit are elevated. The production of the increased red cell mass should be paralleled by an increase in hemoglobin. In a patient with cyanosis and normal iron stores, the hemoglobin also should be elevated so that the red-cell indices are normal.

Iron deficiency

In infancy, iron deficiency is common; it may be accentuated in cyanotic infants because of the increased iron requirements and by the fact that such infants may have a poor appetite and primarily a milk diet. In such infants, the red-cell indices reflect iron deficiency anemia because the hemoglobin value is low relative to the red blood cell count and the hematocrit. In fact, a cyanotic infant may have a hemoglobin value that is normal or even elevated for age and still have iron deficiency.

An example is an infant with a hemoglobin of 16 g/dL and a hematocrit of 66%. The hematocrit value reflects the volume of red cells elevated in response to hypoxemia; the hemoglobin value primarily reflects the amount

> of iron available for its formation. In this infant, the hemoglobin should be 22 g/dL. (Normally, the number for the hemoglobin value should be about one-third of the number of the hematocrit value.)

The mean corpuscular volume is always low in iron deficiency, even if the hemoglobin is normal or above normal. An iron-deficient infant often improves symptomatically following administration of iron. Iron deficiency has been associated with an increased risk of stroke in severely polycythemic patients.

Patients with inoperable cyanotic heart disease should have hemoglobin and hematocrit values measured periodically; discrepancies between the two should be noted and managed with appropriate iron administration. Similar information may be obtained by evaluating a blood smear. Serum iron testing is usually unnecessary.

Hyperviscosity

Vascular resistance varies with blood viscosity, which is affected primarily by hematocrit. The viscosity doubles between a hematocrit of 45% and 75%. The effect on a patient's symptoms is not evident until the hematocrit approaches 65%. In general, adolescents and young adults with inoperable cyanotic heart disease become symptomatic with phlebotomy, probably because of its detrimental effect of lowering oxygen-carrying capacity and temporary reduction of blood volume. Iron deficiency worsens with repeated phlebotomy as iron-containing red blood cells are withdrawn.

Anemia

Anemia may increase the cardiac workload in patients with congestive heart failure and may predispose patients with tetralogy of Fallot to have hypercyanotic spells. In cyanotic patients, severe anemia leads to an important decrease in the oxygen carrying capacity.

Echocardiography

Echocardiography, a powerful noninvasive diagnostic technique, requires a high degree of skill in performance and interpretation of the studies. This method adds considerable information regarding cardiac function and structure to that gained previously from history, examination, electrocardiogram, and chest radiography.

Echocardiography of infants and children is considerably different from that of adults. Special technical performance is required to obtain quality information in uncooperative children. Furthermore, the interpretation emphasizes anatomic relationships, connections, and physiologic principles more than the mere recording of chamber size and ventricular function. In adults, the poor acoustic penetration often makes it difficult to obtain detailed information by transthoracic echocardiography (TTE). Therefore, in adults, transesophageal echocardiography (TEE) is performed, in which the heart is imaged from a probe positioned in the esophagus instead. In most patients of pediatric age, excellent images are obtained using surface (TTE) echocardiograms alone. TEE is used in special circumstances, such as during a cardiac operation, where images from the thoracic wall would be impossible to obtain. Infants and children are not routinely sedated for echocardiography since a complete and high-quality echocardiogram can usually be obtained without sedation.

Echocardiography is based on a familiar principle illustrated by bats, which emit ultrahigh-frequency sound waves that are reflected from surfaces and are received back, allowing the bats to judge their surroundings and to avoid collision with objects. The principles of Doppler determination of the velocity of moving objects are applied to determine the speed and direction of blood flow.

Two-dimensional images

An echocardiogram is recorded by placing a transducer in an interspace adjacent to the left sternal border and at other locations on the chest and abdomen (Figure 1.10). The small transducer contains a piezoelectric crystal that converts electrical energy to high-frequency sound waves. Thus, the transducer emits sound waves into the chest that strike cardiac structures; these sound waves (echoes) are then reflected back to the chest wall. The transducer receives sound (echoes) from the cardiac structures and reconverts them to electrical energy that is then recorded as an echocardiogram.

Because the frequency of the sound waves and the speed of sound in body tissues are constant, the interval between the emission of sound and the receipt of sound indicates the distance into and back from the heart that the sound wave traveled. The ultrahigh-frequency sounds are reflected only from interfaces between structures of different density, such as the interface between the ventricular cavity (blood) and the ventricular septum (muscle). The amount of sound returned depends on the nature of the substances on either side of the interface.

The reflecting surface must be perpendicular to the transducer; when a surface lies tangentially, the sound waves are generally reflected in a different direction and are not received by the transducer. As the sound waves travel into the heart, at each interface some of the transmitted sound returns to the transducer, and some continues to the next structure where more is reflected, while some still continues. In this way, multiple sound waves are reflected at various distances from the surface of the chest; these echoes are used to generate 2D images moving in real time.

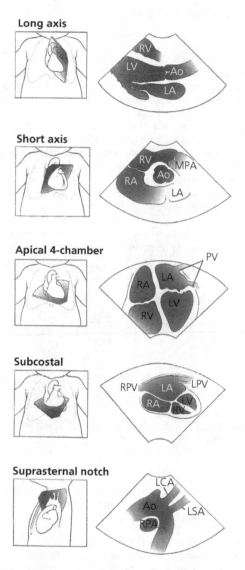

Figure 1.10 Two-dimensional (2D) echocardiography. Five standard views are shown. The illustrations on the left show the sector-shaped plane of the ultrasound beam inscribed on the patient's chest; the illustrations on the right show the corresponding 2D images of the heart and vessels. Ao, aorta; LA, left atrium; LCA, left carotid artery; LSA, left subclavian artery; LV, left ventricle; MPA, main pulmonary artery; PV, pulmonary vein; RA, right atrium. Source: Images courtesy of Philips Healthcare.

M-mode

In an M (movement)-mode echocardiogram (Figure 1.11), the vertical axis represents distance from the transducer on the surface of the chest and the horizontal axis represents time. The movements of cardiac structures can be recorded over several cardiac cycles. A simultaneous electrocardiogram assists in the timing of cardiac events.

Chamber size and left ventricular wall thickness are usually measured by M-mode. Representative normal left heart values are shown in Table 1.8.

Cardiac function is estimated from an M-mode echocardiogram. Although not true measures of contractility, both left ventricular shortening fraction (percentage change in diameter between diastole and systole; normal ≥28%) and ejection fraction (percentage change in estimated volume; normal ≥55%) are often used to describe systolic ventricular function. These values may vary with changes in afterload, preload, or contractility.

Calculation of shortening fraction (SF) and ejection fraction (EF)

$$SF(\%) = \frac{LVEDD - LVESD}{LVEDD} \times 100$$

$$EF(\%) \cong \frac{LVEDD^3 - LVEDD^3}{LVESD^3}\, 100$$

or

$$EF \cong SF \times 1.7$$

Normal: SF ≥28%, EF ≥55%.
LVEDD, left ventricular end-diastolic diameter; LVESD, left ventricular end-systolic diameter.

Doppler

Doppler echocardiography provides information on the direction and speed (velocity) of moving blood. Three main types of Doppler echocardiography are commonly used.

Pulsed wave (PW) Doppler. PW Doppler derives velocity information from discrete packets of ultrasound transmitted and received by the transducer, allowing precise interrogation of small regions of a blood vessel or cardiac chamber. The main limitation of PW Doppler is the compromise between the depth of the

(a)   (b)

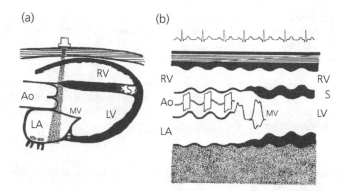

Figure 1.11 Comparison of M-mode echocardiogram and 2D (or cross-sectional) echocardiogram. The transducer beam passing through the cross-sectional view (a) corresponds to the same structures seen in the M-mode (b) during a "sweep" of the transducer from aorta to ventricles. Ao, aorta; LA, left atrium; LV, left ventricle; MV, mitral valve; RV, right ventricle; S, interventricular septum.

structure to be interrogated and the maximum velocity that can be measured – maximum velocity decreases as the distance to the target increases.

Continuous wave (CW) Doppler. Continuous wave (CW) Doppler uses simultaneous continuous transmission and receipt of ultrasound and provides highly

Table 1.8 Echocardiographic upper limits of left ventricular (LV) dimensions by body weight.

Body weight (kg)	LV diastolic diameter (cm)	LV diastolic wall thickness (mm)
4	2.5	5
8	3.0	6
15	3.5	7
30	4.5	9
60	5.0	10

Source: Courtesy of William S. McMahon, MD, based on published data, including Henry, W.L., Ware, J., Gardin, J.M., et al. Echocardiographic measurements in normal subjects: growth-related changes that occur between infancy and early adulthood. *Circulation*, 1978, **57**, 278–285.

accurate estimates of very high-velocity blood flow – for example, through a stenotic aortic valve – but cannot localize the source of the fastest velocities, as PW Doppler can.

Both PW and CW Doppler are commonly used to determine the following:

(1) *Pressure gradient.* Just as river water speeds up on passing through narrow rapids, Doppler velocities can be used to predict pressure gradients between two chambers according to a simplified form of the Bernoulli equation, given a constant flow rate:

$$PG = V^2 \times 4,$$

where *PG* is pressure gradient (mmHg), V^2 is velocity (m/s) of blood flow, and 4 is a constant.

This technique is commonly used to estimate the pressure gradient across a stenotic valve, such as aortic stenosis.

Also, the maximum velocity of blood regurgitating through an AV valve during systole (depending on atrial pressure) gives an approximation of the peak systolic pressure in the ventricle.

(2) *Flow (cardiac output).* In areas where flow is laminar (most of the blood is moving at the same velocity at any given point in time), Doppler can be used to measure the change in this velocity throughout the systolic ejection period. The mean velocity (cm/s) during ejection through a normal semilunar valve of known area (cm^2) can be used to calculate the flow (cm^3/s of ejection) and combined with the heart rate to determine cardiac output (cm^3/s or L/min).

Color (flow velocity mapping) Doppler. Color Doppler allows the generation of a color-coded display of real-time blood flow velocity and direction overlaid on the black-and-white 2D image of the heart. Color Doppler allows the visualization of jets of blood flow, such as through a small VSD, or for grading the degree of regurgitation of a cardiac valve. Physiologic blood flow is easily demonstrated with color Doppler: by convention, flow away from the transducer is represented by blue and flow toward the transducer by red. The colors have no relationship to blood oxygen levels.

Specialized echocardiography

Fetal echocardiography. Cardiac abnormalities can be diagnosed in a fetus by echocardiography. Usually performed by an experienced pediatric cardiologist, major abnormalities of structure or arrhythmias can be identified. Small VSDs and minor valvar anomalies may not be visualized. It is typically performed between 18 and 24 weeks of pregnancy. Whereas general obstetric ultrasound is performed of most fetuses, fetal echocardiography is applied in specific situations including identification of a major extracardiac anomaly or abnormal cardiac structure on screening, presence of an abnormal karyotype, family history of coronary heart disease (CHD), maternal diabetes, or other known risk factors. After identifying the intrauterine position of the fetus, the heart is imaged, the best view being the four-chamber view. The relationship and size of great vessels, the status of cardiac septae, and nature of cardiac valves can be visualized. Cardiac chamber size can be measured and Doppler techniques applied. The information derived can be used to establish a diagnosis, plan care of the infant following birth, and in preparing the parents for the level of care indicated. Frequently, by knowing the seriousness of the cardiac anomaly, the infant can be delivered in a hospital that has prompt access to pediatric cardiac care.

Transesophageal echocardiography. Both TTE and TEE are important diagnostic techniques in children. In general, in infants and children, the range of structures that can be evaluated is greater with TTE and the image quality is comparable to that of TEE. For patients undergoing cardiac surgery or catheterization, TEE is often employed concurrently. TEE usually requires sedation and/or anesthesia, whereas many centers do not routinely sedate children for TTE. The size of the available transesophageal transducer limits the technique to larger infants and children.

Intracardiac echocardiography. Intracardiac echocardiography (ICE) utilizes a catheter-mounted transducer to acquire intravascular and intracardiac image and Doppler data during cardiac catheterization, usually electrophysiologic catheterization. It provides more precise localization of structures than fluoroscopy and angiography.

Tissue Doppler imaging. Tissue Doppler imaging, performed during TTE or TEE, uses Doppler principles to measure the velocity of the ventricular walls, rather than the movement of blood, as in standard Doppler. This provides information about ventricular performance and regional wall motion abnormalities.

Deformational imaging (myocardial strain, speckle tracking). This technique continually analyzes the beat to beat motion of multiple small segments of the ventricular endocardium to assess ventricular performance.

Three-dimensional echocardiography. Three-dimensional echocardiography (3D echo) generates a real-time pseudo-holographic representation of the heart using a "stack" of sequential 2D images. This technique provides enhanced images of complex structures such as AV valves and ventricular outflow tracts.

Magnetic resonance imaging and angiography

Magnetic resonance imaging and angiography (MRI and MRA) generate high-quality static images of the body similar to those of computed tomography (CT) except that ionizing radiation is not used. Rather, a powerful magnetic field surrounds the patient, and the chest is irradiated with radiofrequency pulses that produce alignment of the normally random arrangement of the atomic nuclei of paramagnetic elements. Since hydrogen in water and fat is the most common atom in the body, most MRI images are created using the radiofrequency emitted from these hydrogen nuclei and received as induced current in surrounding coils.

A basic assumption of MRI is that the subject is stationary, a problem partly overcome during cardiac imaging by gating the acquisition of signals to respirations and the electrocardiogram.

Although multiple images can be acquired and combined in a series to create the illusion of movement, considerable time is required to create each image, so "real-time" images, such as those obtained with echocardiography, are not possible (Table 1.9). Since a patient must lie still for the acquisition of multiple images, sedation is required for infants and small children. Although MRI is noninvasive and involves no radiation, sedation increases the relative risk of the procedure.

MRI can provide some data regarding pressure gradients, but the speed and ease of acquisition are not comparable to those with Doppler echocardiography. MRI does provide excellent images in large adolescents and adults where echocardiography is impossible. Patients with certain magnetic implants, such as artificial pacemakers and certain prosthetic devices, cannot be subjected to the intense magnetic field required. Intravenous nonionic contrast agents are often employed, especially with MRA.

Computed tomography

CT for cardiovascular imaging has many of the same advantages and disadvantages of MRI and MRA. Computed tomographic angiography (CTA) utilizes higher resolution and faster CT instruments, along with the intravenous administration of iodinated contrast, to obtain very high-quality images; however, the normally faster heart rates of children limit resolution and hemodynamic data are limited. CTA gated to the patient's electrocardiogram provides higher-resolution images of moving cardiac structures, yet results in significantly higher radiation doses. Table 1.9 compares various imaging techniques.

Cardiac catheterization

Cardiac catheterization requires a staff of trained specialists – pediatric cardiologists, radiologists, laboratory technicians, and nurses. As a diagnostic procedure, it provides detailed information about the heart not found by other techniques. Its use as a diagnostic technique has been reduced by other techniques such as echocardiography, but its application for treatment (intervention) has expanded.

Table 1.9 Comparison of common diagnostic imaging modalities in the evaluation of patients with congenital heart disease.

	CXR	Ba Eso	CT	CTA	MR/MRA	Echo TTE	Echo TEE	Cath
Real time	N	Y/N	N	N	N	Y	Y	Y
Hemodynamics	–	–	–	+	+++	++	++++	++++
Availability	++++	+++	+++	++	+	++	+	+
Interpretation	+	++	+++	++++	++++	++++	++++	++++
Cost	+	++	+++	+++	+++	++	++	++++
Radiation	+	++	+++	++++	–	–	–	+++
Anesthesia and/or sedation	N	N	Y/N	Y/N	Y/N	N/Y	Y	Y
IV contrast	N	N	N/Y	Y	Y	N	N	Y
Heart rate effect	–	–	++	+++	++	–	–	–
Respiratory and movement effect	+	–	+	+	++	–	–	–
Most useful data/condition	Pulmonary blood flow, degree and symmetry	Vascular ring/sling	Rapid assessment aortic dissection; effusions	Detailed images, short acquisition time	Detailed images; best for static structures	Real time, chamber dimension, thickness, hemodynamics, anatomic relationships and situs	Enhanced images when TTE suboptimal, or intraoperative, intracath	Intervention. Diagnosis of PA htn and reactivity
Disadvantages	No direct hemodynamic data	No direct imaging of anomaly	Relatively low resolution	Heart rate, respiratory artifact	Heart rate, respiratory artifact	Acoustic windows become more limiting as patient size increases	Some structures imaged by TTE not seen by TEE	Radiation and contrast load. Vascular entry sites required

CXR, chest radiograph; Ba Eso, barium esophagogram (table refers to fluoroscopically performed examinations; simple studies can be accomplished with barium swallow at the time of an upright CXR in some patients); CT, computed tomography of the chest; CTA, computed tomographic angiography; requires higher-resolution equipment than standard CT; MRI/MRA, magnetic resonance imaging/magnetic resonance angiography; Echo TTE, echocardiogram, transthoracic; Echo TEE, echocardiogram, transesophageal; PA htn, pulmonary hypertension; cath, cardiac catheterization.

Diagnostic cardiac catheterization

With the use of echocardiography and other noninvasive studies, the indications for diagnostic cardiac catheterization have become targeted to acquire specific information: anatomic (e.g. coronary artery anatomy in transposition), functional (e.g. pulmonary vascular resistance in an older child with a VSD), or histologic (cardiac biopsy in a transplant patient).

Interventional therapeutic catheterization

Interventional catheterization began in the 1960s with Rashkind atrial septostomy, in which a spherical latex balloon is withdrawn forcefully through a patent foramen ovale to create a large ASD for palliation of both complete transposition of the great vessels and hypoplastic left ventricle.

Currently, radial balloon dilation with sausage-shaped catheter-mounted balloons is commonly used to relieve obstruction in stenotic semilunar valves and nonvalved pathways (e.g. recurrent coarctation, stenotic pulmonary arteries).

Catheter-based methods for closure of PDA and ASD are used widely, and devices for closure of certain types of VSD are available.

Electrophysiologic catheterization

Electrophysiologic catheterization is performed to define the mechanism and characteristics of arrhythmias.

Radiofrequency ablation or cryoablation may be used to eliminate accessory electrical connections or automatic foci, thus curing certain arrhythmias.

Procedure

Cardiac catheterization is performed in children in a manner that ensures a quiet, controlled, and safe environment for the child, allows minimum discomfort, pain, and anxiety, and also achieves optimum data collection or treatment.

Anesthesia

Two basic approaches are used:

General anesthesia. Anesthesia, usually with endotracheal intubation in neonates, infants, and small children, allows the precise control of airway and ventilation. This avoids elevation of pulmonary vascular resistance that may accompany hypoventilation from oversedation.

Sedation. Sedation alone is used successfully in patients of all ages at many centers. This usually involves a combination of agents, including narcotics, benzodiazepines, phenothiazines, and ketamine.

Vascular access

Both the right and left sides of the heart may be catheterized either by percutaneous puncture (Seldinger technique) or by operative exposure ("cutdown") to major peripheral veins and arteries. The right side of the heart is accessed through veins in the inguinal area or upper body (e.g. internal jugular vein). The left side of the heart can be catheterized through two approaches: a venous catheter passed through the foramen ovale or ASD (or via a tiny defect created with a needle-tipped catheter) into the left atrium; or an arterial catheter inserted into the brachial or femoral artery and passed retrograde across the aortic valve into the left ventricle. Arterial puncture and atrial septum puncture carry more risk than do venous studies.

Technique

Once the catheter has been inserted into the vessel, it can be advanced into the heart and directed into various cardiac chambers and major blood vessels with the aid of fluoroscopy. At any of these sites, pressures can be measured, blood samples obtained, and contrast media injected.

Pressure data. The catheter is connected to a pressure transducer and the values obtained are compared with normal (Table 1.10) to evaluate stenotic lesions or pulmonary hypertension.

Oximetric data. Blood samples from each cardiac site are analyzed for oxygen content or hemoglobin saturation to determine if a shunt is present. Normally, the oxygen saturation in each right-sided cardiac chamber is similar, but an increase in the oxygen saturation in any chamber, compared with the preceding site, may mean a left-to-right shunt at that level. Normal variations in oxygen content occur, so a slight increase may not indicate a shunt. Multiple samples at each site are used to resolve this point.

Table 1.10 Normal cardiac catheterization values.

Site	Oxygen saturation (%)	Pressure (mmHg)
RA	70±5	Mean 3–7
RV	70±5	25/EDP 0–5
PA	70±5	25/10, mean 15
LA, PCW	97±3	Mean 5–10
LV	97±3	100/EDP 0–10
Aorta	97±3	100/70, mean 85

EDP, end-diastolic pressure; LA, left atrium; LV, left ventricle; PA, pulmonary artery; PCW, pulmonary capillary wedge pressure; RA, right atrium; RV, right ventricle.

Normally, the oxygen saturation of blood in the left atrium, the left ventricle, and the aorta should be at least 94%; if less than 94%, a right-to-left shunt is present.

Derived values. The pressure and oximetry data can be used to derive various measures of cardiac function.

Flow (cardiac output). This can be calculated using the Fick principle:

$$\text{Cardiac output }(L/min) = \frac{\text{Oxygen consumption}\left(mLO_2/min\right)}{\text{Arteriovenous oxygen difference}\left(mL/dL\right)\times 10}$$

The patient's rate of oxygen consumption can be determined by analyzing a timed collection of the patient's expired air.

The arteriovenous oxygen difference is obtained by analyzing blood samples drawn from the arterial side of the circulation (aorta or peripheral artery) and from the venous side of the heart (usually the pulmonary artery). The oxygen content (mL O_2/dL whole blood) is used in this calculation (arterial % O_2 saturation − venous % O_2 saturation × O_2 capacity [mL O_2/dL whole blood]) as the percentage hemoglobin saturation alone cannot be used.

Cardiac output determined by the Fick principle is widely used in analyzing catheterization data and has become the standard with which other methods of determining cardiac output, such as thermodilution, are compared.

Many cardiac malformations have either a left-to-right or a right-to left shunt. Therefore, the blood flow through the lungs may differ from that through the body. Since the oxygen consumption in the body equals the oxygen picked up in the lungs, the Fick principle may still be used for such patients:

$$Q_s = \frac{\dot{V}o_2}{SA - MV},$$

where Q_s is systemic blood flow (L/min), $\dot{V}o_2$ is oxygen consumption (mL O_2/min), and $SA - MV$ is systemic arterial − mixed venous oxygen difference (mL O_2/L blood).

$$Q_p = \frac{\dot{V}o_2}{PV - PA},$$

where Q_p is pulmonary blood flow (L/min), $\dot{V}o_2$ is oxygen consumption (mL O_2/min), and $PV - PA$ is pulmonary venous − pulmonary arterial oxygen difference (mL O_2/L blood).

Pulmonary/systemic blood flow ratio (Q_p/Q_s). Without assuming or measuring the oxygen consumption, Q_p can be expressed as a ratio of Q_s:

$$\frac{Q_p}{Q_s} = \frac{SA - MV}{PV - PA},$$

where *SA*, *MV*, *PV*, and *PA* represent oxygen saturations (%).

Except for oxygen saturation (%), all other variables required for oxygen content calculation (e.g. hemoglobin concentration) cancel out of the equation.

Vascular resistance. Systemic and pulmonary vascular resistances can be calculated from the hydraulic equivalent of Ohm's law:

$$R = \frac{P}{Q},$$

where R is resistance, P is mean pressure drop across a vascular bed, and Q is cardiac output. Therefore,

$$R_S = \frac{\overline{SA} - \overline{RA}}{Q_S},$$

where R_S is systemic vascular resistance (mmHg/L/min), $\overline{SA}$ is mean systemic artery (aortic) pressure (mmHg), $\overline{RA}$ is mean systemic vein (right atrial) pressure (mmHg), and Q_S is systemic blood flow (L/min).

$$R_P = \frac{\overline{PA} - \overline{LA}}{Q_P},$$

where R_P is pulmonary vascular resistance (mmHg/L/min), $\overline{PA}$ is mean pulmonary arterial pressure (mmHg), $\overline{LA}$ is mean pulmonary vein (left atrium or pulmonary capillary wedge) pressure (mmHg), and Q_P is pulmonary blood flow (L/min).

The resistance ratio (R_P/R_S) can similarly be calculated from the ratio of the mean pressure differences across the pulmonary and systemic beds, divided by Q_P/Q_S:

$$\frac{R_P}{R_S} = \frac{(\overline{PA} - \overline{LA})/(\overline{SA} - \overline{RA})}{Q_P / Q_S},$$

Normalization of output and resistance. Resistance is normalized to body surface area, either by using cardiac index (CI) expressed as L/min/m² in place of cardiac output in the preceding equations or by multiplying the raw resistance by the patient's body surface area, which yields resistance in mmHg · min/L · m² or Wood units · m² (first described by Paul Wood in the 1950s). Resistance is also expressed as dyne · cm/s⁵, which can be converted from Wood units by multiplying by 80. Normal indexed values are shown in Table 1.11.

Angiocardiography. Radio-opaque contrast material can be injected through the catheter into a cardiac chamber and serial X-ray images obtained digitally or on film (cine angiography). Often two projections are obtained simultaneously (biplane). The imaging system can be rotated around the patient so that angulated projections can be obtained to visualize various structures better (axial angiography).

Table 1.11 Normal derived cardiac catheterization values.

Cardiac index (CI)[a]	3–5 L/min/m²
Pulmonary resistance (R_p)[a]	2 units · m²
Systemic resistance (R_s)[a]	10–20 units · m²
Resistance ratio (R_p/R_s)	0.05–0.10

[a] Values indexed to body surface area.

Cardiac anatomy and blood flow can be defined with high resolution. Satisfactory details may be illustrated by injecting the material into the pulmonary artery and then imaging as the contrast passes through the left side of the heart (levophase).

Complications of cardiac catheterization

As with any procedure, cardiac catheterization is associated with complications; the benefits from cardiac catheterization must clearly outweigh the risks.

Death. Death is extremely uncommon (<0.1%) in children beyond one year of age. The risk is higher in infants, particularly neonates, who are often critically ill and require catheterization so that a lifesaving catheter intervention or operation can be performed.

Vascular complications. Rarely, compromise of blood vessels used for catheter entry occurs. Temporary or permanent occlusion of the femoral vein or entire inferior vena cava may occur, which may cause transient venous stasis and edema in the lower extremities. Seldom dangerous, the major impact is the inability to re-enter these vessels if the patient requires additional catheterization.

Femoral artery injury is more serious, as viability of the limb is at risk. Thrombolytic agents and heparin have been used in the acute management of patients with a pulseless extremity after catheterization.

Rarely, an arteriovenous fistula develops with time between adjacent vessels used for catheter entry and requires an operation.

Arrhythmia. During most cardiac catheterizations, arrhythmias of some type occur, most often premature ventricular contractions. These rarely compromise the patient because they tend to be transient. Occasionally, AV block that lasts for several hours occurs.

Radiation. The ionizing radiation dose received by most patients has fallen over the years because of improved image-intensifier technology, even though procedure times have lengthened for patients having interventional procedures. Short- and long-term complications from radiation are rare.

Exercise testing

This technique is helpful in several situations but requires the cooperation of the child. Hence very young children are not candidates for testing. The authors usually limit exercise testing to children over the age of six years. Dobutamine challenge has been used as an alternative, with assessment of myocardial performance by echocardiography and myocardial perfusion using nuclear scans.

Indications

Preoperative assessment. Preoperative assessment of obstructive lesions (e.g. aortic stenosis) may benefit patients with a borderline gradient because it helps in deciding the timing of intervention. Many patients have a clear indication for intervention (surgery or catheterization) so do not need an exercise study. It can be used to assess symptoms, such as chest pain, palpitations, or syncope, that occur during exercise.

Postoperative assessment. Postoperative assessment of cardiopulmonary function (using maximum oxygen consumption and/or exercise endurance time) helps in symptomatic patients and in those with mild systolic dysfunction. It can also aid in formulating sports or occupational recommendations for adolescents and adults with congenital heart disease.

Evaluation of specific conditions

Myocardial ischemic syndromes. Suspected coronary artery insufficiency (e.g. Kawasaki disease with aneurysm or stenosis or postoperative anomalous coronary artery origin repair) is assessed most sensitively by a combination of electrocardiographic and nuclear perfusion studies done during a maximum exercise study. Echocardiographic views of the left ventricle during an exercise test can be used to identify areas of dyskinesis. Exercise electrocardiography alone has a false-negative rate of 15% in adults.

Arrhythmias

Wolff–Parkinson–White syndrome. Patients with this condition may be at greater risk for life-threatening ventricular tachyarrhythmia if the delta wave persists at sinus rates of >180 bpm.

Premature ventricular contractions. If benign, these usually disappear at fast sinus rates during exercise.

Atrioventricular block. The rate reserve of the patient's natural subsidiary (backup) pacemaker can be assessed during exercise.

Suspected LQTS. Patients with this condition do not show the usual shortening of the QT interval as the heart rate increases.

Tachyarrhythmia. Patients with documented tachyarrhythmia (supraventricular [SVT] or ventricular [VT]) during exercise or those at risk during exercise (e.g. postoperative tetralogy of Fallot) may be candidates for drug treatment; exercise assesses the efficacy of the treatment.

Patients with a history of palpitations usually only have normal exercise tests and are better studied using outpatient electrocardiographic monitoring to document the rhythm during symptoms.

Syncope. Usually, only patients with a history of syncope during exercise need study.

Hypertension. Patients following coarctation repair and some with other forms of systemic hypertension may register as normotensive (or borderline) at rest but may exhibit an exaggerated systolic hypertensive response to exercise.

Procedure
Specialized equipment is used for grading the workload and for continuously recording multilead electrocardiograms.

> Heart rate rises linearly to an age-related maximum (200–210 bpm for normal children and adolescents).
>
> Systolic blood pressure rises to a normal maximum of 180–215 mmHg, whereas diastolic pressure remains constant or falls slightly.

If indicated, pulse oximetry and oxygen consumption are measured.

Stress echocardiography allows the determination of cardiac function or change in gradients but can be technically challenging.

Spirometry before and after exercise is useful if exercise-induced bronchospasm is suspected.

A bicycle ergometer allows more precise setting of the workload but is often limited to larger patients. A treadmill is more common. The Bruce protocol involves increasing treadmill speed and inclination in stages every three minutes; because smaller children are unable to run at the maximum speed (6 mph) of the Bruce protocol, most pediatric laboratories use the modified Bruce protocol, which limits the speed to a maximum of 3.4 mph.

Metabolic exercise testing
While most cardiac testing occurs with a patient in a resting state, exercise testing allows for a quantitative, comprehensive, and sensitive assessment of the patient's

cardiac status. This occurs because typically it is the cardiovascular system that limits exercise, as skeletal muscle is dependent on constant oxygen delivery to endure. Therefore, unless there is serious lung or skeletal muscle disease present, the cardiovascular system eventually cannot continue to meet these increasing demands and exercise must stop. While traditional exercise testing estimates oxygen consumption based on treadmill speed and incline, metabolic testing utilizing a mask and computer analysis measures parameters directly. Metabolic exercise testing is particularly helpful in patients with congenital heart disease, in terms of risk stratification and the ability to measure and quantify the extent of any cardiac limitation present. The tables below list the common metabolic parameters obtained during testing as well as the specific details gleaned from each (Table 1.12) and present a differential diagnosis of a common symptom during exercise, dyspnea (Table 1.13).

Table 1.12 Common metabolic exercise testing parameters.

Parameter	Units	Description
VO_2	mL O_2/kg/min	Peak oxygen consumption rate ($\dot{V}_{O_2}$ max) reflects the maximum ability to take in, transport, and utilize oxygen. It is a measure of maximal cardiorespiratory fitness. Normal values are published and are influenced by age and gender
VE/VCO$_2$ slope	None	Ventilatory efficiency: how well CO_2 is eliminated for any given minute ventilation. Elevated slope (>30) seen in conditions causing V/Q mismatching or in cyanotic heart disease. Extent of elevation reflects severity of cardiorespiratory disease
RER	None	Respiratory exchange ratio: ratio of CO_2 elimination to O_2 consumption. An indicator of effort during testing, with a ratio >1.1 indicating maximal/sufficient patient exertion
O_2 pulse	mL O_2/heart rate	VO_2 for any given HR. Surrogate marker for stroke volume. A low maximal O_2 pulse can indicate cardiac limitation to exercise
PETCO$_2$	mmHg	Partial pressure of end-tidal CO_2. Low values, <35 mmHg, reflect end-tidal air being more significantly comprised from less well-perfused alveoli (decreased CO_2 dropoff). This is an indicator of V/Q mismatching and can indicate pulmonary disease or heart failure
BR	%	Breathing reserve: percentage of maximal minute ventilation that is not used at peak exercise. Lung disease specific parameter, with BR <30% indicating pulmonary limitation to exercise

(*continued*)

Table 1.12 (continued)

Parameter	Units	Description
VT	% of peak VO_2	Ventilatory threshold: graphical point most commonly found by comparing VO_2 to VCO_2 with incremental exercise, expressed as a percentage of the total time to reach peak VO_2. Indicates time during exercise when anaerobic metabolism begins to predominate in order to continue exertion. Reflects lactate production and buffering into CO_2 (and thus disproportionate rise in VCO_2). When reached earlier into exercise (<40–50% of peak VO_2 time), it can indicate deconditioning or heart failure
HRR	bpm	Heart rate reserve: difference between maximal HR during testing and resting HR prior to start of exercise. A blunted HR response to maximal exertion is associated with cardiac limitation to exercise but also can reflect the presence of chronotropic-limiting medications

BR, breathing reserve; CO_2, carbon dioxide; HR, heart rate; HRR, heart rate reserve; O_2, oxygen; PETCO$_2$, partial pressure of end-tidal CO_2; RER, respiratory efficiency ratio; VE/VCO$_2$ slope, minute ventilation to carbon dioxide elimination relationship; VO_2, oxygen consumption; VT, ventilatory threshold.

Table 1.13 Predominant cause of dyspnea based on metabolic exercise testing patterns.

Parameter	Deconditioning	Heart failure or other cardiac limitation	Pulmonary disease
Peak VO_2	Decreased	Decreased	Decreased
VT	Low (<40–50% peak VO_2 time)	Low	Normal
O_2 pulse	Normal	Decreased	Normal
VE/VCO$_2$ slope	Normal	High (>30)	High
BR	Normal	Normal	Decreased
PETCO$_2$	Normal	Low (<35 mmHg)	Low
HRR	Normal	Abnormal	Normal

BR, breathing reserve; CO_2, carbon dioxide; HRR, heart rate reserve; O_2, oxygen; PETCO$_2$, partial pressure of end-tidal CO_2; VE/VCO$_2$ slope, minute ventilation to carbon dioxide elimination relationship; VO_2, oxygen consumption; VT, ventilatory threshold.

Risks

Risks of syncope, arrhythmia requiring immediate treatment, or death are higher in certain conditions, including hypertrophic cardiomyopathy, pulmonary vascular obstructive disease, severe aortic stenosis, uncontrolled hypertension, and severe dilated cardiomyopathy. The potential benefits of exercise testing may not warrant the risk in many of these patients.

ADDITIONAL READING

Driscoll, D.J. (2006). *Fundamentals of Pediatric Cardiology*. Philadelphia: Lippincott Williams & Wilkins.

Eidem, B.W., Johnson, J.N., Cetta, F., and Lopez, L. (ed.) (2020). *Echocardiography in Pediatric and Adult Congenital Heart Disease*, 3e. Philadelphia, PA: Wolters Kluwer.

Moller, J.H. and Hoffman, J.I.E. (ed.) (2012). *Pediatric Cardiovascular Medicine*, 2e. Oxford: Wiley www.mollerandhoffmantext.com (accessed 23 March 2022).

Mullins, C. (2006). *Cardiac Catheterization in Congenital Heart Disease: Pediatric and Adult*. Oxford: Wiley.

Park, M.K. and Salamat, M. (2021). *Park's Pediatric Cardiology for Practitioners*, 8e. Philadelphia, PA: Elsevier.

Chapter 2
Environmental and genetic conditions associated with heart disease in children

Moller's Essentials of Pediatric Cardiology, Fourth Edition.
Walter H. Johnson, Jr. and Camden L. Hebson.
© 2023 John Wiley & Sons Ltd. Published 2023 by John Wiley & Sons Ltd.

This chapter presents the commonest conditions with an association with congenital heart disease. This area is changing rapidly, particularly with the understanding of genetic mutations in conditions that have traditionally been described only clinically.

SYNDROMES ASSOCIATED WITH MATERNAL CONDITIONS

Maternal diabetes mellitus

Maternal diabetes mellitus may result in macrosomic, large-for-gestational-age infants who commonly have hypoglycemia and respiratory distress. Ventricular septal defect (VSD), especially a small muscular VSD, may occur, but the classic cardiac problem of the infant of diabetic mother (IDM) is asymmetric hypertrophy of the interventricular septum. This condition can appear dramatic by echocardiography and result in left ventricular outflow obstruction. It almost always regresses completely, but can take months to occur.

Fetal alcohol syndrome

Fetal alcohol syndrome may result from even a modest consumption of alcohol during early gestation. The clinical spectrum is broad; classical features include unusual triangular facies, thin upper lip, absent philtrum, and small palpebral fissures, often with microphthalmia; hypoplastic nails; and a variety of neurodevelopmental abnormalities. Cardiac anomalies, usually atrial septal defect (ASD), VSD, or tetralogy of Fallot, occur in 15–40% of affected infants and children.

Maternal human immunodeficiency virus infection

Maternal human immunodeficiency virus (HIV) infection has been associated with an increased incidence of congenital malformations, compared with non-HIV-infected mothers. This is independent of antiretroviral therapy during pregnancy. The occurrence of cardiac malformations is about 3% with the usual distribution of anomalies.

Maternal inflammatory (collagen vascular) disease

In the absence of structural cardiac deformities, congenital complete atrioventricular block (CCAVB) is often associated with maternal connective tissue disease, classically systemic lupus erythematosus (SLE). CCAVB may develop from mothers with no history of lupus or related diseases who may have autoantibodies of various types. In clinically well mothers who are antinuclear antibody (ANA) negative, the presence of a Sjogren's syndrome antibody, usually anti-Ro (anti-SS-A), may exist. In these mothers, injury to the developing conduction system and, rarely, the myocardium occurs when these maternal immunoglobulin G (IgG) autoantibodies cross the placenta and bind to fetal cardiac tissue. The risk of a mother with SLE giving birth to an infant with complete heart block has been estimated at 1 in 60; if maternal anti-SS-A antibodies are present, the risk is 1 in 20.

Maternal phenylketonuria

If not properly controlled by diet during gestation, maternal phenylketonuria may result in neurologic abnormality in the neonate. Cardiac malformations, usually tetralogy of Fallot, ASD, or VSD, occur in 20% of these neonates.

Maternal rubella infection

In the first trimester of pregnancy, maternal rubella infection often results in a newborn of low birth weight with multiple anomalies, including microcephaly, cataracts, and deafness. Hepatosplenomegaly and petechiae may be present in infancy. Cardiac lesions are often present, with patent ductus arteriosus (PDA) occurring most commonly, followed by peripheral pulmonary artery stenosis, VSD, and pulmonary valve abnormalities. Maternal immunization prior to pregnancy prevents these problems.

MEDICATIONS AND OTHER AGENTS

Retinoic acid

Retinoic acid, other retinoids, and possibly very large exogenous doses of vitamin A have been associated with various fetal anomalies, including conotruncal defects and aortic arch anomalies.

Lithium

A common therapy for depression, lithium used during early gestation has been associated with Ebstein's malformation of the tricuspid valve, although recent studies show no consistent or a slight association.

Other drugs and environmental exposures

A variety of other therapeutic and nontherapeutic drugs, and also various environmental exposures, have been associated with some increased risk of cardiac malformation, but the strength and consistency of the association are often weak and the amount and quality of the available data are often limited.

Aside from this short list of cardiac teratogens, most cardiac disorders currently have not been consistently associated with specific agents.

It is reasonable to reassure parents of affected children that their child's cardiac problem did not result from some perceived negligence on their part during pregnancy.

In the following sections, diagnostic features of a variety of syndromes are described briefly and include comments on the nature of the associated cardiac anomaly.

SYNDROMES WITH GROSS CHROMOSOMAL ABNORMALITIES

Down syndrome (trisomy 21)

This syndrome involves complete or partial duplication of chromosome 21 in all or some (mosaic) of the body cells of the affected individual.

Features

Features include slanted eyes, thick epicanthal folds, flattened bridge of the nose, thick, protuberant tongue, and a shortened anteroposterior diameter of the head. Common signs are short, broad hands, short, inward-curved fifth fingers, and a single transverse palmar crease (simian crease), together with a generalized hypotonia, joint hyperextensibility, and small stature.

Cardiac anomalies

Anomalies are found in 40–50% of patients. Approximately one-third are VSD, one-third are atrioventricular septal defects (usually the complete form), and the remainder consist almost exclusively of PDA, ASD, and tetralogy of Fallot. It is rare to find cardiac lesions other than these five diagnoses, especially aortic stenosis and coarctation of the aorta.

Pulmonary vascular disease develops more rapidly in patients with Down syndrome than in other patients with a comparable cardiac malformation. Because some of these infants do not have the usual postnatal drop in pulmonary vascular resistance, their cardiac malformation may escape clinical detection until after irreversible pulmonary vascular disease occurs. An echocardiogram is advisable for all Down syndrome infants within a few weeks of birth, even in the absence of clinical findings of cardiac malformation.

Turner syndrome (45, X; monosomy X)

In this syndrome, a complete or partial absence of one of the X chromosomes in all or some (mosaicism) of the body cells is found.

Features

Although children have a female appearance, they also show abnormal gonadal development. Characteristically, they are short in stature throughout childhood and as adults (rarely over 60 inches or 152 cm), have a stocky build, webbing of the neck, a broad chest with widely spaced nipples, cubitus valgus, a low hairline, and edema of the hands and feet (a striking and diagnostic feature in neonates). Renal defects commonly occur, although these anomalies may not explain the majority of systemic hypertension diagnosed in 60% of women with Turner syndrome. Gastrointestinal bleeding occurs rarely but can be catastrophic.

Turner syndrome occurs in 1 in 2500 female live births; it is estimated that 99% of fetuses with 45, X perish in utero.

Cardiac anomalies

Anomalies, almost exclusively obstructive left-sided cardiac lesions, occur in 35–55% of individuals. Coarctation of the aorta occurs in 20% of Turner syndrome patients and accounts for the greatest share (90%) of operations or interventions compared with other defects. Bicuspid aortic valve, with stenosis ranging from minimal to severe, occurs in up to 35% of Turner syndrome patients and may appear without coarctation. Anomalous pulmonary venous connection, hypoplastic left heart syndrome, mitral valve abnormalities, and aortic aneurysm occur less commonly.

> Turner syndrome can be confused with Noonan and related syndromes, but the cardiac findings do not overlap (see later sections).

Trisomy 18 syndrome

Features

Infants with an extra chromosome 18 have low birth weight, multiple malformations, and severe intellectual and developmental disability. Although females live longer than males, infants often die within weeks or months of birth. Overlapping of the flexed middle fingers by the second and fifth digits (camptodactyly) is very characteristic of this condition. Other features include micrognathia, low-set ears, rocker bottom feet, umbilical and inguinal hernias, and generalized hypertonia. Severe anomalies in multiple organ systems may be present and contribute to the high early mortality.

Cardiac anomalies

These are present in virtually all patients who are not mosaic. Usually, a VSD is present, either as an isolated lesion or as a defect associated with the origin of both great vessels from the right ventricle. PDA and bicuspid semilunar valves are commonly associated malformations. Cardiac valves are usually not stenotic or regurgitant yet often have a striking thickened appearance by echocardiography. This appearance is virtually pathognomonic and has been termed polyvalvular dysplasia. Pulmonary vascular disease may occur in infants who survive more than a few weeks.

Trisomy 13 syndrome

Features

Infants with an extra chromosome 13 have low birth weight and severe intellectual and developmental impairment. Central facial anomalies, coloboma, and cleft lip and/or cleft palate are common. Microcephaly, prominent capillary hemangiomas, genitourinary defects, polydactyly, low-set ears, abnormally shaped skull, and rocker bottom feet are other characteristic anomalies.

Cardiac anomalies

These occur in 80% of those neonates with trisomy 13 syndrome. The most frequent lesion is VSD, but ASD, PDA, and cardiac malposition also commonly occur, often coexisting with the VSD.

Despite the large burden of anomalies and high mortality even in those treated, there has been an increasing trend toward offering cardiac surgery for infants with trisomy 13 and trisomy 18.

SYNDROMES WITH CHROMOSOMAL ABNORMALITIES DETECTABLE BY SPECIAL CYTOGENETIC TECHNIQUES

DiGeorge syndrome and velocardiofacial syndrome (22q11.2 deletion)

Features

First defined by the work of DiGeorge, Cooper, and others in the 1960s, DiGeorge syndrome classically involves variable degrees of thymic hypoplasia or aplasia, hypocalcemia from parathyroid hypofunction, and congenital heart malformations.

The syndrome appears to involve failure of proper migration of embryonic neural crest cells into the region of the third and fourth branchial arch clefts, which later form the heart, parathyroid, thymus, and other structures. Proper embryogenesis may depend on one or more genes encoding for embryonically active substances involved in cell migration or differentiation.

An association with the syndrome was noted in some families with gross chromosome 22 defects as early as 1980. A fluorescence in situ hybridization (FISH) probe to detect microdeletions of the q11 region became available only in the early 1990s. This technique is now commonly used and can identify most affected individuals.

Most occur as de novo sporadic deletions, but in approximately 10% of families with an affected child, one parent (usually the mother) is found to have the 22q11 deletion. Many of these parents have few or none of the phenotypic features. Of parents with the deletion, 50% of their offspring have the deletion of chromosome 22q11, consistent with autosomal dominant inheritance. Microarray can also be used to detect the microdeletion.

Physical findings include a bulbous nose, anteverted palpebral fissures, small or low-set ears, cleft palate (many are subtle or submucous), and small stature.

The prevalence of the deletion is estimated to be at least 1 in 4000 live births or 1 in 32 infants with a congenital cardiac malformation.

Immune and endocrine abnormalities that occasionally are problematic in infancy improve with age in most patients with DiGeorge syndrome. When transfusion is indicated, irradiated blood products are recommended to prevent graft-versus-host disease.

Cardiac anomalies

The most common anomalies are the so-called conotruncal malformations: truncus arteriosus, interrupted aortic arch (especially type B), or tetralogy of Fallot with pulmonary atresia. Less common lesions include isolated right aortic arch, left arch with aberrant right subclavian artery, or VSD.

Williams syndrome (Williams–Beuren syndrome)

Features

Almost all patients with Williams syndrome who display the characteristic appearance, neonatal hypercalcemia, and developmental delay have a microdeletion of the long arm of chromosome 7, which is detectable by FISH and microarray but not by standard chromosome analysis. One of the genes missing is responsible for the structural protein elastin.

Some patients with supravalvar aortic stenosis (SVAS) appear normal and test normally for both chromosomes and the FISH probe yet pass the cardiac anomaly in autosomal dominant fashion (first described by Eisenberg in 1964). Presumably, Williams syndrome patients have deletions of the elastin gene and other adjacent genes that may be responsible for their appearance and hypercalcemia, whereas normal-appearing patients with supravalvar aortic stenosis suffer from deletion of a portion of the elastin gene or have a gene that is mutated. In these nonsyndromic patients, sometimes referred to as having Eisenberg type SVAS, clinical testing is not currently available.

The physical findings include a characteristic facial appearance, sometimes called elfin facies, with small, upturned nose with flattened bridge, long upper lip (philtrum), wide cupid-bow mouth, full cheeks, prominent forehead, and a brassy voice. A starburst or lacy pattern in the irises may be seen. The facies become more striking with age. Williams syndrome occurs in about 1 in 10 000 live births.

Cardiac anomalies

The characteristic cardiac lesion is supravalvar aortic stenosis, but patients may also have peripheral pulmonary artery stenosis or systemic arterial stenosis as isolated or combined lesions. Ostial involvement of the coronary arteries can occur. Mitral stenosis may be found. Renal artery stenosis and renal parenchymal dysgenesis can result in systemic hypertension.

OTHER SYNDROMES WITH FAMILIAL OCCURRENCE

Noonan syndrome and related conditions

Features

The chromosomes in most patients with Noonan syndrome are normal by standard karyotype testing. A variety of gene defects have been described, including mutations in a family of genes that regulate basic functions such as cell differentiation, growth, and death (apoptosis), often referred to as RASopathies.

Generally, inheritance is autosomal dominant, but affected individuals vary greatly in the degree of abnormality.

These patients typically present with short stature, hypertelorism, low-set ears, and ptosis, resulting in rather characteristic facies.

Cardiac anomalies

The characteristic anomaly is valvar pulmonary stenosis with thickened "dysplastic" valve leaflets, but ASD and peripheral pulmonary stenosis also occur. The electrocardiogram usually shows a superiorly oriented QRS axis (around −90°). Ventricular tachycardia and a form of hypertrophic cardiomyopathy occur in some.

In contrast to Turner syndrome, left-sided cardiac lesions (other than hypertrophic cardiomyopathy) are not seen.

Related syndromes (RASopathies)

There is phenotypic overlap between Noonan and similar syndromes, including Noonan syndrome with multiple lentigines, cardiofaciocutaneous (CFC) syndrome, and Costello syndrome, and similar gene defects have been reported.

Noonan syndrome with multiple lentigines (previously termed LEOPARD syndrome). Patients show many of the same features as in Noonan syndrome, but skin lesions and deafness distinguish this syndrome. The term LEOPARD derived from the complex of clinical features: multiple lentigines, electrocardiographic conduction abnormalities, ocular hypertelorism, pulmonary stenosis, abnormalities of genitalia, retardation of growth, and sensorineural deafness. As in Noonan syndrome, a consistent genetic pattern of dominant inheritance occurs.

Cardiofaciocutaneous syndrome. This is distinguished by abnormally fragile hair and skin lesions, although the cardiac findings are similar to those for Noonan syndrome. Intellectual and developmental disability is common.

Costello syndrome. At least one-third of these children have atrial arrhythmias, usually a form of automatic atrial tachycardia, often coexisting with pulmonic stenosis and hypertrophic cardiomyopathy.

Limb/heart syndromes

Features
The association of congenital heart disease with deformities of the forearm was pointed out by Birch-Jensen in 1948. Subsequently, cases occurring with deformities of the hand or forearm bones were designated as having the Holt–Oram syndrome (Holt and Oram reported several cases in 1960) or ventriculoradial dysplasia.

Families transmitting Holt–Oram syndrome in autosomal dominant fashion have shown mutations of a gene, *TBX5*, located on the long arm of chromosome 12, but the manifestations are heterogeneous, even among affected members of the same family.

Cardiac anomalies
These usually appear as an ASD in patients with carpal bone deformities and as a VSD in those with a deformed radius. Atrioventricular septal defects can occur in some families.

Syndromes frequently associated with congenital heart malformations are summarized in Table 2.1.

Other diseases related to a gene-determined metabolic defect lead to generalized signs and symptoms in which involvement of the heart may occur. Marfan syndrome, glycogen storage disease type II (Pompe), and Hurler syndrome are discussed in Chapter 9.

Table 2.1 Summary of genetic disorders with cardiac malformations.

Syndrome	Clinical features	Detectable by std chromo?	Detectable by FISH?	Mutation analysis clinically available?	Inheritance	Frequency in live births	Patients with CHD (%)	Most common CHD
Down	Characteristic face, small stature, hypotonia (neonate)	Yes (+21)	–	–	–	1 : 650	40	AVSD, VSD, ASD, PDA, TOF
DiGeorge	Bulbous nose, small ears, small stature ± hypocalcemia	No	Yes (22q11) in 80% of patients	–	Sporadic/AD[a]	1 : 2000–4000 (estimated)	75	TA, IAA, TOF, R Arch
Noonan	Similar to Turner, but male or female	No[b]	No[b]	Yes[b]	Sporadic/AD[a]	1 : 2500	60	PS, HCM
Turner	Female phenotype, "webbed" neck, short stature	Yes (XO)	–	–	–	1 : 5000 (1 : 2500 females)	35–55	COA, Bic Ao, AS, PAPVR, HLHS
Trisomy 18	Rocker bottom feet, overlapping index finger, small stature	Yes (+18)	–	–	–	1 : 3000–5000	>99	VSD, DORV
Trisomy 13	Rocker bottom feet, cleft lip (80%), small stature	Yes (+13)	–	–	–	1 : 10000	>80	VSD, ASD

(continued)

Table 2.1 (continued)

Syndrome	Clinical features	Detectable by std chromo?	Detectable by FISH?	Mutation analysis clinically available?	Inheritance	Frequency in live births	Patients with CHD (%)	Most common CHD
Williams	Elfin face ± hypercalcemia	No	Yes (7q11)	–	Sporadic/ possibly AD[a]	1 : 10000	75	SVAS, branch PA hypoplasia
Holt–Oram	Upper limb defects	No[c]	No[c]	Yes[c]	Sporadic (40%), AD (60%)	1 : 100000	95	ASD, VSD, AVSD

AD, autosomal dominant; AS, aortic stenosis; ASD, atrial septal defect; AVSD, atrioventricular septal defect (AV canal); Bic Ao, bicuspid aortic valve; CHD, congenital heart disease; COA, coarctation; DORV, double outlet right ventricle; FISH, fluorescence in situ hybridization analysis; HCM, hypertrophic cardiomyopathy; HLHS, hypoplastic left heart syndrome; IAA, interrupted aortic arch; PA, pulmonary artery; PDA, patent ductus arteriosus; PS, pulmonary stenosis; R Arch, right aortic arch; std chromo, standard chromosome analysis; SVAS, supravalvar aortic stenosis; TA, truncus arteriosus; TOF, tetralogy of Fallot; VSD, ventricular septal defect.

[a] Most or many new cases are a sporadic mutation but may be transmitted as autosomal dominant.

[b] Clinical testing for gene mutation (PTPN11, KRAS, SOS1, RAF1, etc.) may be clinically available; genetic heterogeneity; 80% of patients with Noonan syndrome or related phenotype have a described gene abnormality.

[c] Clinical testing for gene mutation (TBX5) may be clinically available; genetic heterogeneity; 70% of patients with Holt–Oram syndrome phenotype have a described gene abnormality.

CLINICAL GENETIC EVALUATION

Family history

Often performed in a perfunctory manner, a careful and detailed history of three generations of family members should be sought and a family tree drawn. Therefore, the members of each generation can be easily identified and causes of death, disease conditions, and usual features are shown for each family member.

Genetic testing

A number of tests are available to identify a genetic abnormality. Since these are expensive, it is important to select the test that is most likely to identify the cause of the condition.

Chromosomal analysis (karyotyping) is the oldest of the three techniques presented here, but is still the most commonly used form of genetic testing. The chromosomes can be assessed by karyotyping in which each gene pair is identified and displayed. The chromosomes are banded so that portions of each can be distinguished. The number may vary from the normal of 23 pairs: conditions (e.g. Down syndrome) where the number of chromosomes is 47 or situations where the number is reduced (e.g. Turner syndrome with 45). Deleted, extra, or translocated portions of chromosomes can be identified by the banding pattern or by finding an unequal-sized chromosome of a pair. If a translocation is identified, the parents should be offered genetic testing, so that they can be counseled about the probability of recurrence.

FISH test is a cytogenetic technique to identify the presence or absence of portions of a chromosome. The locations of genes on chromosomes have been identified, and small portions of the chromosome containing small segments of DNA can be isolated and a fluorescent tag applied. This probe is then applied to metaphase chromosomes to identify genes of interest. Examples are the use of this test for the diagnosis of Williams syndrome and identifying deletions of 22q11.

Microarray comparative genomic hybridization (CGH array) is a much more sensitive technique for identifying changes in DNA and can allow the detection of either a gain or a loss of genetic material of a few thousand base pairs (compared with a resolution of approximately 5 million base pairs using conventional karyotyping). This allows the screening of the entire genome for imbalances in genetic material. Since variations in copy numbers occur in all individuals and the function of the identified gene is often unknown, interpretation of the findings may be unclear. Nevertheless, this technique has led to the recognition of "microdeletion" syndromes such as 1p36 deletion and 8p23.1 deletion, both of which commonly are associated with congenital heart malformations. It is useful for children with more than one organ system involved in malformation, particularly when their findings do not appear to fit a classic genetic syndrome. CGH array can also detect the microdeletions present in Williams syndrome and DiGeorge syndrome.

Patients with a clearly defined condition or syndrome should be studied with the appropriate test. For those with dysmorphic facial features, developmental delay, and abnormalities of other organ systems, performing a CGH array may reveal abnormal copy numbers.

Consultation with a clinical geneticist can be essential in directing appropriate genetic testing and in the genetic counseling of patients and their families.

ADDITIONAL READING

Adam, M.P., Ardinger, H.H., Pagon, R.A., et al. (eds.) (1993–2022) GeneReviews® [Internet]. Seattle: University of Washington, Seattle. https://www.ncbi.nlm.nih.gov/books/nbk1116 (accessed 2 February 2022).

Jenkins, K.J., Correa, A., Feinstein, J.A. et al. (2007). Noninherited risk factors and congenital cardiovascular defects: current knowledge. A scientific statement from the American Heart Association. *Circulation* **115**: 2995–3014. https://doi.org/10.1161/circulationaha.106.183216, www.heart.org (accessed 2 February 2022).

Jones, K.L., Jones, M.C., and del Campo, M. (2021). *Smith's Recognizable Patterns of Human Malformation*, 8e. Philadelphia: Elsevier Saunders.

Landstrom, A.P., Kim, J.J., Gelb, B.D. et al. (2021). Genetic testing for heritable cardiovascular diseases in pediatric patients: a scientific statement from the American Heart Association. *Circ. Genomics Precis. Med.* **14** (5): e000086. http://dx.doi.org/10.1161/hcg.0000000000000086, www.heart.org (accessed 2 February 2022).

Online Mendelian Inheritance in Man, OMIM®. (2022) McKusick-Nathans Institute of Genetic Medicine, Johns Hopkins University (Baltimore, MD). www.omim.org (accessed 2 February 2022).

Pierpont, M.E., Brueckner, M., Chung, W.K. et al. (2018). Genetic basis for congenital heart disease: revisited: a scientific statement from the American Heart Association [published correction appears in *Circulation* **138** (21):e713]. *Circulation* (21): 138, e653–e711. https://doi.org/10.1161/CIR.0000000000000606, www.heart.org (accessed 2 February 2022).

Chapter 3
Classification and physiology of congenital heart disease in children

Although congenital cardiac malformations may be grouped in various ways, a clinically useful method is based on two clinical features: the presence or absence of cyanosis and the type of pulmonary vascularity as determined by chest X-ray (increased, normal, or diminished).

Six subgroups of malformations are therefore possible and within each subgroup the malformations result in similar hemodynamic alterations.

The 13 most common cardiac malformations are classified in Table 3.1 and represent the major diagnoses present in 80% of children with congenital heart disease. Certain exceptions to this classification occur in neonates and infants and are discussed in Chapter 8.

Moller's Essentials of Pediatric Cardiology, Fourth Edition.
Walter H. Johnson, Jr. and Camden L. Hebson.
© 2023 John Wiley & Sons Ltd. Published 2023 by John Wiley & Sons Ltd.

Table 3.1 Major cardiac malformations.

Pulmonary vascularity	Acyanotic	Cyanotic (right-to-left)
Increased	*Left-to-right shunts* VSD, PDA, ASD, AVSD	*Admixture lesions* d-TGV, TAPVR, truncus
Normal	*Obstructive lesions* AS, PS, COA *Cardiomyopathy*	None
Decreased	None	*Obstruction to pulmonary blood flow + septal defect* TOF, tricuspid atresia, Ebstein's malformation

AS, aortic stenosis; ASD, atrial septal defect; AVSD, atrioventricular septal defect (AV canal); COA, coarctation; d-TGV, d-transposition of the great vessels; PDA, patent ductus arteriosus; PS, pulmonary stenosis; TAPVR, total anomalous pulmonary venous return; TOF, tetralogy of Fallot; VSD, ventricular septal defect.

PATHOPHYSIOLOGY

Hemodynamic principles

The pathophysiology of these conditions is determined by one of four general hemodynamic principles according to type of lesion: (i) communication at ventricular or great vessel level, (ii) communication at atrial level, (iii) obstructions, and (iv) valvar regurgitation.

In addition, pulmonary hypertension leads to characteristic clinical and laboratory findings.

The first principle concerns conditions with a communication between the great vessels (e.g. patent ductus arteriosus [PDA]) or between the ventricles (e.g. ventricular septal defect [VSD]).

> The direction and magnitude of flow through such a communication depend on the size of the communication and the relative resistances to systemic and pulmonary blood flow.

When the size of the defect or communication approaches or exceeds the diameter of the aortic root (nonpressure-restrictive defects), the systolic pressures in the ventricles and great vessels are equal. Pressures on the right side of the heart are elevated to systemic levels.

In patients with a large communication at either the ventricular or great vessel level, the direction and magnitude of the shunt depend on the relative pulmonary and systemic vascular resistances. These resistances in turn are directly related to the caliber and number of pulmonary and systemic arterioles.

Normally, systemic vascular resistance rises slowly with age, whereas the pulmonary vascular resistance shows a sharp fall in the neonate and a more gradual decline in infancy. This fall in pulmonary vascular resistance is partially related to regression of the thick-walled pulmonary arterioles of the fetal period to the adult pattern of pulmonary arterioles, which have a wide lumen.

Pulmonary vascular resistance falls in all infants following birth, but in infants with a large communication the fall in pulmonary vascular resistance may not be as great but still profoundly affects the patient.

In a patient with a large communication, the systolic pressure of the pulmonary artery (P) remains constant as it is determined largely by the systemic arterial pressure. Therefore, according to the equation $P = R_p \times Q_p$, as the pulmonary vascular resistance (R_p) falls in infancy, pulmonary blood flow (Q_p) increases. If some factor, such as the development of pulmonary vascular disease, increases pulmonary vascular resistance, the pulmonary blood flow decreases, but the pulmonary arterial pressure remains constant.

In defects or communications smaller than the diameter of the aortic root (pressure-restrictive defects), the relative systemic and pulmonary vascular resistances determine the direction of blood flow through the communication, as in large defects; but the size of the defects does not allow pressure equilibration. Therefore, a systolic pressure difference exists across the communication.

The impedance to blood flow through a small defect is a major determining factor governing the magnitude of the blood flow through it. Therefore, if pulmonary and systemic resistances are normal and the aortic and left ventricular systolic pressures are higher than the pulmonary arterial and right ventricular systolic pressures, respectively, then the shunt in these small-sized communications is from the aorta to the pulmonary artery, or from the left ventricle to the right ventricle.

In these conditions, the sizes of the left atrium and left ventricle are enlarged proportionally to the volume of pulmonary blood flow and the right ventricle is hypertrophied to the level of pulmonary artery pressure. Echocardiography is very helpful in identifying the diagnosis and showing the size of the communication. The hemodynamics are accessible by measuring the left ventricular dimensions, which increase as the volume of pulmonary blood flow increases. The left atrial size also increases but often cannot be measured as clearly. Right ventricular pressure can be assessed from tricuspid valve regurgitation, if it is present, according to the simplified Bernoulli equation $PG = V^2 \times 4$, where PG is the pressure gradient and V is the velocity of the tricuspid valve regurgitation.

Communication at the atrial level

The second hemodynamic principle governs shunts that occur at the atrial level. Most atrial communications leading to signs and symptoms are large; hence atrial pressures are equal. Therefore, pressure differences cannot be the primary determinant of blood flow through the atrial communication.

> The direction and magnitude of blood flow through an atrial defect are determined by the relative compliances of the atria and the ventricles.
>
> In contrast to the shunts at the ventricular or great vessel level, which are influenced by the relative resistances of the pulmonary and systemic beds and therefore by systolic events, shunts at the atrial level are governed by factors that influence ventricular filling (diastolic events).

Compliance describes the volume change per unit pressure change. At any given pressure, the more compliant the ventricle, the greater is the volume that it can receive.

Ventricular compliance depends on the thickness of the ventricular wall and on factors, such as fibrosis, that alter the stiffness of the ventricle. Usually a thinner ventricular wall means that the ventricle is more compliant.

Normally, the left ventricle is thicker walled and less compliant than the thin-walled right ventricle. This difference in compliance favors blood flow from the left atrium to the right atrium in patients with atrial communication. In addition, this direction of blood flow is favored because the valveless vena cavae add to the capacitance and compliance of the right atrium.

The direction and volume of an atrial-level shunt can be altered by changes in the degree of thickness of the ventricular walls or by other factors, such as myocardial fibrosis.

Right ventricular compliance increases during infancy as a result of the decrease in pulmonary vascular resistance. During fetal life, the right ventricle develops systemic levels of pressure and ejects a large portion of its output across the ductus arteriosus into the aorta. The right ventricle is thick walled and, at birth, weighs twice as much as the left ventricle. Since ventricular compliance is affected by the thickness of the ventricular wall, the right ventricle is relatively less compliant at birth.

Following birth, the pulmonary vascular resistance decreases and the right ventricular systolic pressure falls to a normal level (25 mmHg). Consequently, the right ventricular wall thins and, by one month, the left ventricular weight exceeds that of the right ventricle. The thinning of the wall is associated with an increase in right ventricular compliance. Although this sequence occurs in every neonate, in those with an atrial septal defect, as right ventricular compliance increases, so does the volume of left-to-right shunt.

The sizes of the right atrium and right ventricle are increased proportionally to the volume of shunt through the communication, whereas the left atrium and left ventricle are relatively normal sized.

Echocardiography, in addition to demonstrating the anatomic details of the malformation, shows features of the hemodynamics. The principal change is an increase in right ventricular size and displacement of the ventricular septum during diastole toward the left ventricle.

Obstructions
The third hemodynamic principle concerns cardiac conditions with obstruction to blood flow.

> In infants and children, the primary response to obstruction is hypertrophy, not dilation. Pressure increases in the chamber proximal to the obstruction, leading to hypertrophy of that chamber.

Beyond the neonatal period, a normal level of pressure is usually maintained distal to the obstruction since the cardiac output is also usually maintained at a normal level. Many of the signs and symptoms of patients with obstruction are related to the pressure elevation proximal to the obstruction, not to low pressure distal to the obstruction. Hence the cardiac chamber, usually the ventricle, is hypertrophied proportionally to the level of pressure elevation.

Echocardiography is useful in measuring the gradient across the obstruction using the modified Bernoulli equation, given in the section "Hemodynamic principles." In addition, the thickness of the ventricular wall proximal to the obstruction is proportional to the level of ventricular systolic pressure.

Valvar regurgitation

The fourth principle governs conditions with valvar regurgitation.

In valvar insufficiency, the chamber on either side of the insufficient valve is enlarged and the volume of blood in each chamber is larger than normal because the chambers are handling not only the normal cardiac output but also the regurgitant volume.

In contrast to conditions with obstruction, where the response is hypertrophy, the response to the increased volume is usually chamber enlargement. The major signs and symptoms in these patients are related to enlargement of the cardiac chambers. The echocardiogram demonstrates the enlarged cardiac chambers of the valve involved. In addition, the velocity of the regurgitant jet can be measured to indicate the gradient across the valve.

Pulmonary hypertension

The term pulmonary hypertension indicates an elevation of pulmonary arterial pressure from whatever cause. As indicated by the equation $P = R \times Q$, pressure (in this case pulmonary arterial pressure) equals the resistance (R_p) to blood flow through the lungs and the volume of pulmonary blood flow (Q_p). Therefore, for any given level of pressure, various combinations of pressure and blood flow may be present. The echocardiogram is useful in determining the level of pulmonary artery pressure by measuring the trans-tricuspid valvar jet and the underlying cause by assessing cardiac chamber size. If chamber size is normal, this indicates that the volume of pulmonary blood flow is limited by the elevated pulmonary resistance; when chambers are enlarged, the blood flow is increased.

Increased pulmonary blood flow (Q)

Pulmonary arterial pressure may be elevated primarily from increased pulmonary blood flow secondary to a left-to-right shunt, as in a large VSD or PDA.

Increased pulmonary vascular resistance (R)

The elevated resistance may occur at either of two sites in the pulmonary circulation: at a precapillary site (usually the pulmonary arterioles) or at a postcapillary site (such as the pulmonary veins, the left atrium, or the mitral valve).

Precapillary site

Pulmonary hypertension from increased pulmonary vascular resistance results from narrowing of the pulmonary arterioles.

Developmental (physiologic) pulmonary hypertension. At birth, the pulmonary arterioles show a thick medial coat and a narrow lumen, so the pulmonary resistance is elevated. With time, the media of the arteriole thins, the lumen widens, and the pulmonary resistance falls. The arterioles of neonates and young infants are responsive to various influences, such as oxygen and acidosis, so that with hypoxia they contract further and with administration of oxygen they dilate. Such responsiveness remains longer in infants with cardiac malformations associated with increased pulmonary blood flow and elevated pressures.

Pathologic pulmonary hypertension. Pulmonary resistance may also be elevated because of acquired lesions in the pulmonary arterioles.

In patients with large pulmonary blood flow and elevated pulmonary arterial pressure, pulmonary vascular obstructive disease develops over time, leading to medial thickening and intimal proliferation.

These changes develop at a variable rate and influence the clinical findings, the operative results, and mortality of patients. If pulmonary vascular resistance is fixed or poorly reactive to maneuvers that usually produce relaxation of pulmonary arterioles, such as hyperventilation or high concentrations of inspired oxygen, the operative risk is high, and the pulmonary resistance remains elevated following operation.

Postcapillary site

Pulmonary arterial pressure can be elevated by malformations that obstruct blood flow beyond the pulmonary capillary (e.g. in the pulmonary veins or left atrium or across the mitral valve). The classic example is mitral stenosis, in which the pulmonary arterial pressure is passively elevated because of elevation of left atrial pressure and the subsequent elevation of pulmonary venous and capillary pressures (Figure 3.1).

Some patients with obstruction at this level show reflex pulmonary arteriolar vasoconstriction, further elevating pulmonary arterial pressure. In such patients without an intracardiac communication, the pulmonary artery systolic pressure may exceed systemic levels. If the obstruction has not been longstanding, pulmonary pressures usually return rapidly to normal postoperatively following relief of the obstruction.

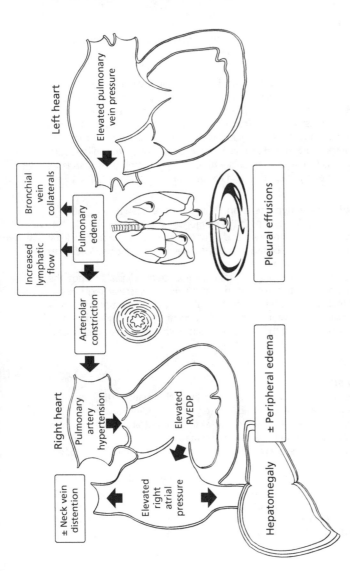

Figure 3.1 Pathophysiology of left ventricular inflow obstruction. Obstruction of pulmonary venous return at any level results in pulmonary venous hypertension. Pulmonary edema results in tachypnea in infants and dyspnea in older children and adults. If increased lymphatic flow is inadequate to compensate, pleural effusions may develop and distend, leading to hemoptysis. Pulmonary arteriolar constriction results in pulmonary artery hypertension and elevated right heart pressures. Right heart failure may result in elevated systemic venous pressure, hepatomegaly in infants, and also jugular venous distension and peripheral edema in older children and adults. Source: Adapted from Lucas RV Jr. (1972) Congenital causes of pulmonary venous obstruction. *Cardiovasc. Clin.* **4**, 19–51. From Johnson, W.H., Jr, Kirklin, J.K. Chapter 27, Left Ventricuar Inflow Obstruction: Pulmonary Vein Stenosis, Cor Triatriatum, Supravalvar Mitral Ring, Mitral Valve Stenosis in *Pediatric Cardiovascular Medicine*, 2nd edn, Moller & Hoffman, eds, Wiley-Blackwell, Oxford, 2012. RVEDP, right ventricular end-diastolic pressure.

Differentiation of these two sites leading to elevated pulmonary arterial pressure can usually be done clinically, although both show right ventricular hypertrophy and a loud pulmonary component of the second heart sound (P_2).

In the postcapillary form, usually signs of pulmonary venous hypertension, such as pulmonary edema and Kerley B lines, are present. Often echocardiography shows an anatomic site of obstruction.

The degree of obstruction can be determined by cardiac catheterization. This also allows differentiation by measurement of the pulmonary capillary wedge pressure. Wedge pressure is obtained by advancing an end-hole catheter as far into the pulmonary artery as possible; as a result, the pulmonary artery is occluded, so the pressure recorded reflects the pressure in the vascular bed beyond the catheter (i.e. pulmonary venous pressure).

In pulmonary hypertension secondary to a postcapillary obstruction, the wedge pressure is elevated, whereas in that of precapillary origin, the wedge pressure is normal.

CLINICAL CORRELATION

During the initial evaluation of patients with cardiac anomalies, a variety of information is obtained clinically. The signs, symptoms, and laboratory data divide conveniently into three categories to permit a better understanding of the physiologic significance of the findings and of the patient's condition. In the first category are findings indicating the cardiac diagnosis; in the second, the severity of the condition; and in the third, features that suggest an etiology.

Diagnosis

The findings, usually auscultatory, that relate directly to the abnormality indicate the diagnosis. These usually stem from the turbulent flow through the defect or abnormality (e.g. the continuous murmur of a PDA or the systolic ejection murmur of aortic stenosis). Once a diagnosis is suspected, other findings from physical examination, electrocardiogram, or chest X-ray can be sought. Examples are the lower blood pressure in the legs compared with arms in coarctation, the left QRS axis in patients with an atrioventricular septal defect, or the appearance of a boot-shaped heart on a chest X-ray in a patient with tetralogy of Fallot. This knowledge can direct further study by echocardiography.

Severity

Findings that reflect the effect of the malformation upon the circulation help in assessing the severity of the malformation. Often symptoms, electrocardiographic and roentgenographic findings, and certain auscultatory findings belong to this category.

Since several malformations have similar effects upon the circulation (e.g. VSD and PDA both place increased volume load on the left atrium and left ventricle), similar secondary clinical features are found in each. Clinical and laboratory evidence will indicate enlargement of these chambers, and the degree of enlargement will roughly parallel the magnitude of symptoms and laboratory changes. For either of these conditions, if the communication is sufficiently large and pulmonary blood flow is excessive, then congestive cardiac failure, apical mid-diastolic murmur, left ventricular hypertrophy, and cardiomegaly are found.

In those with an atrial level shunt, congestive heart failure does not occur because the excess volume from the shunt is ejected by the right ventricle. The shape of the right ventricle and low right ventricular pressure allow it to handle a large volume of blood. The excess flow can be detected by the systolic and diastolic murmurs and evidence of right ventricular enlargement by electrocardiogram and chest X-ray.

The role of the echocardiogram in diagnosis and determining the hemodynamics of various categories of anomalies is considered in Chapter 1, in the section "Echocardiography."

Etiology

The type of cardiac malformation is a useful clue to a possible etiology (e.g. the unequal upper-extremity blood pressures of supravalvar aortic stenosis are common in patients with Williams syndrome).

Certainly, a general knowledge of pediatric conditions, especially genetic, is invaluable in identifying a possible etiology for the cardiac anomaly. Therefore, the examiner should not solely focus on the heart but obtain an overall impression of the patient. Some syndromes associated with a cardiac malformation, such as Down syndrome, are generally easily recognized because of the features and the frequency of the condition. Others that are rarer and with more subtle signs are more difficult to diagnose.

Chapter 4
Anomalies with a left-to-right shunt in children

Moller's Essentials of Pediatric Cardiology, Fourth Edition.
Walter H. Johnson, Jr. and Camden L. Hebson.
© 2023 John Wiley & Sons Ltd. Published 2023 by John Wiley & Sons Ltd.

The combination of increased pulmonary blood flow and absence of cyanosis indicates the presence of a cardiac defect that permits the passage of blood from a left- to a right-sided cardiac chamber.

Four cardiac defects account for most instances of left-to-right shunt and half of all instances of congenital heart disease: (i) ventricular septal defect (VSD), (ii) patent ductus arteriosus, (iii) atrial septal defect of the ostium secundum type, and (iv) atrioventricular septal defect (also called endocardial cushion defect and atrioventricular [AV] canal).

In the first two conditions (VSD and patent ductus arteriosus), the direction and magnitude of the shunt are governed by factors that influence shunts at these sites: relative resistances if the defect is large and relative pressures if the communication is small. In most cases, the resistances and pressures on the right side of the heart and pulmonary arterial system are less than those on the left side of the heart, so that a left-to-right shunt occurs.

In the last two conditions (atrial septal defect and atrioventricular septal defect), since the shunt occurs at the atrial level in these defects, ventricular compliances influence the shunt. The left-to-right shunt occurs because the right ventricle normally is more compliant than the left. In an atrioventricular septal defect with a large ventricular component, vascular resistances are a major influence on pulmonary blood flow.

In certain circumstances, the shunt in each of these four malformations ultimately may become right-to-left because of the development of pulmonary vascular disease. This hemodynamic state, sometimes called Eisenmenger syndrome, will be discussed more fully in Chapter 4.

The clinical and laboratory findings of these conditions vary considerably with the volume of pulmonary blood flow, the status of pulmonary vasculature, and the presence of coexistent cardiac anomalies.

SHUNTS AT VENTRICULAR OR GREAT VESSEL LEVEL

Although most patients with one of these malformations are asymptomatic, poor growth and symptoms of congestive cardiac failure occur in the 5% of patients with greatly increased blood flow. A tendency for frequent respiratory infections and episodes of pneumonia is common in those with a large shunt.

In this chapter, the factors governing flow in a VSD and in a patent ductus arteriosus will be discussed in greater detail. This information should be carefully studied and mastered, as it can be applied for understanding more complex anomalies that also have a communication between the two sides of the circulation.

VENTRICULAR SEPTAL DEFECT

Ventricular septal defect (Figure 4.1), the most frequently occurring congenital cardiac anomaly, is present in at least one-fourth of all patients. Overall, a VSD is a component in half of all patients with a cardiac malformation. An example is the VSD in tetralogy of Fallot.

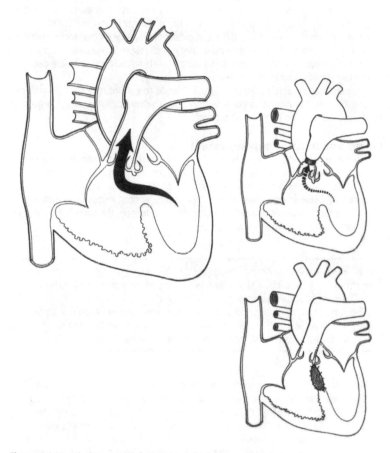

Figure 4.1 Ventricular septal defect. Central circulation and surgical options.

Isolated VSDs causing clinical concern are most frequently located in the perimembranous portion of the ventricular septum. Less frequently they are found either above the crista supraventricularis or in the muscular portion of the septum.

Small defects in the muscular ventricular septum create characteristic murmurs in neonates and young infants as pulmonary resistance falls. It is the most common cardiac "defect" (reported in as many as 5% of neonates, as detected by echocardiography). Most small muscular defects close spontaneously within the first few months of life. Through the defect, blood shunts from the left to the right ventricle. When the size of the defect approaches the size of the aortic annulus, flow is governed by the relative pulmonary and systemic vascular resistances. When the defect is smaller, blood flows from the left to the right ventricle because of the higher left ventricular systolic pressure.

Because two physiologic mechanisms influence the shunt, the clinical findings, natural history, and operative considerations for the two different sizes (large and small) of VSDs will be considered separately.

Large ventricular septal defect

In patients whose VSD approaches the diameter of the aortic annulus, the resistance to outflow from the heart is determined primarily by the caliber of the arterioles of the systemic and pulmonary vascular beds.

Since the systemic arterioles have a thick muscular coat and narrow lumen and the pulmonary arterioles have a thin coat and wide lumen, the systemic resistance is greater than the pulmonary resistance.

In an individual with a normal heart, the difference in systemic and pulmonary resistances is reflected by systemic arterial pressure in the region of 110/70 mmHg and by pulmonary arterial pressure of 25/10 mmHg.

Because the pulmonary and systemic blood flows are identical in a person with a normal heart, the resistance in the pulmonary arteriolar bed is therefore a fraction of that in the systemic vasculature.

Since the flow through a large defect is governed by resistances, any condition that increases resistance to left ventricular outflow, such as coarctation of the aorta or aortic stenosis, increases the magnitude of the left-to-right shunt, whereas any abnormality that obstructs right ventricular outflow, such as coexistent pulmonary stenosis, as in tetralogy of Fallot, or pulmonary arteriolar disease, decreases the magnitude of the left-to-right shunt. If the resistance to right ventricular outflow exceeds the resistance to left ventricular outflow, the shunt is in a right-to-left direction.

Prior to birth, the pulmonary vascular resistance is elevated and is greater than the systemic vascular resistance. In a neonate, the pulmonary arterioles are thick walled and histologically resemble systemic arterioles. The elevation of pulmonary vascular resistance before birth is supported by observations of the fetal circulation: the right ventricular output enters the pulmonary artery, the major portion flows into the aorta through the ductus arteriosus, and only a small portion enters the gasless high-resistance lungs. The systemic vascular bed has relatively low resistance because of the highly vascular placenta. The proportions of flow in utero to each vascular bed depend on the relative resistances.

Immediately after birth, the lungs expand, the pulmonary vascular resistance decreases, and as the placenta is disconnected from the systemic circuit, the systemic resistance nearly doubles. The pulmonary arterioles continue to change gradually. The media becomes thinner and the lumen becomes wider (Figure 4.2). Thus, the pulmonary vascular resistance falls, almost reaching adult levels by the time the child is about eight weeks of age.

Although this sequence occurs in every individual, this decrease in pulmonary vascular resistance has profound effects on patients with a VSD. In those with a large VSD, the medial layer does not undergo regression either as quickly or to the extent of a normal individual. Therefore, at any age the pulmonary vascular resistance is higher than normal yet lower than the systemic resistance.

In patients with a large isolated VSD, the systolic pressures in both ventricles and both great vessels are the same, with the right-sided systolic pressures elevated to the same levels as those normally present on the left side of the heart. Because the aortic systolic pressure is regulated at a constant level by baroreceptors, the pulmonary artery pressure (P) is also relatively fixed. According to $P = R_p \times Q_p$, as the pulmonary vascular resistance (R_p) falls, the volume of pulmonary blood flow (Q_p) increases. This occurrence contrasts with the events that occur in an infant without a shunt, who has constant Q_p; therefore, according to $P = R_p \times Q_p$, as R_p falls following birth, so does P.

Among patients with a large VSD, as the pulmonary resistance falls as a consequence of the maturation of the pulmonary vessels, the volume of pulmonary blood flow increases no matter what the level of the pulmonary arterial pressure is. At birth, flow through the defect is limited, but as the neonate and then young infant grows, the pulmonary blood flow progressively increases.

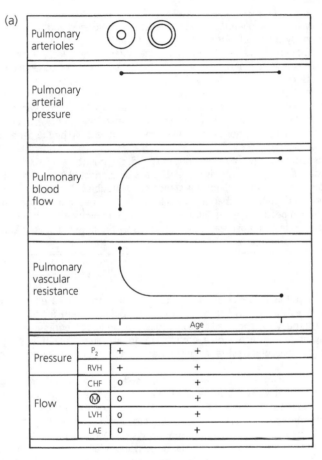

Figure 4.2 Changes in pulmonary arterial pressure, pulmonary blood flow, and pulmonary vascular resistance in (a) an infant with a large VSD and (b) a normal infant. Correlation with major clinical findings reflecting pulmonary arterial pressure and pulmonary blood flow. CHF, congestive heart failure; LAE, left atrial enlargement; LVH, left ventricular hypertrophy; M, murmur; P_2, pulmonary component of second heart sound; RVH, right ventricular hypertrophy.

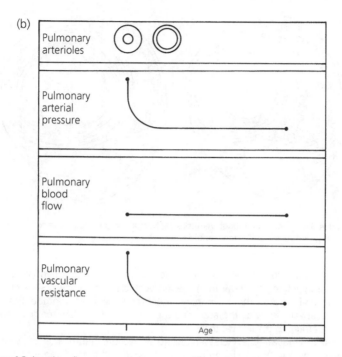

Figure 4.2 (*continued*)

Large VSDs place two major hemodynamic loads upon the ventricles: increased pressure load on the right ventricle and increased volume load on the left ventricle.

In a large defect, the right ventricle develops a level of systolic pressure equal to that of the left ventricle. The right ventricular workload is proportional to the level of pulmonary arterial pressure ($P = R \times Q$); pulmonary arterial hypertension results from either increased pulmonary arterial resistance or increased pulmonary blood flow. Regardless of the origin of pulmonary hypertension, the right ventricle is thick-walled; but its state does not really change from fetal life when it also developed high levels of pressure. Since the pressure remains elevated postnatally, the normal evolution of the right ventricle to a thin-walled, crescent-shaped chamber does not occur. The right ventricle is able to tolerate and to maintain these levels of pressure without the development of cardiac failure.

In a large VSD and left-to-right shunt, volume overload of the left ventricle exists because this chamber not only maintains the systemic blood flow but also

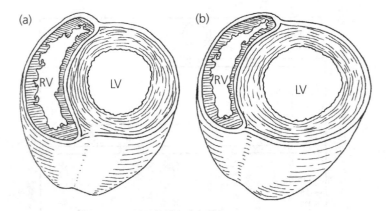

Figure 4.3 Cross-section through ventricles. (a) Normal contour and (b) dilated left ventricle in VSD. LV, left ventricle; RV, right ventricle.

ejects blood through the VSD into the pulmonary vascular bed. When the ventricles contract, the flow from the left ventricle through the VSD is directed almost entirely into the pulmonary artery, and the right ventricle has little additional volume load. The augmented pulmonary blood flow returns through the left atrium to the left ventricle.

To accommodate the increased pulmonary venous return, the left ventricle dilates (Figure 4.3). As dilation occurs, the radius and circumference of the left ventricle increase and the myocardial fibers lengthen. Both the Laplace and Starling laws describe this relationship.

The Laplace relationship (Figure 4.4) states that in a cylindrical object, as the radius (r) increases, the tension (T) in the wall must also increase to maintain pressure ($T = P \times r$). Therefore, as the left ventricle dilates and increases its radius, it must develop increased wall tension to maintain ventricular pressure. If the left ventricle becomes greatly dilated, the myocardium cannot develop sufficient tension to maintain the pressure–volume relationship, causing congestive cardiac failure.

Starling's law states that as myocardial fiber stretches, cardiac function increases up to a certain point only, beyond which function falls.

The signs and symptoms of a large VSD vary with the relative vascular resistances and the volume of pulmonary blood flow. In evaluating a patient with a large VSD, one should seek diagnostic information that permits definition of Q_p and P so that R_p can be estimated.

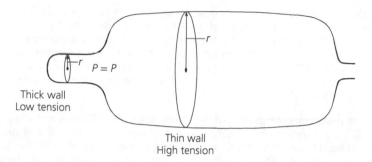

Figure 4.4 Balloon illustrating the Laplace relationship. The pressure (*P*) in both the wide and narrow portions of the balloon is the same, but the wall tension is greater where the radius (*r*) is greater.

History

In many patients with a large VSD, the murmur may not be heard until the first postnatal visit. By that age, the pulmonary vascular resistance has fallen sufficiently that enough blood flows through the defect to generate the murmur.

Patients with a large defect develop congestive cardiac failure by two to three months of age. By this time, the pulmonary arterioles have matured sufficiently to permit a large volume of pulmonary blood flow. As a consequence, left ventricular dilation develops and results in cardiac failure and its symptoms of tachypnea, slow weight gain, and poor feeding.

Physical examination

Holosystolic murmur. The classic auscultatory finding is a loud holosystolic murmur heard best in the third and fourth left intercostal spaces. Usually associated with a thrill, the murmur is widely transmitted. The murmur begins with the first heart sound and includes the isovolumetric contraction period of the cardiac cycle. Since the ventricles are in communication, blood shunts from the left to the right ventricle from the onset of systole. The murmur usually lasts until the second heart sound. The loudness of the murmur does not directly relate to the size of the defect; loudness depends on other factors, such as volume of blood flow through the defect. However, large defects tend not necessarily to produce loud holosystolic murmurs.

Mid-diastolic murmur. In patients with a large VSD and a large volume of pulmonary blood flow, the volume of pulmonary venous blood crossing the mitral valve from the left atrium into the left ventricle during diastole is greatly increased. When the volume of blood flow across the mitral valve exceeds twice normal, a mid-diastolic inflow murmur may be heard, often following the third heart sound. Low pitched, it is best heard at the cardiac apex. The loudness roughly parallels the volume of pulmonary blood flow.

Loud pulmonary component of the second sound (P_2). Patients with a large VSD have pulmonary hypertension related to various combinations of pulmonary blood flow and increased pulmonary vascular resistance. Regardless of etiology, pulmonary hypertension is indicated by an increased loudness of the pulmonary component of P_2. The louder the pulmonary component, the higher is the pulmonary arterial pressure.

In the presence of an apical diastolic murmur, the loud pulmonic valve closure primarily relates to increased pulmonary flow. The absence of a mitral diastolic murmur indicates that the pulmonary hypertension is secondary to increased pulmonary vascular resistance.

Clinical evidence of cardiomegaly. Cardiomegaly is found in patients with increased pulmonary blood flow; it is indicated by a laterally and inferiorly displaced cardiac apex and/or a precordial bulge.

Congestive cardiac failure. Tachypnea, tachycardia, and dyspnea (especially with poor feeding and diaphoresis increasing during feeding in infants) suggest congestive cardiac failure. Cardiomegaly and hepatomegaly support the diagnosis. Peripheral edema and abnormal lung sounds are not typical signs of congestive heart failure in infants.

Electrocardiogram

The electrocardiogram reflects the types of hemodynamic load placed upon the ventricles: left ventricular volume overload related to increased pulmonary blood flow and right ventricular pressure overload related to pulmonary hypertension.

The electrocardiogram varies depending upon the hemodynamics: left ventricular and left atrial enlargement (Figure 4.5) reflects the increased pulmonary blood flow.

Right ventricular hypertrophy indicates elevated right ventricular systolic pressure paralleling the pulmonary arterial pressure level.

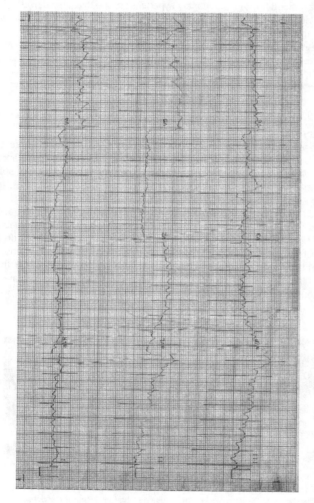

Figure 4.5 Electrocardiogram in VSD. Normal QRS axis. Biphasic P waves in V_1 indicate left atrial enlargement. Pattern of left ventricular hypertrophy/enlargement in a six-week-old infant. Deep Q wave and tall R wave in lead V_6 indicate volume overload of left ventricle.

Biventricular enlargement/hypertrophy exists in patients with a large volume of pulmonary blood flow and pulmonary hypertension due to a large defect.

Isolated right ventricular hypertrophy and right-axis deviation occur in patients with pulmonary hypertension related to increased pulmonary vascular resistance of any cause. The increased pulmonary vascular resistance limits pulmonary blood flow, and therefore a pattern of left ventricular hypertrophy is absent.

Chest X-ray

The chest X-ray (Figure 4.6) shows normal-appearing pulmonary vasculature at birth, but soon thereafter the vascularity increases. The radiographic appearance of the heart varies according to the magnitude of the shunt and the level of pulmonary arterial pressure. Ranging from normal to markedly enlarged, the size varies directly with the magnitude of the shunt.

The cardiac enlargement results from enlargement of both the left atrium and the left ventricle from the increased flow. The left atrium is a particularly valuable indicator of pulmonary blood flow because this chamber is easily assessed on a lateral projection. By itself the right ventricular hypertrophy does not contribute to cardiac enlargement. The pulmonary artery can be enlarged from either the volume of pulmonary blood flow or pulmonary hypertension. There is no characteristic contour of the heart in VSD.

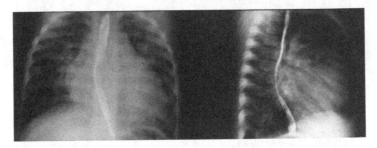

Figure 4.6 Chest X-ray in VSD. Cardiomegaly and increased pulmonary vascular markings. The lateral view shows left atrial enlargement, outlined by barium within the esophagus.

Summary of clinical findings

The primary finding of VSD is a holosystolic murmur along the left sternal border. The secondary features of VSD reflect the components of the equation $P = R \times Q$. P is indicated by the loudness of the pulmonary component of the second heart sound and by the degree of right ventricular hypertrophy on the electrocardiogram. Q is indicated by a history of congestive cardiac failure, an apical diastolic murmur, left ventricular hypertrophy on the electrocardiogram, cardiomegaly, and left atrial enlargement on chest X-ray. The changes with age of the secondary features are shown in Figure 4.2a.

Natural history

An uncorrected large VSD may follow one of three clinical courses.

Pulmonary vascular disease. Pulmonary vascular disease may develop. The initiating factors for the development of medial hypertrophy and later intimal proliferation are unknown, but they are probably related to the arterioles being subjected to high levels of pressure and, to a lesser extent, to elevated blood flow. The pulmonary arteriolar changes can develop in pulmonary arterioles of children as young as one year of age. The early changes of medial hypertrophy are generally reversible if the VSD is closed, but the intimal changes are permanent. The pathologic changes of the pulmonary arterioles usually progress unless the course is interrupted by operation. Children with Trisomy 21 appear to develop irreversible (or, if reversible, a more reactive and problematic) elevation of pulmonary vascular resistance within the first six months of life.

The result of these pulmonary arteriolar changes is progressive elevation of pulmonary vascular resistance (Figure 4.7). The pulmonary arterial pressure does not increase, but instead remains constant because the ventricles are in free communication. Therefore, the volume of pulmonary blood flow decreases.

Eventually, the pulmonary vascular resistance may exceed systemic vascular resistance, at which time the shunt becomes right-to-left through the defect and cyanosis develops (Eisenmenger syndrome).

The progressive rise in pulmonary vascular resistance can be followed clinically by observing the changes in the secondary features of VSD. Those features reflecting elevated pulmonary arterial pressure, right ventricular hypertrophy, and loudness of the pulmonary component remain constant, whereas those reflecting pulmonary blood flow change (Figure 4.7).

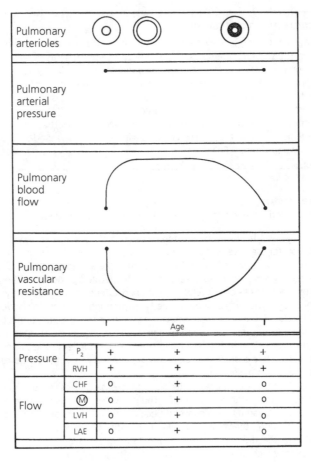

Figure 4.7 Changes in pulmonary arterial pressure, pulmonary blood flow, and pulmonary vascular resistance in a patient with a large VSD who develops pulmonary vascular disease. Correlation with major clinical findings reflecting pulmonary arterial pressure and pulmonary blood flow. CHF, congestive heart failure; LAE, left atrial enlargement; LVH, left ventricular hypertrophy; M, murmur; P_2, pulmonary component of second heart sound; RVH, right ventricular hypertrophy.

The clinical findings reflecting the excessive flow through the left side of the heart gradually disappear. Congestive cardiac failure lessens, the diastolic murmur fades, the electrocardiogram no longer shows the left ventricular hypertrophy, and the cardiac size becomes smaller on a chest X-ray. The heart size eventually becomes normal when the total volume of blood flow is normal. The right ventricle is hypertrophied, but this does not cause enlargement. For many patients with cardiac disease, the disappearance of congestive cardiac failure and the presence of a normal heart size are favorable; but in a large VSD the changes are ominous.

Infundibular pulmonary stenosis. Infundibular pulmonary stenosis may develop. In certain patients with a large VSD, infundibular stenosis develops and progressively narrows the right ventricular outflow tract. The stenotic area presents a major resistance to outflow to the lungs; the pulmonary vascular resistance is often normal (Figure 4.8). The shunt in these patients is influenced by the relationship between the systemic vascular resistance and the resistance that is imposed by the infundibular stenosis. Eventually, the latter may exceed the former so that the shunt becomes right-to-left and cyanosis develops. The clinical picture of these patients then resembles tetralogy of Fallot.

In these patients, the loudness of the pulmonary component becomes normal or is reduced and delayed, but right ventricular hypertrophy persists because the right ventricle is still developing a systemic level of pressure. The features related to pulmonary blood flow – congestive cardiac failure, apical diastolic murmur, left ventricular hypertrophy on the electrocardiogram, cardiomegaly, and left atrial enlargement on a chest X-ray – disappear as the pulmonary blood flow is reduced.

Regardless of whether the resistance to pulmonary blood flow resides in the infundibulum or the pulmonary arterioles, the hemodynamic effects are similar; but the prognosis is different.

Spontaneous closure. Spontaneous closure of the VSD may occur. The exact incidence of spontaneous closure is unknown, but up to 5% of large VSDs and at least 75% of small defects undergo spontaneous closure; others become smaller. The spontaneous closure occurs by two basic mechanisms: either by adherence of the septal leaflet of the tricuspid valve to the ventricular septum which occludes the defect or by closure of a muscular defect by ingrowth of myocardium and then fibrous proliferation. The perimembranous defect may become smaller by the septal tricuspid valve leaflet creating a mobile and partially restrictive so-called aneurysm of the membranous septum.

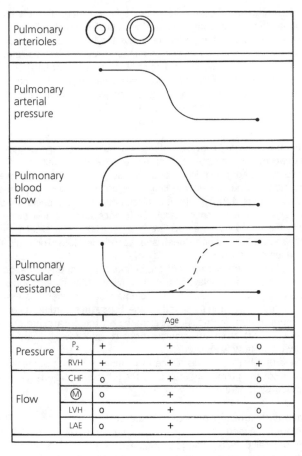

Figure 4.8 Changes in pulmonary arterial pressure, pulmonary blood flow, and pulmonary vascular resistance in a patient with a large VSD who develops infundibular pulmonary stenosis. Correlation with major clinical findings reflecting pulmonary arterial pressure and pulmonary blood flow. Dashed line indicates resistance imposed by infundibular stenosis. CHF, congestive heart failure; LAE, left atrial enlargement; LVH, left ventricular hypertrophy; M, murmur; P_2, pulmonary component of second heart sound; RVH, right ventricular hypertrophy.

Most instances of spontaneous closure occur by three years of age, but may close in adolescents or even adulthood when the pulmonary vascular resistance is still near normal levels.

As the closure of the VSD occurs, the systolic murmur softens, and of the secondary features that reflect pulmonary arterial pressure (Figure 4.9), the pulmonary component becomes normal and the right ventricular hypertrophy disappears. Those features that reflect increased pulmonary blood flow also gradually disappear. Thus, eventually, the systolic murmur disappears and no residual cardiac abnormalities exist, although the heart may remain large for some months. Some liken the gradual resolution of cardiomegaly to the process of a patient "growing into" their own heart size, rather than calling it an active reduction in heart size.

Echocardiogram

A large VSD appears as an area of "dropout" within the septum by cross-sectional two-dimensional (2D) echocardiography.

Perimembranous infracristal defects appear near the tricuspid valve septal leaflet and the right aortic valve cusp.

Small defects, especially those within the trabecular (muscular) septum, may not be apparent by 2D, but color Doppler demonstrates a multicolored jet traversing the septum, representing the turbulent shunt from left to right ventricle.

Inlet VSD, located near the AV valves, is seen in atrioventricular septal defect.

The maximum velocity of the blood traversing the defect, determined by spectral Doppler, is used to estimate the interventricular pressure difference. Large defects that lead to high right ventricular systolic pressure are reflected as low-velocity flow across the defect. In a small defect with normal right ventricular systolic pressure, the shunt is of high velocity, reflecting the large interventricular pressure difference. Small VSDs in neonates may have low-velocity flow, indicating that pulmonary resistance and right ventricular pressure have not yet fallen. Low-velocity shunt, or right-to-left shunt, is seen in older patients with pulmonary vascular obstructive disease or right ventricular outflow obstruction.

In patients with a large VSD, 2D echocardiography reveals left atrial and left ventricular enlargement. Left ventricular systolic function may appear hyperdynamic because of the increased stroke volume associated with a large VSD. The pulmonary systolic pressure can be determined by analysis of the Doppler signal that regurgitates through the tricuspid valve.

Cardiac catheterization

Cardiac catheterization may be indicated in patients with multiple VSDs and congestive cardiac failure, elevated pulmonary vascular resistance, or associated cardiovascular anomalies. The purposes of the procedure are to define the hemodynamics, to identify coexistent cardiac anomalies, and to localize the site(s) of the VSD(s).

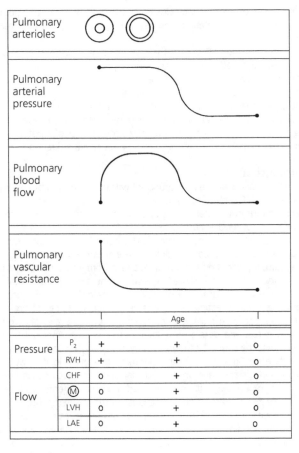

Pressure	P₂	+	+	o
	RVH	+	+	o
Flow	CHF	o	+	o
	Ⓜ	o	+	o
	LVH	o	+	o
	LAE	o	+	o

Figure 4.9 Changes in pulmonary arterial pressure, pulmonary blood flow, and pulmonary vascular resistance in a patient with a large VSD that undergoes spontaneous closure. Correlation with major clinical findings reflecting pulmonary arterial pressure and pulmonary blood flow. CHF, congestive heart failure; LAE, left atrial enlargement; LVH, left ventricular hypertrophy; M, murmur; P₂, pulmonary component of second heart sound; RVH, right ventricular hypertrophy.

A large increase in oxygen saturation is found at the right ventricular level. The pulmonary arterial and right ventricular systolic pressures are identical with those in the aorta and the left ventricle. If the pulmonary vascular resistance is increased, the increase in oxygen saturation at the right ventricular level is not as large as when it is lower. Pulmonary arterial pressure remains at the same level. The left-to-right shunt is not as large.

Left ventriculography is indicated to locate the position of the VSD(s) because location influences operative repair. Aortography may also be performed to exclude a coexistent patent ductus arteriosus, which can be a silent partner to the VSD.

Operative considerations

Patients with a large VSD and congestive cardiac failure should be treated with diuretics, inotropes, and/or afterload reduction and with aggressive nutritional support (discussed in Chapter 11). Fluid restriction (which also means caloric restriction) is usually counterproductive. Although these measures improve the clinical status, many patients frequently show persistent findings of cardiac failure, indicating a need for operative treatment. Two operative procedures are available.

Corrective operation. Corrective operation for closure of the VSD is indicated in infancy for patients with persistent cardiac failure and pulmonary hypertension. Cardiopulmonary bypass is instituted, the right atrium is opened, and, by working through the tricuspid valve, the VSD is closed using a patch of Dacron or pericardium. This technique avoids a transmural scar in the ventricular myocardium. The operative mortality risk in infants is less than 0.25%. The long-term results of the procedure are excellent; virtually no patients who had normal or reactive pulmonary vascular resistance preoperatively develop late pulmonary vascular obstructive disease. Almost no patients develop endocarditis or arrhythmia late postoperatively.

Banding of the pulmonary artery. Banding of the pulmonary artery is a palliative procedure that causes an increase in the resistance to blood flow into the lungs. Therefore, the pulmonary artery pressure and volume of blood flow returning to the left side of the heart are reduced, improving congestive cardiac failure. Pulmonary artery deformity and stenosis may persist after removal of the band.

Because the risk for operative VSD closure is low (usually less than that for banding and subsequent reoperation for debanding with defect closure), corrective surgery is preferable. For some cardiac malformations with a large ventricular communication (e.g. single ventricle), pulmonary artery banding is indicated as temporary or permanent palliation.

Small or medium ventricular septal defects

The size of VSDs varies considerably. The previous section discussed those defects whose diameter approached the size of the aortic annulus. This section discusses smaller VSDs.

The direction and magnitude of blood flow in a small- or medium-sized VSD depend on the size of the defect and the relative resistances of the systemic and pulmonary vascular beds. The pulmonary arterial pressures are lower than the systemic pressures because the defect limits the transmission of left ventricular systolic pressure to the right side of the heart. Such defects are termed "pressure-restrictive."

Whereas in a large VSD the level of pulmonary arterial pressure is determined by the systemic arterial pressure, in a small- or medium-sized defect the pulmonary arterial pressure is determined by a combination of pulmonary vascular resistance and pulmonary blood flow. In most patients, the pulmonary vascular resistance falls normally with age. Pulmonary vascular disease may occur, but appears at a slower rate than with a large defect and only in the few patients who have a large volume of left-to-right shunt despite the pressure-restrictive defect.

In general, the volume of pulmonary blood flow varies with the size of the defect and the level of pulmonary vascular resistance. Since beyond infancy most children have normal pulmonary vascular resistance, the shunt is directly related to the size of the defect. In some patients, the defect is so small that the shunt is undetectable by oximetry data, whereas in patients with a larger defect, the pulmonary blood flow is three times the systemic blood flow.

History

Most of the patients in this category have a small defect which shows little increase in pulmonary blood flow and none in pulmonary artery pressure. Most patients with a small- or medium-sized VSD are asymptomatic. Heart disease is usually detected by the discovery of a murmur either before discharge from the newborn nursery or, more commonly, at the first postnatal visit. The occasional patient with large pulmonary blood flow may have frequent respiratory infections and pneumonia. Relatively few develop congestive cardiac failure. The growth and development of most patients are normal.

Physical examination
Usually no evidence of cardiomegaly is found on physical examination.

There are two categories of murmurs associated with a small VSD. Some murmurs are holosystolic, loud (grades 3/6–4/6), may be accompanied by a thrill, and are heard along the left sternal border. These are more likely from perimembranous VSDs. Other murmurs are softer (grade 2/6), squirty in quality, heard best more toward the apex, and are usually caused by muscular VSDs.

Muscular defects may functionally "close" during each systole as the surrounding myocardium constricts the VSD lumen until the shunt is obliterated in middle to late systole. This results in the murmur being shorter than those associated with membranous VSDs. The "squirty" quality of the murmur is probably due to constantly changing pitch as the blood accelerates through the narrowing defect.

As in patients with a large defect, defining pulmonary arterial pressure by the loudness of the P_2 and defining pulmonary blood flow by the presence of an apical diastolic murmur are important. In patients with a small defect, P_2 is normal and diastole is clear; those with a medium-sized defect may have a slightly accentuated P_2 and a soft apical mid-diastolic murmur.

Electrocardiogram
In many patients in this category, the electrocardiogram is normal, reflecting that the volume of pulmonary blood flow and level of pulmonary arterial pressure are normal or near normal. A pattern of left ventricular hypertrophy indicates an increased volume of pulmonary blood flow with little change in pulmonary arterial pressure. A few patients with elevation of pulmonary arterial pressure and pulmonary blood flow have a pattern of biventricular hypertrophy.

Chest X-ray
The cardiac size, left atrial size, and pulmonary vascularity directly parallel the volume of pulmonary blood flow. The heart and lung fields usually are normal or show some increase in vascularity and size, but not to the extent found in patients with a large VSD and severe pulmonary overcirculation.

Summary of clinical findings

In VSD, the magnitude of the shunt depends on the size of the defect and the relative levels of pulmonary and systemic vascular resistances. A loud, harsh, holosystolic murmur along the left sternal border is the hallmark of VSD. The other clinical and laboratory findings reflect alterations of hemodynamics. Alterations in the second sound, the presence of an apical diastolic murmur, and changes in the electrocardiogram and chest X-ray reflect the magnitude of shunt and the level of pulmonary arterial pressure.

Natural history

Patients with a small- or medium-sized VSD, pulmonary blood flow less than twice systemic blood flow, and normal pulmonary arterial pressure are considered to have a normal life expectancy.

They are at relatively low risk for infective endocarditis. A few patients (<1%) with perimembranous defects develop aortic valve prolapse and regurgitation.

Most patients are not at risk for development of pulmonary vascular disease. Some patients with a larger volume of pulmonary blood flow or with elevated pulmonary arterial pressure may slowly develop pulmonary vascular changes.

The defects do not enlarge, and at least 75% undergo spontaneous closure, usually in early childhood, but it may occur in adulthood.

Echocardiogram

Small VSDs, especially those within the trabecular (muscular) septum, may not be apparent by 2D but are easily viewed using color Doppler. They appear as a multi-colored jet traversing the septum, representing the turbulent flow from left to right ventricle.

The maximum velocity of the blood traversing the defect, determined using spectral Doppler, is used to estimate the pressure difference between the ventricles – a large defect allows elevated right ventricular systolic pressure, reflected as low-velocity flow across the defect. With normal right ventricular systolic pressure, a small defect has a high-velocity Doppler signal, reflecting the large interventricular pressure difference. Small VSDs in neonates may have low-velocity flow, indicating that neither pulmonary resistance nor right ventricular pressure has yet fallen. Low-velocity shunt, or right-to-left shunt, is seen in older patients with pulmonary vascular obstructive disease or right ventricular outflow obstruction.

In patients with a small VSD, 2D echocardiography shows normal left atrial and left ventricular size. Left ventricular and left atrial size may be moderately increased because of the volume overload associated with a moderate-sized VSD.

Cardiac catheterization

In patients with clinical evidence of an obvious, small VSD, cardiac catheterization is not indicated. Cardiac catheterization to verify the diagnosis and to determine the volume of pulmonary blood flow and level of pulmonary arterial pressure may be indicated in patients with a moderate-sized defect and clinical evidence of pulmonary overcirculation and hypertension. Therefore, careful oximetry and pressure data are obtained. Many of these patients may have minimal or no symptoms.

Catheterization is performed before four to five years of age, since spontaneous closure or narrowing of the defect is less likely after that age, yet surgical closure of the defect can be prophylactic against pulmonary vascular disease. Catheterization is performed at an earlier age (within the first year of life) if cardiac failure or other symptoms develop or if risk factors for accelerated pulmonary vascular disease, such as Down syndrome, are present.

Operative considerations

The rate of operative mortality and morbidity for patients with a small defect usually exceeds the rate of problem development in the unoperated patient. Therefore, operation is not recommended for these patients. Patients with either elevated pulmonary arterial pressure or pulmonary blood flow twice normal should have operative closure. Closure, which can be performed at a low risk, eliminates the risk of development of pulmonary vascular disease and bacterial endocarditis. Patients who develop aortic valve prolapse or regurgitation should undergo VSD closure to prevent its progression.

Summary

In VSD, the magnitude of the shunt depends on the size of the defect and the relative levels of pulmonary and systemic vascular resistances. A holosystolic murmur along the left sternal border is the hallmark of VSD. The other clinical and laboratory findings reflect alterations of hemodynamics. Alterations in the second sound, the presence of an apical diastolic murmur, and changes in the electrocardiogram and chest X-ray reflect the magnitude of shunt and the level of pulmonary arterial pressure.

PATENT DUCTUS ARTERIOSUS

Patent ductus arteriosus (Figure 4.10) represents the persistence of the fetal communication between the aorta and the pulmonary trunk. The ductus arteriosus is formed from the embryonic left sixth aortic arch and connects the proximal left pulmonary artery to the descending aorta beyond the left subclavian artery.

Normally, the ductus arteriosus closes functionally by the fourth day of life. Although the mechanisms for closure of the ductus are largely unknown, rising oxygen tension and withdrawal of endogenous prostaglandins are among factors that influence closure.

Pharmacologic ductal closure can be accomplished in premature infants by administration of prostaglandin synthase inhibitors. Ductal patency can be maintained for palliation of certain cardiac malformations by administration of prostaglandin.

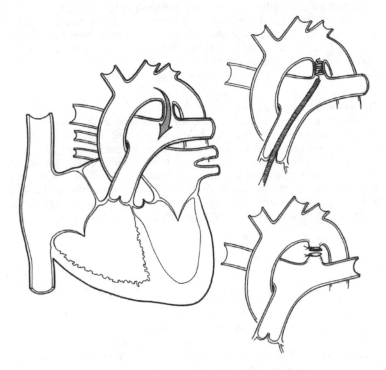

Figure 4.10 Patent ductus arteriosus. Central circulation and closure options.

The direction and magnitude of flow through the ductus depend on the ductus size and the relative systemic and pulmonary vascular resistances.

In fetal life, the ductus is large, and since the pulmonary vascular resistance exceeds systemic vascular resistance, blood flow is from right to left (from pulmonary artery to aorta).

Following birth, if the ductus arteriosus remains patent, the shunt as pulmonary resistance falls changes from the aorta to the pulmonary artery. In patients with a large patent ductus arteriosus, pressures are equal in the aorta and the pulmonary artery, and blood flows into the pulmonary artery because the pulmonary resistance is normally less than systemic resistance. In patients with a smaller ductus arteriosus, the shunt also occurs from left to right because of pressure differences between the great vessels.

The hemodynamics resemble those in VSD. As pulmonary vascular resistance falls following birth, the volume of pulmonary blood flow increases. If the volume of pulmonary blood flow is large, congestive cardiac failure occurs because of the excessive volume load placed upon the left ventricle.

History

Patent ductus arteriosus occurs more frequently in females and in prematurely born infants. The defect is also common in children with Down syndrome. In children whose mothers had rubella during the first trimester of pregnancy, patent ductus arteriosus is the most commonly observed cardiac anomaly. Patent ductus arteriosus occurs more commonly in children born at high altitudes (above 10 000 ft), emphasizing the role of oxygen in closure of the ductus.

The course of patients with patent ductus arteriosus varies, depending on the size of the ductus and the volume of pulmonary blood flow. Many patients are asymptomatic; the ductus is identified only by the presence of a murmur. On the other hand, congestive cardiac failure can develop early in infancy because of volume overload of the left ventricle, although this typically does not occur for at least two to three months. In prematurely born infants, cardiac failure may develop at an earlier age because pulmonary vascular resistance reaches normal levels at an earlier age.

Symptomatic children may also present a history of frequent respiratory infections and easy fatigability.

Physical examination

Continuous murmur

The classical physical finding is a continuous, often machinery-sounding murmur best heard over the upper left chest below the clavicle. The murmur may be associated with a thrill or prominent pulsations in the suprasternal notch. Blood flows through the ductus arteriosus throughout the cardiac cycle because of the pressure or resistance difference between the systemic or pulmonary vascular circuits. The murmur may not continue through the entire cardiac cycle, but generally it does extend well into diastole except in the first few months of life. At this age, the murmur may be confined to systole, perhaps because the diastolic pressure in the pulmonary artery is closer to that in the aorta than at older ages.

Wide pulse pressure

This physical finding resembles that of aortic regurgitation. The aortic systolic pressure is elevated because of an increased stroke volume into the aorta (normal cardiac output + the volume of blood through the shunt) and the diastolic pressure is lowered because of the flow into the pulmonary circuit. Peripheral arterial pulses are prominent. In patients with a small patent ductus arteriosus, the blood pressure readings are normal; however, those patients with a larger flow show wide pulse pressure. Prominent radial arterial pulses in a neonate or small infant suggest either patent ductus arteriosus or coarctation of the aorta. If the femoral pulses are bounding, coarctation is not usually present, but a large ductus can palliate coarctation (e.g. infants with coarctation palliated with prostaglandin are expected to have bounding femoral pulses).

Mid-diastolic murmur and second heart sound

As in VSD, the severity of patent ductus arteriosus may be assessed from two findings: the intensity of the pulmonic component of the second heart sound and the presence of an apical diastolic murmur. The pulmonary component of the second heart sound is accentuated in pulmonary hypertension, either from increased pulmonary blood flow or from increased pulmonary vascular resistance. An apical mid-diastolic murmur suggests a large left-to-right shunt through the patent ductus arteriosus, resulting in a large volume of blood flow crossing a normal mitral valve.

Systolic ejection click

Frequently, an aortic systolic ejection click is heard because the ascending aorta is dilated.

Findings in elevated pulmonary resistance

In an occasional patient (usually older), the pulmonary resistance exceeds the systemic resistance so that blood flow occurs from the pulmonary artery into the aorta. Such patients have a soft systolic murmur, a loud pulmonic second sound, and differential cyanosis involving the lower extremities, a finding almost never appreciated by visual inspection but usually easily demonstrated by comparing upper- and lower-extremity pulse oximetry or arterial blood gases, showing oxygen desaturation in the lower extremities.

Electrocardiogram

The electrocardiographic patterns in patent ductus arteriosus are similar to those in VSD since in both the potential hemodynamic burdens are volume overload of the left ventricle and pressure overload of the right ventricle.

As in patients with VSD, one of four patterns may be present:

Normal. In patients with a small patent ductus arteriosus, a normal electrocardiogram indicates near-normal pulmonary blood flow, pulmonary arterial pressure, and pulmonary vascular resistance.

Left ventricular and left atrial enlargement. In many patients with patent ductus arteriosus, the major hemodynamic burden is volume overload of the left atrium and left ventricle (Figure 4.11). In such patients, pulmonary arterial pressure is near normal. In general, the left ventricular hypertrophy is manifested by a QRS complex in lead V_6 with a sizable Q wave and a very tall R wave followed by a tall T wave.

Biventricular enlargement/hypertrophy. In infants and children with increased pulmonary arterial pressure, right ventricular hypertrophy coexists with the pattern of left ventricular enlargement/hypertrophy. This is manifested by patterns of left and right ventricular hypertrophy or tall (70 mm) equiphasic QRS complexes in the mid-precordial leads.

Isolated right ventricular hypertrophy. Isolated right ventricular hypertrophy may be present in those patients with a major elevation of pulmonary vascular resistance secondary to pulmonary vascular disease. The elevated resistance reduces pulmonary blood flow so that left ventricular enlargement/hypertrophy is not present.

Chest X-ray

In patent ductus arteriosus, the chest X-ray (Figure 4.12) reveals increased pulmonary vascularity and left atrial and left ventricular enlargement; however, cardiac and left atrial size vary from normal to greatly enlarged, depending on the volume of shunt. A normal-sized heart is found in patients either with a small ductus or with markedly increased pulmonary vascular resistance. Usually, both the aorta and the pulmonary trunk are enlarged, although in infants the thymus may obscure the aortic knob.

Patent ductus arteriosus is the only major cardiac malformation with a left-to-right shunt causing aortic enlargement. The aorta is enlarged because it carries not only the systemic output but also the blood to be shunted through the lungs.

In each of the other cardiac malformations discussed in this section on left-to-right shunts, the aorta is normal or appears small.

Therefore, if a distinctly enlarged aorta is present and a left-to-right shunt is suspected, patent ductus arteriosus must receive serious consideration.

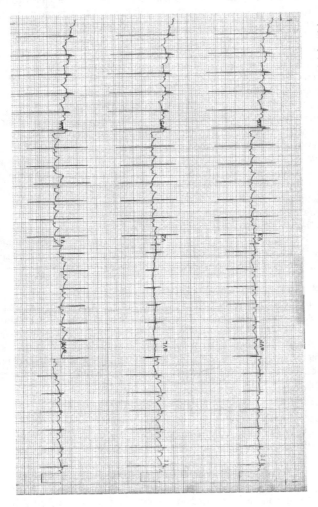

Figure 4.11 Electrocardiogram in patent ductus arteriosus. Normal QRS axis. Biphasic P waves in V_1, consistent with left atrial enlargement. Left ventricular hypertrophy/enlargement manifested by deep Q wave and tall R wave in lead V_6.

Summary of clinical findings

The primary features of patent ductus arteriosus include the continuous murmur and the findings associated with a wide pulse pressure. The secondary features are explained by the relationship $P = R \times Q$. Pulmonary arterial pressure is indicated by the intensity of the pulmonic component of the second heart sound and by the degree of right ventricular hypertrophy on the electrocardiogram. Flow is reflected by electrocardiographic evidence of left ventricular hypertrophy, the chest X-ray findings of cardiomegaly and left atrial enlargement, or the development of congestive cardiac failure. The presence of an apical diastolic murmur also reflects increased flow but may be obscured by the continuous murmur.

Natural history

The course of patients with patent ductus arteriosus resembles that described previously for patients with VSD.

Patients with a small- or medium-sized patent ductus arteriosus do well and have few complications.

(a)

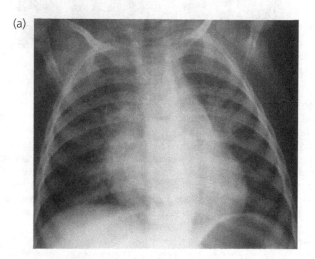

Figure 4.12 Chest X-ray in patent ductus arteriosus. Cardiomegaly, left atrial enlargement, and increased pulmonary vasculature. (a) Frontal and (b) lateral projections.

(b)

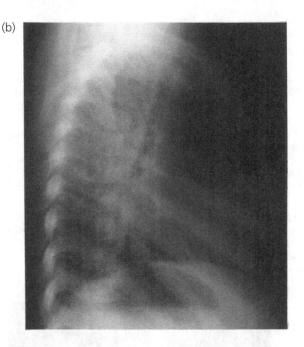

Figure 4.12 (*continued*)

Pulmonary vascular disease can develop in patients with a large patent ductus arteriosus and in those with elevated pulmonary arterial pressure and blood flow. As pulmonary vascular resistance rises, the volume of pulmonary blood flow falls. Eventually, the pulmonary vascular resistance can exceed the systemic vascular resistance, so the shunt becomes right-to-left. Such patients have differential cyanosis manifested by cyanosis of the lower extremities and normal color of the upper extremities.

Similar to patients with VSD who develop pulmonary vascular disease, the congestive cardiac failure improves, the diastolic murmur fades, and the left ventricular hypertrophy and cardiomegaly disappear as the pulmonary vascular resistance increases.

Echocardiogram
The patent ductus may appear fairly large by 2D echocardiography, with a diameter exceeding that of the individual branch pulmonary arteries or aortic arch, especially in newborn infants who are ill or who are receiving prostaglandin.

In such a large ductus, the velocity of the shunt is low, less than 1 m/s, because little pressure difference exists between the great vessels. The direction of shunting, however, provides important clues to the physiology.

In infants with a normal postnatal fall of pulmonary vascular resistance, the shunt is continuous from aorta to pulmonary artery, without a demonstrable shunt from pulmonary artery to aorta.

In infants with abnormally high pulmonary resistance, such as those with "primary pulmonary hypertension of the newborn," or obstruction to pulmonary venous return, as in some types of total anomalous pulmonary venous connection, the ductal shunt is predominantly from pulmonary artery to aorta. A to-and-fro, or "bidirectional," shunt is commonly seen in situations where pulmonary vascular resistance and systemic vascular resistance are similar, when a large ductus coexists with complete transposition (elevated pulmonary resistance), or large systemic arteriovenous malformation (decreased systemic vascular resistance).

A small ductus in an older patient may appear as a narrow jet of multicolored echoes, representing high-velocity turbulent flow, from aorta to pulmonary artery. In patients with normal pulmonary artery pressure, Doppler shows a continuous signal from aorta to pulmonary artery at high velocity; the maximum velocity helps in estimating the pulmonary artery systolic pressure when one calculates the pressure difference between this and the measured systolic blood pressure (equivalent to aortic pressure).

Treatment

Prostaglandin synthase inhibitors (indomethacin, ibuprofen, and acetaminophen)

For a patent ductus arteriosus in a premature infant, closure is usually accomplished by oral or intravenous administration of a prostaglandin synthase inhibitor. Three doses of indomethacin (dosed every 12 hours) or ibuprofen (every 24 hours) achieve ductal closure in more than 80% of premature infants, although subsequent medication courses can improve success. Acetaminophen (every 6 hours) achieves similar results, possibly with less risk. Renal insufficiency and thrombocytopenia are relative contraindications to these medications.

In patients older than two weeks, drug therapy is usually unsuccessful, but a variety of other techniques are available for closure. In asymptomatic infants, some have suggested delay in closure until the child is one year old; although the risk of waiting is extremely low, the potential occurrence of spontaneous closure is extremely unlikely. The ductus should be closed regardless of age and patient size if it causes congestive cardiac failure. In older children it should be closed when recognized, although a tiny "silent ductus," too small to result in a continuous murmur, may not need closure.

Operative division and ligation of the ductus arteriosus

This is the time-honored treatment, first performed in 1938 by two groups of surgeons in the United States and Europe who were working independently.

Classically, the procedure involves a left lateral thoracotomy and does not involve cardiopulmonary bypass. The risk of ligation and division of patent ductus arteriosus is extremely small; the results are generally excellent. The operation can be performed in the smallest of prematures who fail to respond to indomethacin treatment.

Thorascopic (endoscopic) closure of the ductus has been performed in patients past late infancy to avoid thoracotomy, but surgical closure of both types has largely been replaced by transcatheter closure.

Transcatheter closure

Using a variety of implantable devices, transcatheter closure has become a standard therapy. Occlusion of the ductus with catheter-delivered spring wire coils covered with thrombogenic Dacron strands (Gianturco coils) has been a widely and successfully used nonsurgical technique.

Incomplete closure, embolism of dislodged coils to distant sites (requiring an extended procedure for retrieval), and prolonged radiation exposure remain the most frequent complications. Long-term efficacy data suggest that the results and the risks are at least as good as those for surgical closure.

Because of advancements in the size of the closure devices and delivery catheters the technique is being increasingly used in smaller patients less than 2 kg in body weight; the length and shape of the ductus arteriosus are factors in successful coil occlusion.

Otherwise, for patients having operative closure of patent ductus arteriosus, cardiac catheterization and angiocardiography are not indicated because the physical and laboratory findings are so characteristic of the disease. In infants, however, aortography may be required in order to rule out suspected associated defects, such as aortic arch obstruction, vascular rings or sling, or aorticopulmonary window, which may be difficult to exclude by clinical means and echocardiography.

Summary

Patent ductus arteriosus is an abnormal communication between the aorta and the pulmonary artery. It occurs more frequently in prematurely born infants and term infants with respiratory disease, Down syndrome, or congenital rubella syndrome. The hemodynamics and many clinical findings resemble those of VSD because both lesions place an excessive volume load on the left ventricle and may elevate pulmonary arterial pressure. The characteristic finding is a continuous murmur, combined with findings reflecting the flow and pressure characteristics. Closure of the ductus is indicated in almost all patients and is associated with low risk.

ATRIAL SEPTAL DEFECT

Atrial septal defect (Figure 4.13) is usually located in the area of the fossa ovalis and termed ostium secundum-type defect.

Less frequently, atrial septal defect is of the sinus venosus type when it is located immediately below the entrance of the superior vena cava into the right atrium. This type may be associated with partial anomalous pulmonary venous connection of the right upper pulmonary veins to the right atrium or superior vena cava.

Atrial septal defect is distinguished from patent foramen ovale, a small opening or potential opening between the atria in the area of the fossa ovalis. In many infants and one-fourth of older patients, the foramen ovale is not anatomically

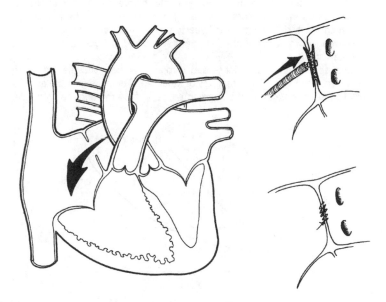

Figure 4.13 Atrial septal defect. Central circulation and closure options.

sealed and remains a potential communication. In conditions that raise left atrial pressure or increase left atrial volume, the foramen ovale may stretch open to the point of incompetence, resulting in a communication that permits a left-to-right shunt because of the higher left atrial pressure. A right-to-left shunt may occur through a patent foramen ovale if the right atrial pressure is elevated.

Atrial septal defect is usually large and allows equalization of the atrial pressures. During diastole, pressure is equal in the atria and the ventricles so that the direction and the magnitude of the shunt depend only on the relative compliances of the ventricles.

Ventricular compliance is determined by the thickness and stiffness of the ventricular wall. Normally, the right ventricle is more compliant (i.e. more distensible than the left ventricle), since it is much thinner than the left ventricle. At any filling pressure, the right ventricle accepts a greater volume of blood than the left ventricle (Figure 4.14).

In most patients with atrial septal defect, the relative ventricular compliances allow a left-to-right shunt so that the pulmonary blood flow is often three times the systemic blood flow. Factors altering ventricular compliance affect the magnitude and direction of the shunt. For example, myocardial fibrosis of the left ventricle, developing from coronary arterial disease, increases the left-to-right shunt. In contrast, right ventricular hypertrophy, as from associated pulmonary stenosis, reduces the volume of left-to-right shunt and, if significant, leads to a right-to-left shunt.

In atrial septal defect, the right-sided cardiac chambers and the pulmonary trunk are enlarged. The clinical features of atrial septal defect reflect the enlargement of these chambers and the augmented blood flow through the right-sided

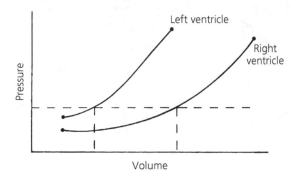

Figure 4.14 Schematic illustration of right and left ventricular compliance.

cardiac chambers and lungs. In patients with atrial septal defect, the pulmonary arterial pressure is usually normal during childhood.

History

Several factors obtained in the history may be useful in diagnosing atrial septal defect.

Ostium secundum atrial septal defect occurs two to three times more frequently in females than males.

Most children are asymptomatic and rarely develop congestive cardiac failure during infancy and childhood because the major hemodynamic abnormality, volume overload of the right ventricle, is well tolerated.

The right ventricle is crescent shaped and therefore has a large surface area for its resting volume. By altering its shape, the right ventricle can increase its volume with little change of myocardial fiber length.

According to the Laplace law, $T = P \times r$, ventricular wall tension (T) varies directly with increasing pressure (P) and radius (r).

In the right ventricle, the systolic pressure is relatively low and the radius is relatively large. Therefore, although the volume increases the radius, in comparison with the already large radius this increase adds relatively little to the level of tension required to maintain the pressure–volume relationship.

With an increased volume, the right ventricle is better able to maintain its pressure–volume relationship than the left ventricle.

On occasion, relatively asymptomatic neonates with atrial septal defect show mild cyanosis in the first week of life and subsequently become acyanotic. The other condition that typically gives such a history is Ebstein's malformation of the tricuspid valve. The transient neonatal cyanosis indicates a right-to-left shunt at the atrial level. Right ventricular compliance in the neonate is decreased because the right ventricle is thick-walled, since before birth the right ventricle has developed systemic pressure. The right ventricular hypertrophy alters compliance (Figure 4.14) and leads to the right-to-left shunt. As pulmonary resistance falls, right ventricular compliance and architecture change, so the shunt becomes left-to-right.

Atrial septal defect may first be recognized during a preschool physical examination or even in adulthood because the murmur is soft and is mistaken for a functional murmur or is obscured during the examination of an active or fearful toddler.

Physical examination

The major cardiac findings are related to increased blood flow through the right side of the heart. Enlargement of the right ventricle may cause a precordial bulge.

The auscultatory features of atrial septal defect are usually diagnostic.

Accentuated first heart sound

Accentuated first heart sound is found in the tricuspid area.

A systolic ejection murmur

A systolic ejection murmur related to turbulence from the increased output of the right ventricle is located in the pulmonary area. The murmur varies from grade 1/6 to 3/6 and is rarely associated with a thrill. The systolic murmur of atrial septal defect resembles a functional pulmonary flow murmur but can be distinguished by the classic characteristics of the second heart sound and the presence of a diastolic murmur.

Abnormalities of the second heart sound

Abnormalities of the second heart sound are important for diagnosis of atrial septal defect. Classically, wide and fixed splitting of the second heart sound are present.

Wide splitting

Wide splitting results from delay of the pulmonic component because right ventricular ejection is prolonged from the increased volume of blood that it must eject. Any condition in which the right ventricle ejects a larger quantity of blood has wide splitting.

Fixed splitting

Fixed splitting means that the degree of splitting does not vary between inspiration and expiration. Fixed splitting indicates the presence of a major left-to-right shunt through an atrial communication regardless of its anatomic form. Because the degree of shunt is determined by the relative ventricular compliances, the relative volume of blood entering each ventricle is constant regardless of the total amount of blood entering the atria from the systemic and pulmonary veins. During inspiration, systemic venous return increases the total volume of blood in the atria, so during this respiratory phase, less blood flows from left to right. During expiration, systemic venous return diminishes, so the left-to-right shunt increases. In each respiratory phase, the relative blood volume entering the ventricles is constant, so the duration of ejection for each ventricle is also constant.

Mid-diastolic murmur

A mid-diastolic murmur is present along the lower left and right sternal border from the increased blood flow across the tricuspid valve.

Electrocardiogram

Although the electrocardiogram may be normal in patients with an ostium secundum atrial septal defect, it usually reveals abnormalities.

The right atrium and right ventricle are enlarged in atrial septal defect and the electrocardiogram reflects these anatomic changes:

(1) Right atrial enlargement.
(2) Right axis deviation, usually +120° to +150°.
(3) Right ventricular enlargement/hypertrophy.
(4) An RSR' pattern in lead V_1.

The pattern of the QRS complex in lead V_1 is important in the diagnosis of atrial septal defect (Figure 4.15). In 95% of patients with atrial septal defect, an RSR' pattern is present in lead V_1, with the R' being tall and broad. Lead V_6 shows a QRS pattern with a prominent and broad S wave. Diagnosing atrial septal defect clinically is difficult without this electrocardiographic finding.

This particular QRS pattern has also been called incomplete right bundle branch block, but in this circumstance, it reflects the increased right ventricular volume. No anatomic abnormality of the conduction system is present. An RSR' pattern with an r' that is neither tall nor broad may be found in lead V_1 of normal children and in some children with forms of congenital cardiac anomalies without right ventricular enlargement. A rule of thumb for electrocardiographic diagnosis of right ventricular enlargement is that the R' must be taller than the R wave and taller than 5 mm. This sign is less reliable in infants less than two months of age.

Chest X-ray

The chest X-ray shows increased pulmonary vascularity and enlargement of the right side of the heart (Figure 4.16). On the posteroanterior view, the pulmonary trunk is prominent, as is the right cardiac border (right atrium). On the lateral view, the right ventricle is enlarged. The left atrium is not enlarged since it is readily decompressed by the atrial communication. Therefore, the absence of displacement of the esophagus or other signs of left atrial enlargement in the presence of increased pulmonary blood flow indicates an atrial communication.

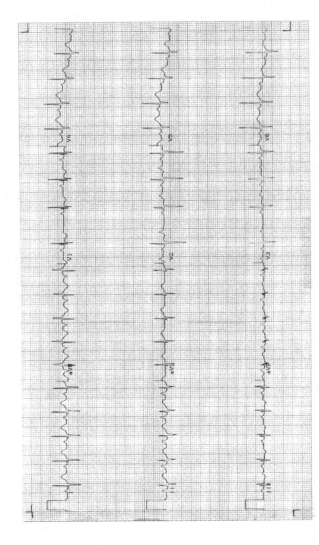

Figure 4.15 Electrocardiogram in atrial septal defect. Right atrial enlargement shown by tall P waves. The RSR' pattern in lead V_1 indicates incomplete right bundle branch block. Right ventricular hypertrophy/enlargement manifested by large R' wave in lead V_1 and deep S wave in lead V_6.

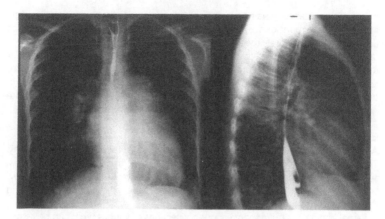

Figure 4.16 Chest X-ray in atrial septal defect. Left: posteroanterior view. Cardiomegaly and increased pulmonary blood flow; enlarged pulmonary artery segment. Right: lateral view. Enlargement of right ventricle indicated by obliteration of retrosternal space. As outlined by barium in the esophagus, left atrial enlargement is not present.

Summary of clinical findings

In atrial septal defect, the fixed splitting of the second heart sound indicates the presence of an atrial communication. The other findings – pulmonary ejection murmur, tricuspid diastolic murmur, RSR' on electrocardiogram, cardiomegaly, and increased pulmonary blood flow – each reflect the augmented volume of flow through the right side of the heart. In virtually all patients with a large atrial septal defect, the flow through the right side of the heart is usually three times normal, and the pulmonary arterial pressure is normal. Thus, assessment of the severity of the condition is of less concern than in the case of most other forms of left-to-right shunts.

Natural history

Children with atrial septal defect rarely develop pulmonary arterial hypertension and usually remain asymptomatic. The absence of symptoms stems from the fact that excessive pulmonary blood flow returning to the left atrium passes from left to right across the atrial defect. Therefore, since the left ventricle does not receive excess blood flow, congestive heart failure does not develop as in VSD. The excess volume load is carried entirely by the right ventricle, which, because of its adaptable shape, tolerates volume overload much better than the left ventricle. As long as pulmonary resistance remains normal, the right ventricular pressure is also normal. In adulthood, the incidence of pulmonary vascular disease increases with each decade, although it rarely reaches the extent found in patients with VSD or patent ductus arteriosus. Ultimately, pulmonary hypertension leads to right ventricular dysfunction, right heart failure, atrial arrhythmias, and development of right-to-left shunt. The average life span of those with untreated atrial septal defect is in the mid-50s. Infectious endocarditis is rare in atrial septal defect, because there are neither jet lesions nor a significant pressure gradient between the atria.

Echocardiogram
An area of "dropout" can be seen in the atrial septum by 2D echocardiography. This is best seen when the transducer is placed over the epigastrium, giving a subcostal view that profiles the atrial septum and shows the fossa ovalis. Low-velocity left-atrium-to-right-atrium shunt is demonstrated by Doppler, reflecting the presence of similar atrial pressures.

Partial anomalous pulmonary venous connections of various types can be associated with secundum atrial septal defect and must be excluded using color Doppler. Sinus venosus atrial septal defects are located cephalad and distinct from the fossa ovalis; the defect appears close to the entrance of the superior vena cava into the right atrium. Partial anomalous pulmonary venous connection is frequently associated with sinus venosus atrial septal defect. The right upper pulmonary vein joins the superior vena cava at its right atrial junction and may be viewed by color Doppler.

The right atrium, right ventricle, and pulmonary arteries are all dilated with a large atrial septal defect, yet the left heart remains normal in size.

When "physiologic" tricuspid regurgitation and pulmonary valve insufficiency are present, the right ventricular and pulmonary artery pressures are measured as normal.

Echocardiography is useful in excluding possible associated anomalies such as persistent left superior vena cava.

Cardiac catheterization
In most patients, cardiac catheterization is not performed as the diagnosis is easily made by other means. Catheterization is reserved to answer specific anatomic or hemodynamic questions, or usually to perform interventional closure of this defect. In most children with an ostium secundum defect, cardiac catheterization is not indicated unless device closure is planned. Patients with suspected partial anomalous pulmonary venous connection, particularly those with a sinus venosus defect, may benefit from catheterization.

Cardiac catheterization reveals a large increase in oxygen saturation at the atrial level from the left-to-right shunt; the elevated oxygen level is maintained throughout the right side of the heart. In children, the pulmonary arterial pressure is usually normal. A pressure gradient of 10–20mmHg from increased blood flow, not right ventricular outflow tract obstruction, may appear between the right ventricle and the pulmonary artery. The atrial pressures are equal, with left atrial pressure lower than normal.

If contrast material is injected into the pulmonary artery, the pulmonary veins fill after two to three seconds. This can identify coexistent anomalous pulmonary venous connection, although determination of the precise site of connection may be difficult since pulmonary overcirculation dilutes the contrast material in pulmonary veins.

Operative considerations

In most children with clinically recognizable atrial septal defect, the defect should be closed, either surgically or by transcatheter (device) techniques.

Patients with a smaller atrial septal defect and pulmonary blood flow less than twice normal may not require closure. The optimum age for closure is by approximately three to five years, since many secundum defects have either closed or narrowed sufficiently by that age to preclude intervention. Spontaneous closure is unlikely after that age.

Surgical closure

Although the operation requires cardiopulmonary bypass, the operative risk is very low, and usually the hospital stay is brief. The most common short-term complication is postpericardiotomy syndrome. Few patients experience long-term complications.

Catheter-delivered devices

The devices used to close a defect are formed from fabric with a support skeleton of metal and usually resemble umbrellas or double umbrellas linked in a dumbbell configuration. Catheter-delivered devices have become a standard option for many children with ostium secundum atrial septal defects.

Current devices can be deployed through a relatively small catheter. The risk of vascular injury can be minimized by planning for closure after infancy, yet few infants have indications for closure, especially since at an early age the defect may become smaller.

Multiple defects or those defects that are not surrounded by a complete rim of atrial septum are unsuitable for closure with standard devices. Children with partial anomalous pulmonary venous return are not candidates for device closure and should have surgery. Transesophageal echocardiography at the time of catheterization is helpful in identifying children with these anatomic barriers to device closure.

Long-term safety and efficacy data for catheter-delivered devices are comparable to those for surgical closure.

Summary

Atrial septal defect occurs more frequently in females, may remain undiscovered until later in life than most forms of congenital heart disease, and rarely results in cardiac failure in childhood. Physical examination, electrocardiogram, chest X-ray, and echocardiography are usually sufficient to diagnose the condition in preparation for closure. Large atrial septal defects should be closed by operation or interventional catheterization during childhood to prevent complications in adulthood.

ATRIOVENTRICULAR SEPTAL DEFECT

Atrioventricular septal defect (endocardial cushion defect or AV canal defect) (Figure 4.17) is a term encompassing a spectrum of cardiac malformations with a range of anomalies in the formation of the endocardial cushions. Developmentally, the endocardial cushions contribute to the lower portion of the atrial septum, the upper portion of the ventricular septum, and the septal leaflets of the mitral and tricuspid valves. Therefore, defective development of various portions of the endocardial cushions results in several types of malformations representing a spectrum of defects.

The simplest malformation, incomplete atrioventricular septal defect (ostium primum defect or incomplete AV canal), consists of an atrial septal defect located low in the atrial septum, adjacent to the mitral valve annulus, which is often associated with a cleft in the anterior leaflet of the mitral valve that leads to mitral regurgitation.

In other cases, the ostium primum defect is continuous with a larger defect in the adjacent ventricular septum. In these instances, the resultant defect crosses both the mitral and tricuspid valvar annulae, causing deficiencies of both septal valve leaflets. This forms complete atrioventricular septal defect.

In some forms of complete atrioventricular septal defect, one of the ventricles and its portion of the AV valve leaflets are hypoplastic, leading to a condition termed unbalanced AV canal. In its extreme forms, it must be managed similarly to single ventricle defects.

Three major hemodynamic abnormalities are found in atrioventricular septal defect.

The first abnormality is right atrial and right ventricular volume overload and pulmonary overcirculation, as in an atrial left-to-right shunt. Even if the atrioventricular septal defect involves portions of the ventricular septum, a sizable shunt occurs above the level of the AV valves at the atrial level.

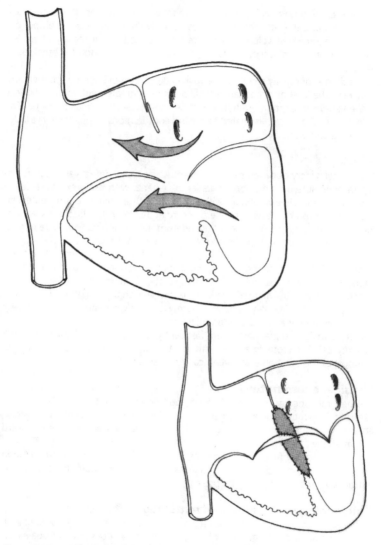

Figure 4.17 Atrioventricular septal defect (endocardial cushion defect or AV canal defect). Central circulation and surgical repair.

The second abnormality is mitral regurgitation. This increases left ventricular volume because the left ventricle handles not only the normal cardiac output but also the regurgitated volume. In contrast to isolated mitral regurgitation, left atrial enlargement is absent because it is decompressed through the atrial septal defect.

The third abnormality relates to the varying degrees of pulmonary hypertension. Generally, the level of pulmonary arterial pressure is greater with more deficiency of the ventricular septum, even though little ventricular shunt may be found. The pulmonary hypertension is related to varying contributions of pulmonary vascular resistance and blood flow.

History

The clinical history of patients with atrioventricular septal defect varies considerably. In general, symptoms appear earlier in patients with more extensive septal defects and mitral valve abnormalities. Infants with a complete atrioventricular septal defect usually develop congestive cardiac failure in the first few weeks or months of life. Patients with the ostium primum defect with little mitral regurgitation may be asymptomatic, as in an ostium secundum defect.

Symptoms are usually those of congestive cardiac failure: poor growth and frequent respiratory infections. Mild cyanosis may be found related to right-to-left shunt from considerable pulmonary overcirculation with intrapulmonary right-to-left shunting, the streaming of inferior vena caval blood through the defect, or the development of pulmonary vascular disease. Frequently, the murmur is heard early in life, even if the patient is asymptomatic.

Atrioventricular septal defects are frequently associated with Down syndrome (trisomy 21). Therefore, in a child with this trisomy and cardiac disease, the first diagnostic consideration is atrioventricular septal defect.

Physical examination

The general appearance of the child may be normal, but infants with congestive cardiac failure may be scrawny, dyspneic, and tachypneic. In patients with cardiac enlargement, the precordium bulges and the cardiac apex are displaced leftward and inferiorly.

The auscultatory findings vary, but characteristically reflect mitral regurgitation and an atrial left-to-right shunt. In patients with ostium primum defect and cleft mitral valve, five findings may be present.

Apical holosystolic murmur of mitral regurgitation

This apical holosystolic murmur radiates to the axilla and may be associated with a thrill. The absence of a murmur of mitral regurgitation does not preclude a cleft mitral valve.

Apical mid-diastolic murmur

This apical low-pitched mid-diastolic murmur is present in patients with larger amounts of mitral regurgitation and reflects the increased antegrade flow across the mitral valve.

Pulmonary systolic ejection murmur

This murmur is similar in characteristics and origin to the pulmonary flow murmur of an ostium secundum defect. It is related to increased blood flow and not obstruction through the right ventricular outflow area.

Wide, fixed splitting of S_2

The second heart sound reveals these characteristic findings of an atrial communication. The pulmonic component of the second sound may be accentuated and the splitting narrower if pulmonary hypertension coexists.

Tricuspid mid-diastolic murmur

Because of the left-to-right shunt at the atrial level, a large blood flow crosses the tricuspid valve.

Although these five are the expected findings, a murmur of VSD is found in some patients.

Surprisingly, a few patients with pulmonary vascular disease have a soft murmur, but the pulmonary second heart sound is accentuated.

Electrocardiogram

The electrocardiogram in atrioventricular septal defect is diagnostic (Figure 4.18). Five features are commonly observed:

(1) Left-axis deviation. This is from the abnormal position of the conduction system in the ventricle. The bundle of His displaced inferiorly by the septal defect enters along the posterior aspect of the ventricular septum. Ventricular depolarization proceeds inferiorly to superiorly and generally leftward. This leads to left-axis deviation. The QRS axis ranges from 0° to −150°; greater degrees of left-axis deviation occur in patients with increasing degrees of right ventricular hypertrophy secondary to elevated pulmonary arterial pressure.
(2) Prolonged PR interval. This is probably related to the longer course of the bundle of His and the developmentally abnormal AV node.
(3) Atrial enlargement.
(4) Ventricular enlargement/hypertrophy. Often biventricular enlargement/hypertrophy is present; left ventricular hypertrophy indicates excess volume in the left ventricle, and right ventricular enlargement/hypertrophy arises from combinations of

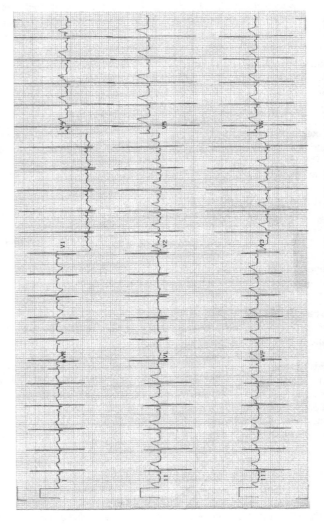

Figure 4.18 Electrocardiogram of atrioventricular septal defect. QRS axis of −75°. Biventricular hypertrophy/enlargement in a two-month-old infant. RSR' pattern in lead V_1.

excess right ventricular volume and increased pulmonary arterial pressure. Despite the abnormal ventricular conduction sequence, the precordial leads accurately predict ventricular hypertrophy.
(5) RSR' pattern. An RSR' pattern is found in lead V_1 because of increased right ventricular volume. The height of the R' reflects the level of right ventricular pressure.

The last three features reflect the cardiac hemodynamics and vary according to the relative volume and the pressure loads on the respective ventricles. They are therefore helpful in assessing the hemodynamic characteristics of the particular anomaly.

Chest X-ray
In addition to the increase in pulmonary vascularity, varying degrees of cardiomegaly are observed. Cardiac size increases because of both the left-to-right shunt and the mitral regurgitation leading to left ventricular enlargement. Because of mitral regurgitation, cardiac size may be greater than expected from the increased pulmonary vascular markings (Figure 4.19). Left atrial enlargement may be present, although it is not as prominent as that observed in a VSD with a comparable-sized shunt. The right-sided cardiac chambers are enlarged.

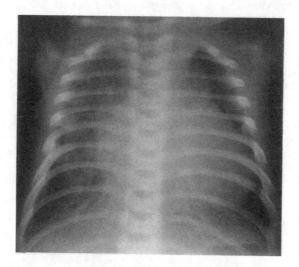

Figure 4.19 Chest X-ray in atrioventricular septal defect. Cardiomegaly and increased pulmonary vasculature.

> *Summary of clinical findings*
>
> Although the clinical and laboratory findings vary considerably, the electrocardiographic features are the most diagnostic for endocardial cushion defect. The auscultatory, electrocardiographic, and chest X-ray findings reflect the three potential hemodynamic abnormalities: mitral regurgitation, pulmonary hypertension, and left-to-right atrial shunt.

Natural history

Patients with complete atrioventricular septal defect develop intractable cardiac failure in infancy, which prompts medical management in preparation for an operation. They also develop pulmonary vascular disease during childhood. Patients with an ostium primum defect and mild mitral regurgitation are asymptomatic into adulthood, although pulmonary vascular disease may develop or mitral regurgitation may worsen progressively.

Echocardiogram

The 2D echocardiogram is easily interpreted in complete atrioventricular septal defect: a four-chamber or apical view demonstrates that both AV valves have a large common central leaflet that spans a large "dropout" in both atrial and ventricular septae (Figure 4.20). Unbalanced ventricular size is usually obvious if present. The degree of AV valve regurgitation can be judged using color Doppler. Associated lesions, such as persistent left superior vena cava or patent ductus arteriosus, can be ruled out in this view.

Partial forms of atrioventricular septal defect may show two apparently discrete AV valve rings. The normal "offset" of the septal leaflets created by the slightly more apical position of the tricuspid annulus is not present. Partial atrioventricular septal defects vary in severity from a large "primum" defect to a solitary cleft of the anterior leaflet of the mitral valve, which may produce mitral regurgitation.

In atrioventricular septal defect and excessive pulmonary blood flow, the left atrium and left ventricle do not appear dilated unless considerable mitral regurgitation coexists. The right atrium and right ventricle are dilated. The right ventricle is hypertrophied because of pulmonary hypertension.

Cardiac catheterization

Cardiac catheterization is not always performed if the anatomy and physiology can be clearly illustrated by an echocardiogram. A large increase in oxygen saturation is found at the atrial level. Occasionally, an additional increase is found at the ventricular level, but the atrial increase is often so large that it obscures the ventricular component of the shunt. A slight right-to-left shunt may be detectable, either at

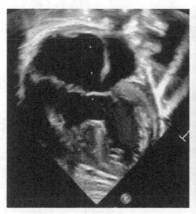 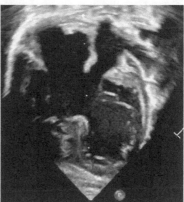

Figure 4.20 Echocardiogram in atrioventricular septal defect. The left panel shows an apical four-chamber view in systole; the common AV valve is closed and the leaflets bridge across the septal defect. The right panel is a diastolic view of the open common AV valve; the size of the atrioventricular septal defect and the lack of any tissue separating the VSD from the primum ASD are best appreciated in this view.

the atrial level or at the intrapulmonary level (because of pulmonary overcirculation and edema). A large right-to-left shunt suggests pulmonary resistance exceeding systemic resistance or an associated anomaly (e.g. a communication between the coronary sinus and left atrium). The pulmonary arterial pressure ranges from normal to systemic levels, the latter suggesting a complete atrioventricular septal defect.

Left ventriculography reveals a characteristic abnormality of the left ventricle termed "gooseneck deformity." The medial border of the left ventricle, when viewed on an anteroposterior film, appears scooped out because of the lower margin of the endocardial cushion defect and the presence of abnormal chordal attachment to the septum. Mitral regurgitation is also demonstrated by the study. In a left anterior oblique projection or four-chamber view of a left ventriculogram, the common AV valve can be outlined.

Operative considerations

In patients with an ostium primum defect and a cleft mitral valve who are asymptomatic or who have few symptoms, operation can be delayed beyond infancy and can be performed at a low risk. The defect is closed, and the cleft of the mitral valve is sutured, which greatly reduces the degree of mitral regurgitation.

In patients with complete atrioventricular septal defect, corrective operation can be indicated in very young symptomatic infants who often respond poorly to medical management. The authors routinely send infants for a corrective operation at two to three months of age. The risk of pulmonary vascular disease developing within the first six to nine months of life is high, especially in patients with Down syndrome.

The operative results are good in almost all cases, although some infants have such deficient mitral valve anatomy that prosthetic replacement is required. Surgically induced AV block is uncommon but is more likely than with closure of perimembranous VSD. Banding of the pulmonary artery is beneficial in a few instances, especially for patients with greatly unbalanced ventricular or AV valve size.

Summary

Atrioventricular septal defect encompasses a group of anomalies involving specific portions of the atrial and ventricular septa and adjacent AV valves. The clinical and laboratory findings reflect the atrial left-to-right shunt and the mitral regurgitation. The electrocardiogram showing left axis deviation, atrial and ventricular hypertrophy, and incomplete right bundle branch block is quite diagnostic. X-ray studies reveal enlargement of each cardiac chamber. The anatomic details of the anomaly are clearly identified by echocardiography. The anatomic features of the defect complicate operative correction.

Summary of left-to-right shunts

Certain generalizations can be made concerning the cardiac conditions with a left-to-right shunt that aid in understanding their hemodynamics and that can be applied to other lesions, such as those with admixture, discussed in Chapter 6.

Shunts occurring distal to the mitral valve (VSD, patent ductus arteriosus) have certain general characteristics. The flow through the defect depends on either the size of the defect or the relative resistances of the pulmonary and systemic vascular systems. Therefore, systolic events influence the shunt primarily. Volume load is placed on the left side of the heart and can lead to congestive cardiac failure. Left atrial enlargement, apical diastolic murmur, and left ventricular hypertrophy are other manifestations of the excess volume in the left side of the heart.

Table 4.1 Summary of defects with acyanosis and increased pulmonary blood flow (left-to-right shunt).

Malformation	History				Physical examination			
	Gender prevalence	Major associated syndrome	Congestive cardiac failure	Age murmur first heard	Pulse pressure	Thrill	Murmur	Degree splitting of S_2
Atrial septal defect	F>M	Holt–Oram	Rare	5 years	Normal	Rare	Grade I–III systolic ejection murmur, pulmonary area; tricuspid mid-diastolic rumble	Fixed, wide splitting
Ventricular septal defect	M>F	Trisomy 21, 13, 18	± Onset 1–2 months	6 weeks	Normal	Precordial	Grade IV harsh holosystolic, left sternal border; mitral mid-diastolic rumble	Normal
Patent ductus arteriosus	F>M	Low birth weight, rubella	± Onset 1–2 months	Infancy	Wide	Upper precordial (±); SSN (±)	Continuous (older) or systolic ejection (neonate); apical mid-diastolic rumble	Normal
Atrioventricular septal defect	F = M	Trisomy 21	± Onset 1–2 months	Infancy	Normal	Apical (±)	Grade I–IV apical holosystolic murmur; systolic ejection murmur, pulmonary area; mid-diastolic rumble	Fixed, wide splitting

(*continued*)

Table 4.1 (*continued*)

Malformation	Axis (QRS)	Electrocardiogram			Chest X-ray	
		Atrial enlargement	Ventricular hypertrophy/ enlargement	Other	Left atrial enlargement	Aortic enlargement
Atrial septal defect	Normal or right	None or right	Right	Incomplete RBBB (RSR' in V_1)	Absent	Absent
Ventricular septal defect	Normal or right	None or left	None (small defect); left (medium defect); biventricular (large defect); right (high R_p)		Present	Absent
Patent ductus arteriosus	Normal	None or left	None (small defect); left (medium defect); biventricular (large defect); right (high R_p)		Present	Present
Atrioventricular septal defect	Left	Right, left, or both	Biventricular	Incomplete RBBB (RSR' in V_1)	Present	Absent

F, female; M, male; RBBB, right bundle branch block; R_p, pulmonary vascular resistance; S_2, second heart sound; SSN, suprasternal notch; ±, may be present or absent.

Shunts occurring proximal to the mitral valve (atrial septal defect) have other characteristics. The shunt depends on the relative compliance of the ventricles and therefore is influenced predominantly by diastolic events. Congestive heart failure is uncommon in uncomplicated cardiac anomalies because the volume load is placed on the right ventricle. Left atrial enlargement is absent. The electrocardiogram shows a pattern of right ventricular volume overload, and a tricuspid diastolic murmur may be present.

The features and classic findings of the four major acyanotic conditions associated with increased pulmonary blood flow are presented in Table 4.1.

Chapter 5
Conditions obstructing blood flow in children

Although conditions leading to obstruction of blood flow from the heart are common in children, those causing inflow obstruction, such as mitral stenosis, are rare in comparison. In this chapter, therefore, the emphasis is on coarctation of the aorta, aortic stenosis, and pulmonary stenosis.

Each of these obstructive conditions has two major effects upon the circulation:

(1) Blood flow through the obstruction is turbulent, leading to a systolic ejection murmur and dilation of the great vessel beyond the obstruction.
(2) Systolic pressure is elevated proximal to the obstruction, leading to myocardial hypertrophy proportional to the degree of obstruction.

Moller's Essentials of Pediatric Cardiology, Fourth Edition.
Walter H. Johnson, Jr. and Camden L. Hebson.
© 2023 John Wiley & Sons Ltd. Published 2023 by John Wiley & Sons Ltd.

The severity of obstruction varies considerably among patients. The smaller the orifice size of the obstruction, the greater is the level of systolic pressure required to eject the cardiac output (CO) through the obstruction. This principle is represented by the following equation:

$$\text{Orifice size} = \text{Constant} \times \frac{\text{Cardiac output}}{\sqrt{\text{Pressure difference across obstruction}}}$$

> The primary response to the obstruction is myocardial hypertrophy, not ventricular dilation.

During childhood, the heart usually maintains the elevated ventricular systolic pressure without dilation. Eventually, ventricular enlargement may appear because myocardial fibrosis develops. The fibrotic ventricular changes occur from an imbalance between the myocardial oxygen demand and supply. In most children, coronary arterial blood flow is normal, but with ventricular hypertrophy, myocardial oxygen requirements are increased.

Myocardial oxygen requirements are largely devoted to the development of myocardial tension and therefore are related directly to the level of ventricular systolic pressure and the number of times per minute the heart must develop that level of pressure. Thus, elevated ventricular systolic pressure and tachycardia increase myocardial oxygen consumption considerably.

With exercise, myocardial oxygen requirements increase even more in an obstructive lesion for two reasons: (i) CO increases; so according to the relationship shown in the equation above, ventricular systolic pressure also increases; and (ii) with exercise, the heart rate increases.

If the increased myocardial oxygen requirements cannot be met, myocardial ischemia occurs and ultimately leads to myocardial fibrosis. These myocardial changes occur with time and lead to signs and symptoms. With the development of sufficient fibrosis, the contractile properties of the ventricle are affected so that ventricular dilation and cardiac enlargement develop and diastolic dysfunction may occur.

As a group, the obstructive conditions are associated with normal pulmonary vascularity because the CO is equal and normal on both sides of the heart and there is no shunting.

Children with obstructive lesions usually show few symptoms, but severe degrees of obstruction lead to congestive cardiac failure in neonates and young infants.

COARCTATION OF THE AORTA

Coarctation of the aorta (Figure 5.1) is a narrowing of the descending aorta that occurs opposite the site of the ductus arteriosus.

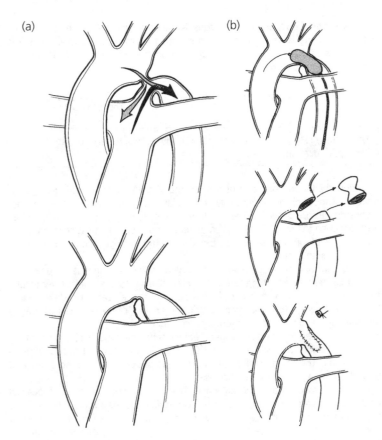

Figure 5.1 Coarctation of the aorta. (a) Central circulation before and after ductal closure; (b) repair options.

Aortic coarctation has traditionally been defined by its relationship to the ductus arteriosus, whether patent or ligamentous. This relationship has been described as either preductal or postductal. However, virtually all coarctations of the aorta are located juxtaductal (i.e. occurring in the wall of the aorta opposite the ductus arteriosus).

Coarctation may occur either as a localized constriction of the aorta or as tubular hypoplasia of the aortic arch and proximal descending aorta. In general, patients with tubular hypoplasia of the aortic arch develop cardiac failure in the neonatal period or early infancy. The coarctation in older children is usually discrete and is located distal to the origin of the left subclavian artery. Preoperative treatment and correction depend more on the associated lesions, such as arch hypoplasia, than on the precise relationship of the coarctation to the ductus.

The descending aorta beyond the coarctation usually shows poststenotic dilation. At least 50% of patients have a coexistent bicuspid aortic valve.

Coarctation of the aorta presents mechanical obstruction to left ventricular output. The pressure proximal to the coarctation is elevated, whereas that beyond the obstruction is either normal or lower than normal; this blood pressure difference is the major diagnostic feature of coarctation. In response to the pressure difference between the proximal and distal compartments of the aorta, collateral arteries develop between the high-pressure ascending and the low-pressure descending aorta.

Collateral vessels develop in any vascular system when a pressure difference exists. These vessels represent enlargement of naturally occurring small arteries bridging the high- and low-pressure components. Blood flows through these bridging vessels, and the volume of flow slowly increases, leading to the eventual dilation of the vessels. The internal mammary and intercostal arteries are the most frequently occurring collateral vessels in coarctation of the aorta.

Left ventricular hypertrophy develops in response to the elevated systolic pressure proximal to the coarctation.

History

Although most children with coarctation of the aorta are asymptomatic throughout childhood, 10% develop congestive cardiac failure during the neonatal period or early infancy. In the latter group, recognition of the lesion is important because proper management can be lifesaving.

Older children rarely develop congestive cardiac failure; instead, they have complaints such as headaches, related to the systolic hypertension in the upper portion of the body. The very common childhood and adolescent symptom of chest pain, benign in most youngsters, occurs occasionally in coarctation patients and may be an ominous sign of myocardial ischemia secondary to severe left ventricular hypertrophy.

Coarctation of the aorta predominates in males at a ratio of 1.5 : 1. When coarctation of the aorta occurs in a female, Turner syndrome should be considered and chromosome analysis performed when appropriate. Some Turner syndrome patients exhibit very subtle findings and often escape clinical detection.

If coarctation of the aorta does not lead to congestive cardiac failure, the condition may be unrecognized until preschool age, when a murmur is heard, or later with the detection of hypertension.

Physical examination

Most patients show normal growth and development; many have an athletic physique. In neonates or infants, the signs of congestive cardiac failure may be present and profound. Mild degrees of acrocyanosis and mottling of the skin may be present because of pulmonary edema and poor perfusion, but these signs are common in healthy infants when cold.

Clinical diagnosis of coarctation of the aorta rests on identifying a blood pressure difference between the upper and lower extremities. This information may be gathered by palpation of both the radial and femoral arteries. If a substantial difference between the two is found, coarctation of the aorta should be suspected.

In addition, finding very sharp and brisk radial pulses in infants should lead one to consider coarctation of the aorta; radial pulses are ordinarily difficult to palpate in this age group.

Regardless of whether the femoral pulses feel diminished or not, the blood pressure should be taken in both arms and a leg in every child with a murmur. Coarctation of the aorta has been missed in many patients because the "femoral arteries were palpable."

The blood pressure should be obtained either by direct auscultatory means or with automated devices (see Chapter 1). Blood pressure cuffs of appropriate width must be used. The largest cuff that fits the extremity should be used. In a patient without cardiac disease, the blood pressure should be the same in the upper and lower extremities. If the blood pressure is higher in the arms than in the legs by 20 mmHg or more, the difference is considered significant and indicates coarctation of the aorta. Using an inadequate-sized leg cuff can artifactually increase the leg pressures and lead to failure to detect a significant systolic pressure difference when one exists.

In infants with congestive cardiac failure secondary to severe coarctation of the aorta, the blood pressure values may be similar in the arms and legs, but at low levels at both sites, because CO is so reduced. Following stabilization of such infants, however, the pressure difference between the upper and lower extremities usually becomes apparent.

An open ductus, either native or from prostaglandin administration, palliates a neonate with coarctation and equalizes upper- and lower-extremity pulses because the aortic end of the ductus provides a bypass around the obstruction.

The examination of the heart may reveal cardiac enlargement. Palpation in the suprasternal notch reveals a prominent aortic pulsation and perhaps a thrill in patients with a coexistent bicuspid aortic valve. An ejection-type murmur is present along the sternal border, at the apex, and over the back between the left scapulae and the spine in the fourth interspace. The murmur is generally grade 2/6 to 3/6. It is rare for an older patient with coarctation not to have a murmur over the left back along the spine. This is a valuable diagnostic clue.

An aortic systolic ejection click is often heard, indicating dilation of the ascending aorta from a coexistent bicuspid aortic valve. The loudness of the aortic component of the second heart sound may be increased. In an infant with congestive cardiac failure, auscultatory findings may be muffled until cardiac performance is improved.

Electrocardiogram
The electrocardiographic findings vary with the age of the patient.

Neonate
In the neonatal and early infancy periods, the electrocardiogram usually reveals right ventricular hypertrophy.

Several explanations have been offered for this seemingly paradoxical finding. If the ductus arteriosus remains patent, the right ventricle, because of its communication through the pulmonary artery and ductus arteriosus, continues to work against the resistance imposed by the systemic circulation. In other patients with coarctation of the aorta and patent ductus arteriosus, the left ventricle is hypoplastic, so the electrocardiogram shows a pattern of right ventricular hypertrophy. Right ventricular hypertrophy has also been explained by the development of pulmonary hypertension secondary to left ventricular failure. The load placed on the fetal right ventricle, normally about 60% of the combined output from both fetal ventricles, may increase because less blood is able to traverse the left ventricle and to pass through the narrowed aortic isthmus.

Regardless of its origin, the typical pattern of coarctation of the aorta in a symptomatic infant is right ventricular hypertrophy, and severe "strain" may be reflected in inverted T waves in the left precordial leads. Subsequently, the electrocardiogram shifts to a pattern of left ventricular hypertrophy.

Older infants
In older infants with severe coarctation of the aorta or in those with coexistent aortic outflow obstruction and endocardial fibroelastosis (representing subendocardial scarring) of the left ventricle, a pattern of left ventricular hypertrophy, inverted T waves, and ST depression in the left precordial leads is present. These ventricular repolarization abnormalities are often signs of a poor prognosis.

Older patients
In the older patient with coarctation of the aorta, the precordial leads show either left ventricular hypertrophy or a normal pattern.

Chest X-ray

In symptomatic infants, significant cardiac enlargement is present, with the cardiomegaly consisting primarily of left ventricular and left atrial enlargement. The lung fields show a diffuse reticular pattern of pulmonary edema and pulmonary venous congestion.

In older children, cardiac size and pulmonary vasculature are usually normal.

The appearance of the descending aorta is often diagnostic of coarctation of the aorta by showing poststenotic dilation. The barium swallow shows an E sign. The upper portion of the E is formed by the segment of the aorta proximal to the coarctation, and the lower portion of the E is formed by the deviation of the barium from the poststenotic dilation. On plain chest X-rays, often the left side of the thoracic aorta shows soft-tissue densities in the form of the number 3 that mirror the barium sign. The upper portion of the 3 sign represents the aortic knob, and the lower portion represents the poststenotic dilation. These findings help in identifying the extent of the coarctation.

The ascending aorta may be prominent with coexistent bicuspid aortic valve.

Rib notching (Figure 5.2) may be apparent in older children and adolescents, but its absence does not rule out the diagnosis of coarctation. The inferior margins of the upper ribs show scalloping caused by pressure from enlarged and tortuous intercostal arteries serving as collaterals.

Summary of clinical findings

Whether the patient is an infant in congestive cardiac failure or is asymptomatic, the clinical diagnosis rests upon the demonstration of a blood pressure difference between the arms and leg. Other findings, such as those on the electrocardiogram and chest X-ray, reflect the severity of the condition. Prominence of the ascending aorta on chest X-ray and an apical systolic ejection click indicate a coexistent bicuspid aortic valve.

Natural history

The anastomotic site following coarctation repair may not grow in proportion to aortic diameter growth. Therefore, recoarctation may develop, often necessitating a second operation when the patient is older. This need occurs more frequently among children with a very hypoplastic aorta who were operated upon in infancy. Follow-up of all operated patients includes periodic determination of blood pressure in both the upper and lower extremities.

Since half of the patients with coarctation of the aorta have a bicuspid aortic valve, they are at some increased risk for development of endocarditis compared with persons with a normal aortic valve; however, antibiotic prophylaxis is no

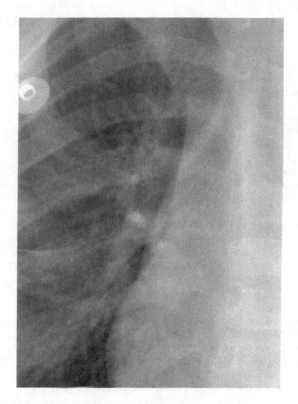

Figure 5.2 Chest X-ray in coarctation. Detail of rib notching.

longer advised for most patients (see Chapter 12). The long-term course of patients with bicuspid aortic valve is variable as the valve may become slowly regurgitant or stenotic with age and eventually require valvar surgery.

Following operation, some patients have persistent hypertension in both the arms and the legs. The reasons are not well understood, but it does not seem to be related to elevated levels of renin and angiotensin. Abnormal vascular reactivity has been demonstrated in patients with well-repaired coarctation. After repair, some patients with normal resting blood pressure have an exaggerated hypertensive response to exercise. This hypertension requires management. Delay in diagnosis and corrective surgery until an older age in childhood increases the risk of permanent systemic hypertension.

Echocardiogram

Cross-sectional images of the aortic arch, usually best obtained with the transducer positioned near the suprasternal notch, reveal narrowing at the site of coarctation. In some patients, hypoplasia of the transverse segment of the aortic arch extends to the coarctation. The proximal thoracic descending aorta just distal to the coarctation may be normal in size or may be slightly dilated, representing poststenotic dilation.

Color Doppler shows a disturbed (turbulent) signal at the stenosis, and spectral Doppler shows high-velocity flow from the transverse aortic arch to the descending aorta with a continuous pattern (extending from systole into diastole).

In neonates, the diagnosis may be difficult as long as the ductus arteriosus remains large. Flow through a neonatal ductus in coarctation is bidirectional, often predominantly right to left (pulmonary artery to aorta). This is an important echocardiographic clue to the diagnosis.

The echocardiogram provides rapid assessment of left ventricular hypertrophy, size, and function and also allows diagnosis of possible associated lesions, such as bicuspid aortic valve, mitral valve malformations, and ventricular septal defect.

Cardiac catheterization and angiography

Usually, the clinical findings and echocardiogram are sufficient to diagnose coarctation of the aorta. Diagnostic catheterization and angiography are unnecessary, unless performed in conjunction with balloon dilation.

Oximetry data are usually normal, except in neonates with a large ductus. Pressure measurements demonstrate systolic hypertension proximal to the coarctation and a gradient at the site of the coarctation, often dramatically shown by pullback of the catheter across the lesion during pressure recording.

Treatment

Medical management prior to gradient relief

Infants with a coarctation of the aorta who develop congestive cardiac failure usually respond to medical management within a few hours and then undergo successful repair. Infants who fail to respond promptly to medical management or to reopening of the ductus with prostaglandin may require emergency repair. The operative risk is higher in these patients.

Assessment in preparation for gradient relief

To make appropriate operative decisions, the exact location of the coarctation of the aorta must be known. This is done by integrating information from the physical examination, and by directly imaging the lesion by echocardiography, angiography, magnetic resonance imaging (MRI)/magnetic resonance angiography (MRA), or computed tomography angiography (CTA).

The distal extent of the coarctation can be recognized by the identification of poststenotic dilation, and the proximal extent by the blood pressure in the two arms. Usually, the recordings are similar in both arms, indicating that the coarctation is located distal to the left subclavian artery. Occasionally, the blood pressure of the left arm is lower than that of the right arm, indicating that the coarctation of the aorta involves a longer segment of the aorta: hypoplasia of the transverse aortic arch and possibly the origin of the left subclavian artery.

Echocardiographic images are often limited by the size of older patients. MRI/MRA and CTA are particularly useful imaging techniques in adolescents and adults with coarctation, since the coarcted segment of the aorta has little motion throughout the cardiac cycle.

In an infant in cardiac failure, the diagnosis may be difficult, in which case aortography, MRI/MRA, or CTA may be helpful.

Surgery

Two major types of operation for coarctation have been widely used:

- **Excision and end-to-end anastomosis**. A discrete coarctation is excised and the two ends of the aorta are reanastomosed. An elliptical incision is made to minimize narrowing that may accompany growth of the patient and/or shrinkage of the anastomotic scar.
- **Subclavian flap repair**. In patients with a very hypoplastic aorta or long-segment stenosis, the repair site can be augmented by transecting the left subclavian artery distally and opening it linearly to create a flap of living tissue. Early attempts to augment the arch repair with synthetic or pericardial patch material often led to late aneurysm formation.

Although long-term surgical results are very good, no operative technique is free from the risk of late restenosis. Operation should be performed on most patients with coarctation of the aorta when the defect is diagnosed, except perhaps in a small, premature infant who can be palliated with prostaglandin infusion and allowed to grow to near-term weight. Doing this improves the efficacy of repair and minimizes the risk of late restenosis. The operative mortality risk is low (less than 1 in 400) in patients with an uncomplicated coarctation.

Infants with severe associated anomalies, such as a very large ventricular septal defect, small left ventricular outflow tract, and associated left ventricular failure from volume and pressure overload, may benefit from a staged repair.

Repair of the coarctation and pulmonary artery banding first often leads to rapid improvement in the left ventricular dysfunction and eventual growth of the outflow tract. Several weeks or months later, removal of the band and closing of the ventricular septal defect follow. The operative mortality for primary one-stage neonatal repair of such infants can be higher than that of a staged approach, although currently many centers employ primary repair with low operative risk.

Interventional catheterization

Balloon dilation of coarctation at the time of cardiac catheterization has been successful for native (previously unoperated) coarctation and for postoperative restenosis.

In postoperative restenosis, the results of gradient relief are good and the risk of balloon dilation is low, possibly due to the external buttressing of the dilated region by the old operative scar. Reoperation for restenosis carries increased risk compared with balloon dilation, partly because of the operative scarring, which must be dissected to achieve exposure.

Balloon dilation of native coarctation avoids some operative disadvantages, but, compared with operative repair, it involves a greater chance of immediate complications such as extravasation and of late complications of aneurysm formation or restenosis. The age and size of the patient at the time of balloon dilation influence the risks and long-term outcomes: younger and smaller patients have higher risk.

Implantation of a metallic stent at the time of balloon dilation may lessen the risk of aneurysm formation, but in small patients the stents do not allow for growth; hence repeat balloon dilation of the stented region is usually needed.

Summary

Coarctation of the aorta is usually an easily diagnosed condition. In most patients it requires treatment, as it can lead to several problems: congestive cardiac failure, hypertension, and left ventricular dysfunction. In most patients, either operation or balloon dilation is used to relieve the obstruction. Despite the apparent anatomic success of intervention, recoarctation, persistent hypertension, and a coexistent bicuspid aortic valve are long-term problems following successful gradient relief.

AORTIC STENOSIS

Aortic stenosis can occur at one of three anatomic locations (Figure 5.3). Usually, aortic stenosis is caused by a stenotic congenital bicuspid or unicuspid valve. Obstruction to left ventricular outflow may also occur below the aortic valve,

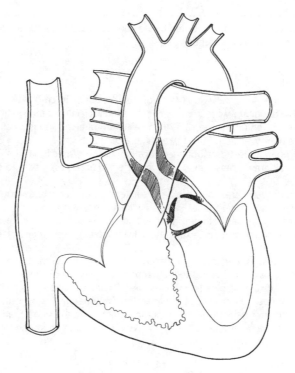

Figure 5.3 Aortic stenosis. Composite drawing showing three types of left ventricular outflow obstruction: subvalvar (fibromuscular ridge or membrane), valvar, and supravalvar aortic stenosis.

either as an isolated fibrous ring (discrete membranous subaortic stenosis) or as septal hypertrophy (idiopathic hypertrophic subaortic stenosis [i.e. hypertrophic cardiomyopathy]) (see Chapter 9). Rarely, aortic stenosis is located in the proximal ascending aorta (supravalvar aortic stenosis).

Regardless of the site of obstruction, the effect upon the left ventricle is similar. Because of the stenosis, the left ventricular systolic pressure rises to maintain a normal CO.

This relationship can be illustrated by the equation used to calculate the severity of valvar aortic stenosis:

$$AVA = \frac{AVF}{K\sqrt{LV - AO}}$$

where AVA is aortic valve area (area of stenotic orifice in cm^2), AVF is aortic valve flow (blood flow occurring during the systolic ejection period in mL/s), LV is mean left ventricular pressure during ejection (mmHg), AO is mean aortic pressure during ejection (mmHg), and K is a constant.

This equation uses data obtained at catheterization, specifically the mean pressure difference between the left ventricle and aorta, essentially to derive velocities.

The aortic valve area may also be calculated by Doppler echocardiography in a more direct fashion, since velocity is directly measured.

The mean velocities both proximal and distal to the aortic valve are measured by integrating the area under the respective Doppler curves (the velocity time integral, or VTI).

By measuring the diameter of the left ventricular outflow tract, the cross-sectional area proximal to the stenosis can be easily calculated.

Volume (V) (cm^3) can be found when the VTI (cm) is multiplied by area (cm^2).

The Continuity Principle states that as flow (volume/time) is the same through the normal left ventricular outflow tract as via the stenotic aortic valve, in the same amount of time, one systolic ejection period, the following equation can be derived:

$$AVA = \frac{\left(\pi d^2 / 4\right) \times VTI_{LVOT}}{VTI_{Ao}},$$

where AVA is aortic valve area (cm^2), d is left ventricular outflow tract diameter (cm), VTI_{LVOT} is the velocity time integral of the left ventricular outflow tract flow (mean velocity in cm), and VTI_{Ao} is the velocity time integral of the aortic valve flow (mean velocity in cm).

In practice, the Doppler maximum velocities in the left ventricular outflow tract and in the aorta are sometimes substituted for the mean velocities. In patients without shunts, alternative methods of estimating the flow per beat (the stroke volume in cm^3 or mL) are often employed, including M-mode and 2D or 3D echo techniques to determine the change in ventricular volume during a single systole. The following equation yields the valve area:

$$AVA = \frac{Stroke\ volume}{VTI_{Ao}}$$

In patients with more severe aortic stenosis (smaller aortic valve area) for a given CO, left ventricular systolic pressure is higher. Similarly, when the patient exercises, since the aortic valve area is fixed, as the CO rises, the left ventricular systolic pressure increases as a squared function (Figure 5.4).

The primary effect upon the heart of each type of aortic stenosis is elevation of left ventricular systolic pressure, resulting in left ventricular hypertrophy. Many of the clinical and laboratory features of aortic stenosis are related to the left ventricular hypertrophy and its effects. Because of the elevated left ventricular systolic pressure, the myocardial oxygen demands are increased. During exercise, the oxygen demands are further increased because both heart rate and left ventricular systolic pressure increase. If these oxygen needs are unmet, myocardial ischemia may occur and lead to syncope, chest pain, or electrocardiogram changes. Recurrent myocardial ischemic episodes can lead to left ventricular fibrosis, which can ultimately progress to cardiac failure and cardiomegaly.

Other clinical features of aortic stenosis are related to the turbulence of blood flow through the stenotic area, manifested by a systolic ejection murmur, and in valvar aortic stenosis, manifested by poststenotic dilation of the ascending aorta.

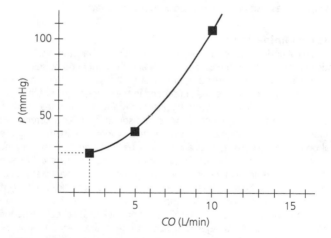

Figure 5.4 Effect of exercise on the gradient in aortic stenosis. Hypothetical values are shown. At rest, cardiac output is 2 L/min and the systolic gradient is 25 mmHg. Two levels of exercise are shown. At moderate exercise, cardiac output is 5 L/min and the gradient is 40 mmHg; but at maximum exercise, the cardiac output is 10 L/min and the gradient exceeds 100 mmHg. *P*, pressure; *CO*, cardiac output.

Aortic valvar stenosis

Aortic valvar stenosis is related to either a unicuspid valve (most often presenting in infants) or a congenitally bicuspid valve (usually presenting in older children and adults) (Figure 5.3). The orifices of the abnormal valves are narrowed, accompanied by various degrees of regurgitation in some patients.

History

Aortic stenosis is commonly associated with a significant murmur at birth. In most cardiac anomalies, the murmur is often first recognized later in infancy. Aortic stenosis occurs two to three times more frequently in males.

Patients with aortic stenosis are usually asymptomatic throughout childhood, even when stenosis is severe. Only 5% of children with aortic stenosis develop congestive cardiac failure in the neonatal period, but it can develop later in children whose severe stenosis was not relieved. Exercise intolerance may occur so gradually that it is unnoticed by parents and teachers. Some asymptomatic children, as they approach adolescence, may develop episodes of anginal chest pain. These episodes signify myocardial ischemia and may precede sudden death.

Syncope, another serious symptom of aortic stenosis, may occur upon exercise. This symptom has also been associated with sudden death.

Physical examination

Several clinical findings suggest the diagnosis of aortic valvar stenosis. With severe stenotic lesions, the pulse pressure is narrow and the peripheral pulses feel weak, but in most patients the pulses are normal. A thrill may be present in the aortic area along the upper right sternal border and in the suprasternal notch.

An aortic systolic ejection murmur begins shortly after the first heart sound and extends to the aortic component of the second sound. In older children the murmur is located in the aortic area, but in infancy it is more prominent along the left sternal border; because of this location it may be confused with the murmur of ventricular septal defect. The murmur of aortic stenosis characteristically transmits into the carotid arteries. However, in normal children a functional systolic carotid arterial bruit may be heard; therefore, a murmur in the neck does not, by itself, prove the diagnosis of aortic valvar stenosis.

The murmur usually follows a systolic ejection click that reflects poststenotic dilation of the aorta. Aortic ejection clicks are heard best at the cardiac apex when the patient is reclining and may also be heard over the left lower back. The click is generally present in mild aortic stenosis and may be absent in severe stenosis.

In about 30% of children with aortic stenosis, a soft, early diastolic murmur of aortic insufficiency is heard along the mid-left sternal border.

Electrocardiogram

The electrocardiogram (Figure 5.5) generally reveals a normal QRS axis, but in a few patients left axis deviation, suggesting severe left ventricular hypertrophy, is observed. The prominent finding is left ventricular hypertrophy, usually manifested by deep S waves in lead V_1 and normal or tall R waves in lead V_6.

Attention should be directed to changes in the ST segment and T waves in precordial leads V_5 and V_6. The development of T-wave inversion and ST-segment depression indicates increasingly significant left ventricular hypertrophy and strain. Left ventricular strain is a warning; the few children with aortic stenosis who die suddenly usually manifest these electrocardiographic changes of abnormal ventricular repolarization.

Occasionally in infants and less frequently in older children, left atrial enlargement occurs.

Chest X-ray

The cardiac size is normal in most children with aortic stenosis because the volume of blood in the heart is normal. Cardiomegaly occurs in infants with severe stenosis and congestive cardiac failure. It rarely occurs in older children; when present, it indicates left ventricular myocardial fibrosis. Severe stenosis may be present with normal cardiac size. The ascending aorta is prominent because of poststenotic dilation. The pulmonary vasculature is normal, unless marked left ventricular dysfunction has occurred, at which point pulmonary venous markings are increased.

Summary of clinical findings

An aortic ejection murmur, often associated with a thrill in the suprasternal notch, indicates that the site of the obstruction is in the left ventricular outflow area. Prominent ascending aorta on chest X-ray and the presence of a systolic ejection click reflect poststenotic dilation of the ascending aorta. The electrocardiogram shows left ventricular hypertrophy. Chest pain, syncope, ST- and T-wave changes, and cardiomegaly are serious findings, indicating inadequate myocardial oxygen supply, and should prompt relief of the stenosis.

Natural history

Aortic valvar stenosis progresses. Two processes account for this: the development of myocardial fibrosis and the absolute or relative (because of differential growth) decrease in size of the stenotic aortic valvar orifice by cartilaginous changes and ultimately by valvar calcification.

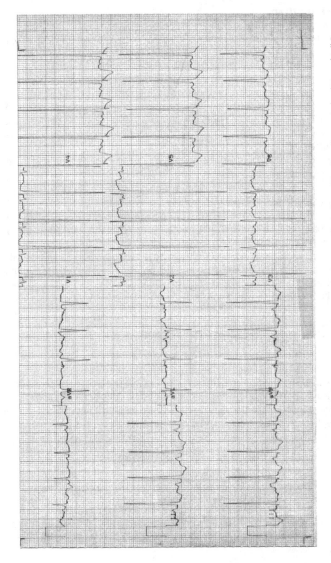

Figure 5.5 Electrocardiogram in valvar aortic stenosis. Left ventricular hypertrophy indicated by deep S wave in lead V_1, and tall R wave in lead V_5. Inverted T waves in left precordial leads. Biphasic P waves in V_1, indicate left atrial enlargement.

Patients with mild congenital aortic stenosis may live 50 years or more before symptoms develop, representing the calcific aortic stenosis syndrome of adulthood.

Echocardiogram

The architecture of the aortic valve can usually be determined with great accuracy by cross-sectional echocardiography. A normal aortic valve has three leaflets that appear thin, open completely in systole, and close (coapt) fully, without prolapse, in diastole. In contrast, stenotic aortic valves are often bicuspid or unicuspid with thick-appearing, highly echo-reflective leaflets that do not open fully in systole, producing the appearance of a dome at their maximum excursion. These stenotic valves rarely show prolapse.

Color Doppler provides a highly sensitive means for detecting aortic regurgitation, often when it cannot be detected by auscultation.

Spectral Doppler allows highly accurate estimation of the pressure gradient across a stenotic valve. The gradient estimated using the maximum velocity represents a peak instantaneous systolic gradient that is usually 25–30% more than the peak-to-peak systolic gradient obtained at cardiac catheterization. A Doppler mean gradient may more closely approximate the values obtained by catheterization.

Aortic valve area can be estimated using Doppler and 2D measurements of the area of the normal outflow tract proximal to the obstructed valve.

Echocardiography allows the precise measurement of left ventricular function, enlargement, and hypertrophy. The presence of mitral valve regurgitation, even in the absence of a holosystolic murmur, suggests left ventricular dysfunction.

Neonates with severe aortic obstruction may have highly echo-reflective endocardium (so-called endocardial fibroelastosis) representing scarring from intrauterine subendocardial ischemia.

Cardiac catheterization

Cardiac catheterization may be indicated when children become symptomatic or develop electrocardiographic or echocardiographic changes. It is used for balloon dilation of the aortic valve stenosis.

The oxygen data are usually normal. The important finding is a systolic pressure difference across the aortic valve (Figure 5.6a). This gradient reflects the degree of obstruction. To assess the severity adequately, CO must be measured, as the gradient depends upon it also.

During cardiac catheterization, the measurements of both the pressures and the CO can be made simultaneously; with this information, the size of the stenotic orifice (AVA) can be calculated according to the previously shown equation (stroke volume divided by VTI).

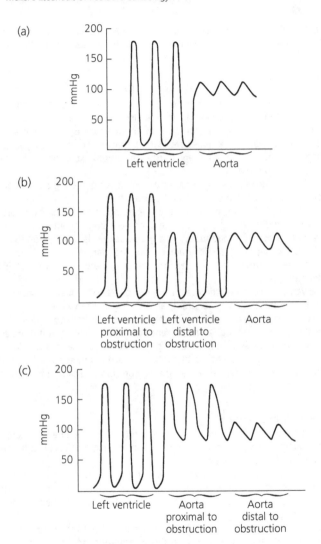

Figure 5.6 Pressure tracings in different types of aortic stenosis as the catheter is withdrawn from the left ventricle to the aorta. (a) Valvar aortic stenosis; (b) subvalvar aortic stenosis; (c) supravalvar aortic stenosis.

Aortography or left ventriculography is routinely performed to show the details of the aortic valve and the surrounding vascular and cardiac structures. The aortogram may be used to grade coexistent aortic valvar regurgitation.

Balloon dilation is commonly performed to reduce the gradient. A fluid-filled catheter-mounted balloon with inflated diameter similar to the measured aortic valve annulus diameter is positioned across the aortic valve and rapidly inflated and deflated. Balloon dilation may result in valvar regurgitation Provided that pre-dilation aortic regurgitation was not severe, any increase is usually well tolerated.

Operative considerations
Relief of the aortic stenosis gradient, by either balloon dilation or cardiac surgery, is indicated for patients with significant symptoms or for those whose catheterization data or echocardiogram indicate moderate or severe stenosis.

Aortic stenosis gradient – indications for intervention

Echocardiogram – Doppler
  Peak instantaneous systolic gradient (PISG) = 70–80 mmHg
  Mean gradient = 45–50 mmHg
Catheterization
  Peak-to-peak systolic pressure gradient = 50–60 mmHg
Catheterization or echocardiogram – Doppler
  Aortic valve area (AVA) ≤0.5–0.7 cm²/m²

These criteria are not absolute; the decision to intervene varies between cardiac centers, with the diagnostic modality used, and depending on the age and condition of the patient.

In children, the stenotic valve is usually pliable enough for valvotomy or valvuloplasty so that an aortic valve replacement with a prosthesis or homograft (cadaveric human valve) is not required. Ultimately, children who have undergone aortic valvotomy may require a prosthesis or homograft in adulthood if the valve becomes calcified or rigid, or sooner if the valve develops important regurgitation.

No currently available replacement valve is perfect: mechanical prostheses are long-lived but thrombogenic, so anticoagulation is required; homograft valves, although free from thrombogenic complications, are often shorter-lived because of destruction by calcification at an unpredictable rate.

An alternative is the Ross autograft procedure, in which the patient's normal pulmonary valve is excised and placed in the aortic position. A homograft valve is placed in the pulmonary position, where performing balloon dilation or future surgical revision is less risky because of its more accessible anterior location and presence on the pulmonary side of the circulation. Higher operative risk and longevity of the patient's native pulmonary valve functioning in the aortic position have been limitations with the Ross operation.

Summary

In aortic valvar stenosis, a suprasternal notch thrill is present, associated with a systolic ejection murmur in the aortic area and with an aortic systolic ejection click. The chest X-ray may show cardiomegaly but usually appears normal. The electrocardiogram may show left ventricular hypertrophy and repolarization abnormalities. The echocardiogram is the most crucial laboratory examination for following the course of the patient. The echocardiographic estimate of the degree of obstruction or symptoms, such as chest pain or syncope, alerts the provider that further diagnostic studies and intervention are warranted. Relief of the obstruction by valvotomy or valvuloplasty can be done at low risk in children with moderate or severe stenosis.

Discrete membranous subaortic stenosis

This is the second most common form of left ventricular outflow obstruction but much less frequent than aortic valvar stenosis. This obstruction is a fibromuscular membrane with a small central orifice located in the left ventricle, usually within 1 cm of the aortic valve (Figure 5.3). A jet of blood passes through the orifice and strikes the aortic valve. Because the jet strikes the aortic valve, the energy of the jet is dissipated so that poststenotic dilation of the ascending aorta rarely occurs; however, problems with aortic valve regurgitation frequently result from alterations in the aortic valve.

History

A murmur is usually recognized in infancy. Congestive cardiac failure is rare. The symptoms of chest pain and syncope may occur in patients with severe obstruction, but most patients are asymptomatic.

Physical examination

The prominent physical finding is an aortic systolic ejection murmur heard best along the left sternal border, often lower than in patients with valvar aortic stenosis. A suprasternal notch thrill is uncommon. Systolic ejection clicks rarely occur because the ascending aorta is usually normal in size.

An aortic early diastolic murmur of aortic regurgitation is present in about 70% of patients.

Electrocardiogram

The electrocardiogram shows findings similar to those of valvar aortic stenosis: left ventricular hypertrophy and ST- and T-wave changes that may indicate ischemia. Some patients have an RSR' pattern in lead V_1 and an RS pattern in lead V_6. The reason for these findings is unknown.

Chest X-ray

Heart size is normal without enlargement of the ascending aorta. Pulmonary vasculature is normal.

Natural history

Discrete membranous subaortic stenosis progresses, not usually because of increasing subaortic stenosis but because of aortic valvar regurgitation. The aortic regurgitation develops and progresses from trauma of the jet on the aortic valve.

Echocardiogram

A discrete subaortic ridge can usually be seen projecting from the septum into the left ventricular outflow tract. In contrast to valvar aortic stenosis, the disturbed color Doppler signals indicating turbulent flow begin at the site of the membrane, proximal to the valve itself. The maximum velocity of flow through the outflow tract is used to estimate the gradient. Some patients with a relatively unimportant gradient, less than 40 mmHg, have important aortic valvar regurgitation.

Cardiac catheterization

Cardiac catheterization is not needed in making a decision whether to treat surgically if echocardiography indicates important progressive obstruction and/or regurgitation.

Oxygen data are normal. A systolic pressure gradient is found below the level of the aortic valve within the left ventricle (Figure 5.6b). Aortic regurgitation, if severe, causes a wide aortic pulse pressure and an elevated left ventricular end-diastolic pressure. Left ventriculography may identify the location of the membrane but is less helpful than echocardiography. If aortic regurgitation is present, it is best shown by aortography.

Operative considerations

Excision of the membrane is indicated in most patients, unless the gradient is small. Balloon dilation of the subaortic membrane has been unsuccessful in reducing the gradient. The purposes of operation are relief of the elevated left ventricular systolic pressure and reduction of the aortic valve trauma.

The operative risk, which is minimal, approaches that of operation for valvar aortic stenosis. The major hazard of the operation is damage to the septal leaflet of the mitral valve, since the membrane is often attached to this leaflet. The results are generally very good, with near-normal left ventricular systolic pressure postoperatively. The degree of aortic valve regurgitation is lessened and progression is generally halted. Regrowth of the subaortic membrane can occur, but this risk is virtually eliminated by removal of a shallow layer of myocardium forming the base of the membrane's attachment to the left ventricular walls.

Summary

Discrete membranous subaortic stenosis clinically resembles valvar aortic stenosis in many respects, but it lacks the clinical and chest X-ray findings of poststenotic dilation of the aorta.

Supravalvar aortic stenosis

Obstruction to left ventricular outflow can also result from supravalvar stenosis. In most patients, the ascending aorta narrows in an hourglass deformity (Figure 5.3). Although usually limited to the ascending aorta, other arteries, such as the brachiocephalic and the renal arteries, may also be narrowed. Peripheral pulmonary arterial stenosis and hypoplasia may coexist and represent the most important cardiovascular problem.

The systolic pressure is elevated in the ascending aorta proximal to the obstruction; therefore, the coronary arteries are subjected to this elevated pressure. The elevation can lead to tortuosity of the coronary arteries and to premature atherosclerosis. The coronary artery ostia may be narrowed by the same obstructive process operating in the aorta and other large vessels and has a poor prognosis.

Two factors have been implicated in the etiology of this condition. The first is Williams syndrome, in which a defect in the elastin gene is present. The second is familial supravalvar aortic stenosis, which occurs in patients who do not have Williams syndrome, but who carry a mutated elastin gene (see Chapter 2).

History

Most patients are asymptomatic; cardiac disease is identified by either the presence of a murmur or the facial characteristics of Williams syndrome. Congestive cardiac failure or growth retardation is rare, as in other forms of aortic stenosis, but sudden death can occur. The risk might even be higher because of acquired abnormalities of the coronary arteries.

Physical examination

The general physical characteristics of the child, particularly the facies, suggest the diagnosis of supravalvar aortic stenosis (see Chapter 2). However, many children appear normal.

Careful blood pressure recording in both arms and legs can lead to suspicion of supravalvar aortic stenosis if a blood pressure discrepancy of 20 mmHg or more is found between the arms (Coanda effect). This effect is related to either a narrowing of a subclavian artery or the pressure effect of the jet from the supravalvar aortic stenosis directed into the right subclavian artery. In the latter circumstance, the blood pressure is higher in the right arm.

An aortic systolic ejection murmur is the prominent cardiac finding and, in contrast to valvar stenosis, is located maximally beneath the right clavicle, not along the left sternal border. A systolic ejection click is not present because poststenotic dilation does not occur. Diastole is silent, as valvar regurgitation does not occur.

Electrocardiogram

The electrocardiogram usually shows features similar to those of valvar aortic stenosis, including left ventricular hypertrophy. Some patients, for unknown reasons, show an RSR' pattern in lead V_1 and an RS in lead V_6, without criteria of left ventricular hypertrophy. ST-segment and T-wave changes may be present, reflecting myocardial ischemia that is possibly accentuated by coronary arterial abnormalities.

Chest X-ray

The cardiac size is normal, with the absence of poststenotic dilation.

Natural history

The narrowing in affected arteries may progress. The major change over the course of this disease is the development of myocardial ischemia and fibrosis and its consequences, although findings of right heart hypertension predominate in peripheral pulmonary artery stenosis. In following the patient, attention must be directed to the history of syncope or chest pain and to electrocardiographic changes in the ST segment and T waves.

Echocardiogram

Cross-sectional views of the ascending aorta parallel to its long axis show discrete and often severe narrowing at the sinotubular junction and, at times, more diffuse narrowing into the distal ascending aorta. Unlike valvar aortic stenosis, flow acceleration and turbulence begin at the supravalvar narrowing. The gradient is estimated using spectral Doppler. Associated lesions, such as branch pulmonary artery hypoplasia and stenosis, are readily detectable by cross-sectional echo; the presence of tricuspid and pulmonary valve regurgitation allows the estimation of right-sided cardiac pressures.

Cardiac catheterization

The oxygen data are normal. The diagnosis is established by measuring a systolic pressure difference within the ascending aorta (Figure 5.6c) and/or the pulmonary arteries. Angiography demonstrates the anatomic details of the obstruction and, more importantly, identifies associated lesions – involvement of coronary, brachiocephalic, and peripheral pulmonary arteries – which is usually difficult by echocardiography. Because a greater risk of coronary artery compromise exists, contrast injection into individual coronary arteries is usually avoided in favor of aortography.

Operative considerations

Operative relief of the obstruction may be indicated for a lesser gradient, 30–40 mmHg, compared with aortic valvar stenosis, or if symptoms related to myocardial ischemia are present. A longitudinal incision is made across the stenotic area, which is widened by placement of a diamond-shaped patch. During the operation, the coronary ostia are inspected, but rarely is coronary arterial bypass indicated. The operative risk for supravalvar aortic stenosis is higher than for valvar aortic stenosis. Over the long term, reobstruction can occur because of progressive medial thickening of affected vessels.

Summary

Supravalvar aortic stenosis differs from valvar aortic stenosis since findings of poststenotic dilation are absent. The lesion can progress and may involve multiple arteries. Characteristic facies and abnormal chromosome probe are seen in Williams syndrome, which occurs sporadically, whereas other patients appear normal and have a normal chromosome probe but usually have multiple family members who are affected. Relief of the obstruction in the ascending aorta can be accomplished by surgical widening of the narrowing with a patch.

PULMONARY STENOSIS

Pulmonary stenosis (Figure 5.7) occurs at three sites in the outflow area of the right ventricle: below the pulmonary valve (infundibular), at the level of the valve (valvar), or above the valve (supravalvar). Infundibular pulmonary stenosis rarely occurs as an isolated lesion. Supravalvar stenosis or stenosis of the individual pulmonary arteries is uncommon after early infancy. In most patients, obstruction occurs at the level of the pulmonary valve.

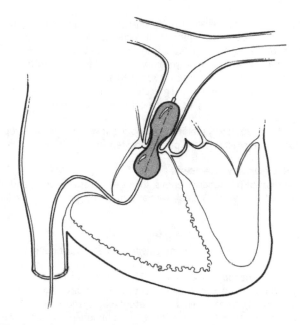

Figure 5.7 Valvar pulmonary stenosis. Balloon dilation via catheter.

Regardless of the anatomic type of stenosis, the results are similar. Blood flow through the stenotic area is turbulent and leads to a murmur. The other major effect is an increase in right ventricular systolic pressure. This effect is illustrated by the equation for calculating the area of the stenotic pulmonary valve orifice:

$$PVA = \frac{PVF}{K\sqrt{RV - PA}},$$

where PVA is pulmonary valve area (area of stenotic orifice in cm^2), PVF is pulmonary valve flow (blood flow occurring during the systolic ejection period in mL/s), RV is mean right ventricular pressure during ejection (mmHg), PA is mean pulmonary artery pressure during ejection (mmHg), and K is a constant.

Because of the restricted orifice, the level of right ventricular systolic pressure increases to maintain a normal CO. With the elevation of right ventricular systolic pressure, right ventricular hypertrophy develops, the degree of which parallels the level of pressure elevation. With significant hypertrophy, right ventricular compliance is reduced, elevating right atrial pressure and causing right atrial enlargement. Because of the right atrial changes, the foramen ovale may be stretched open, leading to a right-to-left shunt at the atrial level. Right ventricular compliance may be reduced by myocardial fibrosis, secondary to the inability to meet augmented myocardial oxygen requirements.

A second complication of right ventricular hypertrophy is the development of infundibular stenosis that may become significant enough to pose a secondary area of obstruction.

The clinical and laboratory manifestations of right ventricular hypertrophy serve as indicators of the severity of the pulmonary stenosis.

Valvar pulmonary stenosis

In the usual form of pulmonary stenosis, the valve cusps are fused, and the valve appears domed in systole. A small central orifice and poststenotic dilation are found.

History

No gender predominance in pulmonary stenosis exists. Most patients are asymptomatic during childhood, but those with more severe degrees of pulmonary stenosis complain of fatigue on exercise. The murmur of pulmonary stenosis is frequently heard in the neonatal period; critical pulmonary stenosis may present with cyanosis. Rarely, older patients may present with cyanosis and cardiac failure. This combination of cyanosis and failure in pulmonary stenosis with intact ventricular septum usually occurs early in the first year of life, although it may occur at any age, and indicates severe stenosis and decompensation of the right ventricle.

Physical examination

Most children appear normal, although cyanosis and clubbing exist in the few with right-to-left atrial shunt. Usually, the cardiac apex is not displaced. Often, a systolic thrill is present below the left clavicle and upper left sternal border and, occasionally, in the suprasternal notch.

A systolic ejection murmur, heard along the upper left sternal border and below the clavicle, transmits to the left upper back. Usually, the murmurs are loud (grade 4/6) because the volume of flow across the valve is normal, but in patients with severe stenosis, particularly with cyanosis or cardiac failure, the murmur is softer because of reduced CO.

The quality and characteristics of the second heart sound give an indication of the severity of the stenosis. In severe stenosis, the pulmonary valve closure sound is delayed and soft (i.e. it can be so soft that the second heart sound seems single).

If a pulmonary systolic ejection click is present, it indicates pulmonary artery poststenotic dilation. This finding is present in mild to moderate pulmonary stenosis, but it may be absent in severe pulmonary stenosis.

Electrocardiogram

The electrocardiogram (Figure 5.8) is useful in estimating the severity of the pulmonary stenosis. In mild pulmonary stenosis, the electrocardiogram may appear normal. With more severe degrees of stenosis, right-axis deviation and right ventricular hypertrophy are found, with a tall R wave in lead V_1 and a prominent S wave in lead V_6. The height of the R wave roughly correlates with the level of right ventricular systolic pressure.

Right atrial enlargement commonly occurs, reflecting elevated right ventricular filling pressure.

In patients with severe stenosis, a pattern of right ventricular strain develops, manifested by ST-segment depression and deep inversion of T waves in the right precordial leads. Inverted T waves in leads V_1–V_4 do not indicate strain in and of themselves because this pattern is normal in younger children.

Chest X-ray

Usually, cardiac size is normal because the right heart volume is normal. Cardiac enlargement is found with congestive cardiac failure or cyanosis because of the increased volume of the right heart chambers. Except in patients with cyanosis, the pulmonary vascularity appears normal, not decreased, because patients with pulmonary stenosis have normal systemic output and a normal quantity of blood passes through the pulmonary valve.

A distinctive feature of pulmonary valvar stenosis is poststenotic dilation of the pulmonary trunk and left pulmonary artery (Figure 5.9). This appears as a prominent bulge along the upper left cardiac border. In patients with severe stenosis, this finding can be absent.

Summary of clinical findings

The systolic ejection murmur indicates the turbulence of flow through the stenotic pulmonary valve. Poststenotic dilation is indicated by the pulmonary systolic ejection click and the roentgenographic findings of an enlarged pulmonary trunk. The electrocardiogram is the best indicator of the degree of right ventricular hypertrophy. Right atrial enlargement, cyanosis, and congestive cardiac failure are indicators of altered right ventricular compliance resulting from severe right ventricular hypertrophy and/or fibrosis.

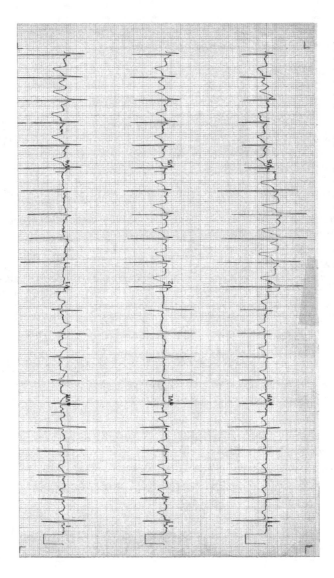

Figure 5.8 Electrocardiogram in pulmonary stenosis. Tall R wave in V_1 and right-axis deviation indicate right ventricular hypertrophy.

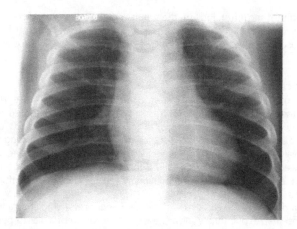

Figure 5.9 Chest X-ray in pulmonary stenosis. Normal-sized heart and pulmonary vasculature. Poststenotic dilation of pulmonary artery.

Natural history

The orifice of the stenotic pulmonary valve increases as a child grows, meaning that the degree of obstruction usually does not increase with age. The deterioration of the clinical status in some patients results from altered right ventricular myocardial performance related to fibrosis. This complication occurs in infancy and in adulthood, but rarely in the mid-childhood years. Occasionally, an infant or toddler has progression of infundibular stenosis without apparent change in the degree of valvar stenosis.

Echocardiography

Cross-sectional echocardiography shows thickened and doming pulmonary valve leaflets. Poststenotic dilation of the main pulmonary artery and ductus "diverticulum" can be dramatic. Doppler recording reveals turbulent high-velocity flow through the pulmonary valve; the maximum velocity allows the estimation of the pressure gradient between the right ventricle and the pulmonary artery. Right ventricular hypertrophy may occur, but quantitation is more difficult than in left ventricular hypertrophy, because of both right ventricular geometry and opposition between the right ventricular wall with the chest wall. Differentiation of the boundary between the two structures is problematic.

Hypertrophy of the infundibulum, the tubular right ventricular outflow tract, can become severe and is easily demonstrated by cross-sectional echocardiography; as the muscular walls squeeze, the pathway is virtually closed by the end of each systole.

Cardiac catheterization
Oximetry data are normal except in an occasional patient with a right-to-left shunt at the atrial level. The right ventricular systolic pressure is elevated, whereas pulmonary arterial pressure is normal or low. Both pressure and CO data are needed to assess the severity of the stenosis. This is done by calculating the pulmonary valve area, although in children with normal CO the pressure gradient may be used to determine the indications for intervention. Right ventricular angiography outlines the details of the pulmonary valve and associated infundibular narrowing.

Balloon dilation is the procedure of choice to reduce the gradient. Any patient with dome-shaped pulmonary valvar stenosis and a right ventricular-to-pulmonary artery systolic pressure gradient greater than 35 mmHg should undergo consideration for balloon valvotomy. This low-risk procedure almost always results in a favorable outcome and reduces right ventricular systolic pressure to normal or near normal. Even though pulmonary valvar regurgitation may increase following valvuloplasty, it is usually mild and well tolerated because the pulmonary arterial pressure is low.

In patients with a significant infundibular component, this procedure may not produce an immediate fall in right ventricular pressure; the infundibular stenosis usually resolves over several weeks.

Operative considerations
Since the development of catheter balloon dilation, operative valvotomy may be considered for those patients who have failed dilation (e.g. patients with Noonan syndrome with dysplastic valves) or who are not candidates for balloon dilation (e.g. the neonate with critical stenosis and an extremely hypoplastic pulmonary annulus instead requires outflow tract widening by use of a patch). Infundibular narrowing may require excision in some patients.

Summary
Pulmonary stenosis can usually be diagnosed on the basis of clinical and laboratory findings. Cardiac catheterization is required to determine precisely the severity and to perform balloon valvotomy in patients with moderate or severe stenosis; it can be performed at low risk and with excellent results.

Pulmonary stenosis secondary to dysplastic pulmonary valve

This distinctive form of pulmonary stenosis accounts for less than 10% of valvar pulmonary stenosis. Anatomically, the commissures of the pulmonary valve leaflets are not fused as in most examples of stenotic valves. Rather, the commissures are open, but each leaflet is greatly thickened and redundant. The valvar obstruction is caused by the bulk of valvar tissue within the pulmonary annulus. The pulmonary annulus can also be reduced in diameter. Poststenotic dilation usually does not occur.

History

The history is similar to that of patients with pulmonary stenosis with a dome-shaped pulmonary valve.

Physical examination

In many patients, a dysplastic pulmonary valve is associated with various syndromes, such as Noonan syndrome (see Chapter 2). Auscultation shows a pulmonary systolic ejection murmur, usually grades 2/6 to 4/6. Poststenotic dilation and a systolic ejection click are not found. The P_2 is soft and delayed.

Electrocardiogram

The electrocardiogram is distinctive. The QRS axis is almost always superiorly directed ($-60°$ to $-150°$) and distinguishes the dysplastic from dome-shaped pulmonary stenosis, in which the QRS axis rarely exceeds $+180°$. The reason for this alteration of the QRS axis is unknown, but it may represent an abnormal location of the conduction system.

Right ventricular hypertrophy is present, its degree reflecting the level of right ventricular systolic pressure. Right atrial enlargement may appear.

Chest X-ray

The heart size is normal, as is the vascularity. The pulmonary arterial segment is of normal size compared with dome-shaped valvar pulmonary stenosis.

Natural history

In this form of pulmonary stenosis, the stenotic valve orifice probably grows in relation to the growth of the child. Changes that occur with age are related to the effects of the elevated right ventricular systolic pressure and right ventricular hypertrophy upon the right ventricle, to the frequent development of severe infundibular stenosis, and perhaps to changes in the pliability of the thickened valve leaflets themselves.

Echocardiogram
In patients with a so-called dysplastic valve, the leaflets may be so thick that they appear globular, with very little motion or opening during systole. Some patients have biventricular hypertrophy disproportionate to the degree of outflow obstruction. Although this finding may represent a form of hypertrophic cardiomyopathy for patients with Noonan syndrome, it has a more benign natural history than in patients with hypertrophic cardiomyopathy from the more common sarcomeric protein mutations.

Cardiac catheterization
The data resemble those obtained in dome-shaped pulmonary stenosis. Angiography confirms the dysplastic nature of the valve as the leaflets appear thickened and immobile. The pulmonary artery may be only slightly enlarged. Balloon dilation is not effective in most patients.

Operative considerations
The indications for operation are similar to those for dome-shaped pulmonary stenosis; however, the operative approach is different. Valvotomy cannot be performed because commissural fusion is not present. One or two leaflets must be excised, and in some patients a patch must be placed across the annulus to widen this area of right ventricular outflow. Resection of infundibular muscle often accompanies valvotomy.

Peripheral pulmonary artery stenosis
Stenosis also occurs in the pulmonary artery branches. One or more major branches may be involved, usually showing a long area of narrowing, or the entire pulmonary arterial tree may be hypoplastic.

- Physiologic. The most common type is neonatal pulmonary artery stenosis which is normal. The branch pulmonary arteries are small in relation to the pulmonary trunk, so there is mild obstruction from a discrepancy in size. Over the first three to six months of life, the branches increase in size and evidence of the flow acceleration (murmur) disappears. It is unusual to hear a murmur from physiologic branch pulmonary artery flow in infants older than a year of age.
- Pathologic. Peripheral pulmonary artery stenosis occurs in other conditions, including congenital rubella syndrome and supravalvar aortic stenosis, and particularly in patients with Williams syndrome and Alagille syndrome (with a clinical presentation similar to biliary atresia). Hypoplastic pulmonary arteries frequently accompany tetralogy of Fallot with pulmonary valve atresia and these patients often have DiGeorge syndrome.

History
Most patients with this condition are asymptomatic unless other conditions, such as Williams syndrome, are present.

Physical examination
Features of one of the syndromes mentioned above may be discovered. In normal neonates with auscultatory findings of peripheral pulmonary artery "stenosis," the murmur disappears with time (see Chapter 1), and the pulmonary arteries are, in fact, normal.

The classic finding is a systolic ejection murmur present under the clavicles that is well heard throughout the lung fields and the axillae. Typically, either no murmur or only a soft murmur is heard over the precordium. The second heart sound is normal, and a systolic ejection click is not heard because the pulmonary artery is not dilated.

Electrocardiogram
No features distinguish peripheral pulmonary artery stenosis from valvar pulmonary stenosis. Right ventricular hypertrophy exists proportional to the degree of stenosis.

Chest X-ray
This usually appears normal. Pulmonary blood flow appears symmetric because most children have symmetric stenoses.

Natural history
The prognosis is variable.

- Physiologic. Since the degree of stenosis is often mild and does not increase with age in most patients, it is essentially a benign condition, a form of functional murmur.
- Pathologic. In some conditions, including Alagille syndrome, apparent growth of the pulmonary arteries may occur in some patients, resulting in clinical and laboratory features becoming more normal with age. Rarely, especially in patients with Williams syndrome, stenosis may progress in severity and can cause suprasystemic right ventricular pressure and eventually right heart failure.

Echocardiogram
The proximal few centimeters of each branch pulmonary artery are easily seen on the cross-sectional echocardiogram, particularly in young infants, and precise diameter measurements can be made. Doppler is used to estimate pressure

gradients within the branch pulmonary arteries; however, the Bernoulli equation is more applicable to discrete stenoses, so gradient estimates of long tubular (or serial) stenoses are often inaccurate.

Cardiac catheterization
Oxygen data are normal. Pressure tracings show a systolic gradient within the pulmonary arteries. Diastolic pressures are identical proximal and distal to the obstruction. The anatomic details are shown by pulmonary arteriography.

Catheter balloon dilation, sometimes with placement of endovascular metal stents, is widely used, although with variable results that depend greatly on the etiology and severity of the stenosis.

Operative considerations
Most patients do not require operation, as the degree of stenosis is not severe. In patients with severe obstruction, operation often cannot be performed because anatomic features, such as diffuse hypoplasia of the pulmonary arteries or multiple areas of stenosis, preclude an operative approach and are best served by having catheter balloon dilation.

Summary of obstructive lesions

In each of the conditions discussed, turbulence occurs through a narrowed orifice, causing a systolic ejection murmur. Beyond the obstruction, poststenotic dilation occurs; this is evidenced either by chest X-ray findings or by an ejection click. The restricted orifice leads to elevation of systolic pressures proximally and to ventricular hypertrophy. The clinical and laboratory findings reflecting this hypertrophy permit assessment of the severity of the condition (Table 5.1). In patients with moderate or severe obstruction gradient, relief can be performed successfully by operative and catheterization means.

Table 5.1 Summary of obstructive lesions.

Malformation	History					Physical examination			
	Major syndrome	Gender	Age murmur	Congestive cardiac failure	Symptoms	Blood pressure	Thrill	Murmur	Systolic ejection click
Coarctation of aorta	Turner	M > F	Infancy	±	None, or headache	Upper extremity hypertension	Suprasternal notch	Systolic, precordium and back	Aortic (if bicuspid valve present)
Aortic stenosis	Williams (supravalvar aortic stenosis)	M > F	Birth	±	None, or chest pain, syncope, sudden death	Normal, or narrow pulse pressure	Suprasternal notch and/or aortic area	Systolic ejection, aortic area and left sternal border	Aortic
Pulmonary stenosis	Noonan	M = F	Birth	±	None, or exercise intolerance. variable cyanosis (neonates)	Normal	Pulmonic area	Systolic ejection, pulmonic area and left back	Pulmonic

Malformation	Electrocardiogram				Chest X-ray			
	Axis (QRS)	Atrial enlargement	Ventricular hypertrophy/enlargement	Other	Aortic enlargement	Pulmonary artery enlargement	Chamber enlargement	Other
Coarctation of aorta	Normal	None or left	Right (neonate and infant), left (older child)	Strain pattern if severe	Absent unless bicuspid valve	Absent	± Left ventricle	Poststenotic dilatation descending aorta
Aortic stenosis	Normal	None or left	Left	Strain pattern if severe	Present	Absent	± Left ventricle	None
Pulmonary stenosis	Normal or right	Normal or right	Right	Strain pattern if severe	Absent	Present	± Right ventricle	None

F, female; M, male; ±, may be present or absent.

Chapter 6
Congenital heart disease with a right-to-left shunt in children

In most patients with cyanosis related to congenital cardiac abnormalities, an abnormality permits a portion of the systemic venous return to bypass the lungs and enter the systemic circulation directly. Therefore, this creates a right-to-left shunt and results from two general types of cardiac malformations: (i) admixture of the systemic and pulmonary venous returns or (ii) a combination of an intracardiac defect and obstruction to pulmonary blood flow. The first group shows increased pulmonary vascularity, but the second shows diminished pulmonary vascularity. Therefore, the most common conditions resulting in cyanosis are divided between these two categories (Table 6.1).

Regardless of the type of cardiac malformation leading to cyanosis, a risk of polycythemia, clubbing, slow growth, and brain abscess exists. The first three findings related to tissue hypoxia have been discussed in Chapter 1. Brain abscess results from the direct access of bacteria to the systemic circuit from the right-to-left shunt of venous blood.

Moller's Essentials of Pediatric Cardiology, Fourth Edition.
Walter H. Johnson, Jr. and Camden L. Hebson.
© 2023 John Wiley & Sons Ltd. Published 2023 by John Wiley & Sons Ltd.

Table 6.1 Physiologic classification of cyanotic malformations.

Admixture lesions (increased pulmonary vascularity):
  Complete transposition of the great arteries
  TAPVC
  Persistent truncus arteriosus
Obstruction to pulmonary blood flow and an intracardiac defect (decreased pulmonary vascularity):
  Tetralogy of Fallot
  Tricuspid atresia
  Pulmonary atresia with intact ventricular septum
  Ebstein's malformation of the tricuspid valve

These cyanotic conditions usually present in the early neonatal period and need prompt recognition and management. Most can be palliated by prostaglandin administration until the patient can be transferred to a center or stabilized in the center in preparation for an operation.

Early recognition, careful stabilization, and timely operation are the keys to an excellent outcome.

ADMIXTURE LESIONS

The combination of cyanosis and increased pulmonary blood flow indicates an admixture lesion. In most cardiac malformations classified in this group, a single cardiac chamber receives the entire systemic and pulmonary venous blood flows as they return to the heart. These two blood flows mix and then the mixture leaves the heart into both the aorta and pulmonary artery. The admixture of blood can occur at any cardiac level: venous (e.g. total anomalous pulmonary venous connection [TAPVC]), atrial (e.g. single atrium), ventricular (e.g. single ventricle), or great vessel (e.g. persistent truncus arteriosus).

Near-uniform mixing of the two venous returns occurs. Complete transposition of the great arteries is included in the admixture group because patients are cyanotic with increased pulmonary blood flow. They have, however, only partial admixture of the two venous returns; this incomplete mixing leads to symptoms of severe hypoxia.

The hemodynamics of the admixture lesions resemble those of the left-to-right shunts that occur at the same level. The direction and magnitude of blood flow in TAPVC and single atrium are governed, as in isolated atrial septal defect, by the relative ventricular compliances. Relative resistances to systemic and pulmonary flow determine the distribution of blood in patients with single ventricle and persistent truncus arteriosus, similarly to ventricular septal defect. Thus, the natural history and many of the clinical and laboratory findings of the admixture lesions resemble those of similar left-to-right shunts, including the development of pulmonary vascular disease.

In an admixture lesion, the systemic arterial oxygen saturation is a valuable indicator of the volume of pulmonary blood flow, since the degree of cyanosis is inversely related to the volume of pulmonary blood flow.

In patients with large pulmonary blood flow, the degree of cyanosis is slight because large amounts of fully saturated blood return from the lungs and mix with a relatively smaller volume of systemic venous return (Figure 6.1). If the patient develops pulmonary vascular disease or pulmonary stenosis that limits pulmonary blood flow, the amount of fully oxygenated blood returning from the lungs and mixing with the systemic venous return is reduced, so the patient becomes more cyanotic and the hemoglobin and hematocrit values rise.

Complete transposition of the great arteries (d-TGA); or transposition of the great vessels (d-TGV).

This is the most frequently occurring condition with cyanosis and increased pulmonary blood flow.

The term *transposition* indicates an anatomic reversal in anteroposterior, not left–right relationships. Normally, the pulmonary artery lies anterior to and slightly to the left of the aorta. In complete transposition of the great arteries (Figure 6.2a), the aorta lies anterior to the pulmonary artery. Normally, the anterior blood vessel arises from the infundibulum, which is the conus portion of the right ventricle. The aorta in complete transposition arises from the infundibulum of the right ventricle. The pulmonary trunk, on the other hand, originates posteriorly from the left ventricle.

Because of the transposition of the great arteries and their anomalous relationship to the ventricles, two independent circulations exist. The systemic venous blood returns to the right atrium, enters the right ventricle, and is ejected into the aorta, while the pulmonary venous blood flows through the left side of the heart into the pulmonary artery and returns to the lungs.

A communication must exist between the left and right sides of the heart to allow bidirectional shunting between of these two venous returns. The communication exists in one or more of the following: patent foramen ovale, atrial septal defect, ventricular septal defect, or patent ductus arteriosus. In about 60% of patients, the ventricular septum is intact and the shunt occurs at the atrial level.

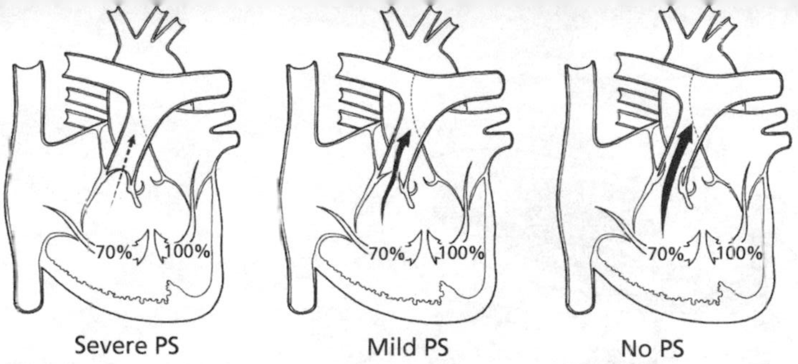

	Severe PS	Mild PS	No PS
	$\dfrac{Q_P}{Q_S}=\dfrac{0.5}{1}=0.5$	$\dfrac{Q_P}{Q_S}=\dfrac{1}{1}=1$	$\dfrac{Q_P}{Q_S}=\dfrac{4}{1}=4$
Pulmonary venous blood (100% saturation)	0.5 part	1 part	4 parts
Plus			
Systemic venous blood (70% saturation)	1 part	1 part	1 part
Equals			
Systemic artery saturation	80%	85%	94%

Figure 6.1 Estimation of the pulmonary blood flow in admixture lesions. Using a single ventricle, three clinical examples are shown, each with different degrees of pulmonary stenosis and pulmonary blood flow. Cyanosis is inversely related to the pulmonary blood flow. Assuming healthy lungs and complete mixture of the pulmonary and systemic venous return, the systemic arterial oxygen saturation represents the average of the contribution of the pulmonary blood flow (Q_P), represented by the pulmonary venous return, and the systemic blood flow (Q_S), represented by the systemic venous return. Q_P/Q_S can be estimated from the pulse oximetry value. PS, pulmonary stenosis; Q_P/Q_S, ratio of pulmonary blood flow to systemic blood flow.

(a)

(b)

(c)

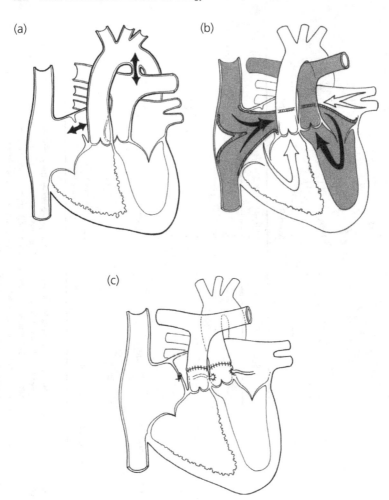

Figure 6.2 Complete transposition of the great vessels (d-TGV). (a) Central circulation. Surgical options: (b) venous switch; (c) arterial switch.

In the other 40%, a ventricular septal defect is present. Pulmonary stenosis, often valvar and subpulmonic, may coexist.

In patients with an intact ventricular septum, the communication (either a patent foramen ovale or a patent ductus arteriosus) between the two sides of the circulation is often small. As these communications follow the normal neonatal course and close, neonates with transposition and an intact septum develop profound cyanosis. Because a greater degree of mixing usually occurs in patients with a coexistent ventricular septal defect, cyanosis is mild in such infants with transposition and diagnosis is sometimes delayed.

History
Complete transposition of the great arteries occurs more frequently in males. Cyanosis becomes evident shortly after birth. Without intervention, almost all infants exhibit dyspnea and other signs of cardiac failure in the first month of life; infants with intact ventricular septum develop cardiac symptoms in the first two days of life and are more intensely cyanotic than those with coexistent ventricular septal defect. In the absence of operation, death occurs, usually in neonates, and in nearly every patient by six months of age. Patients with ventricular septal defect and pulmonary stenosis are often the least symptomatic because the pulmonary stenosis prevents excessive pulmonary blood flow and enhances the flow of fully saturated blood through the ventricular septal defect into the aorta; these patients resemble those with tetralogy of Fallot.

Physical examination
Infants may be large for gestational age. Setting aside cyanosis and congestive cardiac failure, physical findings vary with the coexistent defect associated with the complete transposition. Neonates on the first day of life are often asymptomatic, except for cyanosis, but quickly develop tachypnea.

With an intact ventricular septum and an atrial shunt, either no murmur or a soft, nonspecific murmur is present. With an associated ventricular septal defect, a louder murmur is present. The second heart sound is single and loud along the upper left sternal border, representing closure of the anteriorly placed aortic valve. Although the murmur does not diagnose complete transposition, it can indicate the type of associated defect. If pulmonary stenosis coexists, the murmur often radiates to the right side of the back.

Electrocardiogram
Since the aorta arises from the right ventricle, its pressure is elevated to systemic levels and is associated with a thick-walled right ventricle. The electrocardiogram reflects this by a pattern of right-axis deviation and right ventricular hypertrophy.

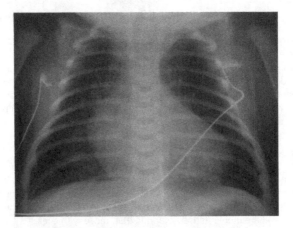

Figure 6.3 Chest X-ray in complete transposition of the great vessels: cardiomegaly, narrow mediastinum, and increased pulmonary vasculature.

The latter is manifested by tall R waves in the right precordial leads. Right atrial enlargement is also possible. In neonates it may be indistinguishable from normal for the age.

Patients with a large volume of pulmonary blood flow, as with coexistent ventricular septal defect, also may have left ventricular enlargement/hypertrophy because of the volume load on the left ventricle.

Chest X-ray

Cardiomegaly is generally present. The cardiac silhouette has a characteristic egg-shaped appearance (Figure 6.3); the superior mediastinum is narrow because the great vessels lie one in front of the other; the thymus is usually small. Left atrial enlargement exists in the unoperated patient.

Summary of clinical findings

The diagnosis of complete transposition is usually indicated by a combination of rather intense cyanosis in the neonatal period, chest X-ray findings of increased pulmonary vasculature, and characteristic cardiac contour.

Echocardiogram

The key to the echocardiographic diagnosis of complete transposition is the recognition of an anteriorly arising aorta and a posteriorly arising pulmonary artery. In views parallel to the long axis of the left ventricle, both arteries course parallel to each other for a short distance. This appearance is not seen in a normal heart, where the great arteries cross each other at an acute angle. In views profiling the short axis of the left ventricle, the aorta is seen arising anterior and rightward of the central and posterior pulmonary artery (hence the term d-transposition, or dextro-transposition). A cross-sectional view of the aortic root allows demonstration of the origins, branching, and proximal courses of the coronary arteries.

In neonates with transposition, the interventricular septum usually has a flat contour when viewed in cross-section; however, as the infant ages, the septum gradually bows away from the right (systemic) ventricle and bulges into the left (pulmonary) ventricle.

Ventricular septal defect represents the most important associated lesion diagnosed by echocardiography; the shunt through it and any atrial septal defect or ductus is bidirectional, consistent with the physiology of transposition described earlier. The atrial septal defect may be small and restrictive (Doppler signals are high velocity) before balloon septostomy; after, it is typically large and unrestrictive, with a mobile flap of the torn fossa ovalis waving to and fro across the defect. Balloon septostomy may be performed under echocardiographic guidance.

Cardiac catheterization

Since echocardiography shows the diagnosis, the primary purpose of cardiac catheterization is the performance of interventional creation of an atrial septal defect (Rashkind procedure). In patients with an intact septum, oximetry data show little increase in oxygen saturation values through the right side of the heart and little decrease through the left side. Among those with coexistent ventricular septal defect, larger changes in oxygen values are found. The oxygen saturation values in the pulmonary artery are higher than those in the aorta, a finding virtually diagnostic of transposition of the great arteries.

In all patients, right ventricular systolic pressure is elevated. When the ventricular septum is intact, the left ventricular pressure may be low; but in most patients with coexistent ventricular septal defect or in those with a large patent ductus arteriosus, the left ventricular pressure is elevated and equals that of the right (systemic) ventricle.

Angiography confirms the diagnosis by showing the aorta arising from the right ventricle and the pulmonary artery arising from the left ventricle, and it identifies coexistent malformations. Aortic root injection demonstrates coronary artery anatomy in preparation for surgery. A left ventricular injection is indicated to demonstrate ventricular septal defect(s) and pulmonic stenosis.

Palliative procedures

Hypoxia, one of the major symptoms of infants with transposition of the great vessels, results from inadequate mixing of the two venous returns, and palliation is directed toward improvement of mixing by two means. Unless hypoxia is treated, it becomes severe, leading to metabolic acidosis and death.

Intravenous prostaglandin. This substance opens and/or maintains patency of the ductus arteriosus and improves blood flow from the aorta to the pulmonary artery.

Rashkind balloon atrial septostomy procedure. Patients with inadequate mixing benefit from the creation of an atrial septal defect (enlargement of the foramen ovale). At cardiac catheterization or by echocardiographic guidance, a balloon catheter is inserted through a systemic vein and advanced into the left atrium through the foramen ovale. The balloon is inflated and then rapidly and forcefully withdrawn across the septum, creating a larger defect and often improving the hypoxia.

Infants who do not experience adequate improvement of cyanosis despite a large atrial defect and patent ductus are rare. Factors responsible in these neonates include nearly identical ventricular compliances, which limits mixing through the atrial defect, and elevated pulmonary vascular resistance, which limits the ductal shunt and pulmonary blood flow. Increased intravenous fluids may benefit the patient by increasing blood volume.

Surgical atrial septectomy. Rarely, an atrial defect is created surgically by atrial septectomy, an open-heart procedure. A closed-heart technique, the Blalock–Hanlon procedure, was used previously, but frequently resulted in scarring of the pulmonary veins.

Corrective operation

Atrial (venous) switch. The first successful corrective procedure was performed by Senning in the 1950s and later modified by Mustard. These procedures invoke the principle that two negatives make a positive. Since the circulation of transposition is reversed at the arterial level, these operations reverse it at the atrial level. This procedure involves removal of the atrial septum and creation of an intra-atrial baffle to divert the systemic venous return into the left ventricle and thus to the lungs, whereas the pulmonary venous return is directed to the right ventricle and thus to the aorta (Figure 6.2b).

It can be performed at low risk in patients with an intact ventricular septum and at a higher risk in patients with ventricular septal defect. Serious complications, stroke, or death can occur in infants before an atrial (venous) switch procedure, which is usually done after three to six months of age.

The long-term results of the atrial switch procedure have been identified. Arrhythmias, the most frequent long-term complication, are often related to abnormalities of the sinoatrial node and of the atrial surgical scar. Sometimes these are life threatening, although the exact mechanism of sudden death in the rare child who succumbs is not usually known. Scarring can also cause systemic or pulmonary obstruction of the venous return. The most common significant complication is not sudden death but progressive dysfunction of the right ventricle, leading to death from chronic heart failure in adulthood. This complication is related to the right ventricle functioning as the systemic ventricle. Predicting which patients will develop failure and at what age postoperatively is not possible.

Arterial switch (Jatene). This operation, developed in the 1970s, avoids the complications inherent with the atrial (venous) switch and involves switching the aorta and pulmonary artery to the correct ventricle (Figure 6.2c). The great vessels are transected and reanastomosed, so blood flows from the left ventricle to the aorta and from the right ventricle to the pulmonary arteries. Since the coronary arteries arise from the aortic root, they are transferred to the pulmonary (neoaortic) root. Certain variations of coronary artery origins or branching make transfer more risky. The arterial switch operation must occur early in life (within the first two weeks) before the pulmonary resistance falls and the left ventricle becomes "deconditioned" to eject the systemic pressure load.

Arterial switch is not free from complications: coronary artery compromise may result in left ventricular infarct or failure; pulmonary artery stenosis can result from stretching or kinking during the surgical repositioning of the great vessels; and the operative mortality may be higher, partly because of the risks of neonatal open-heart surgery.

The short- and long-term outcomes favor those receiving the arterial switch procedure.

Summary

Complete transposition of the great arteries is a common cardiac anomaly that results in neonatal cyanosis and ultimately in cardiac failure. Many neonates are initially asymptomatic but quickly become cyanotic. The physical findings and electrocardiogram vary with associated malformations. The chest X-ray reveals cardiomegaly and increased pulmonary vascularity. Palliative and corrective procedures are available.

Total anomalous pulmonary venous connection/return (TAPVC or TAPVR)

The pulmonary veins, instead of entering the left atrium, connect with a systemic venous channel that delivers pulmonary venous blood to the right atrium (Figure 6.4). Developmentally, this anomaly results from failure of incorporation of the pulmonary veins into the left atrium, so that the pulmonary venous system retains earlier embryologic communications to the systemic venous system.

In the embryo, the pulmonary veins communicate with both the left and right anterior cardinal veins and the umbilical vitelline system, both precursors of the systemic veins. If the pulmonary veins, which form with the lungs as outpouchings of the foregut, are not incorporated into the left atrium, the result is anomalous pulmonary venous connection to one of the following structures: right superior vena cava (right anterior cardinal vein), left superior vena cava (distal left anterior cardinal vein), coronary sinus (proximal left anterior cardinal vein), or the infradiaphragmatic site (umbilical-vitelline system), usually a tributary of the portal system.

Therefore, the right atrium receives not only the entire systemic venous return, but also the entire pulmonary venous return. The left atrium has no direct venous supply. An obligatory right-to-left shunt exists at the atrial level through either a patent foramen ovale or usually an atrial septal defect.

The volume of blood shunted from the right to the left atrium and the volume of blood that enters each ventricle depends upon their relative compliances. Ventricular compliance is influenced by ventricular pressures and vascular resistances. Right ventricular compliance normally increases following birth as pulmonary vascular resistance and pulmonary arterial pressure fall. Therefore, in most patients with TAPVC, pulmonary blood flow becomes considerably greater than normal; systemic blood flow is usually normal. Since a disparity exists between the volume of blood being carried by the right and left sides of the heart, the right side becomes dilated and hypertrophied, whereas the left side is relatively smaller but near-normal size.

In patients with TAPVC, the degree of cyanosis inversely relates to the volume of pulmonary blood flow. As the volume of pulmonary blood flow becomes larger, the proportion of the pulmonary venous blood to total venous blood returning to the right atrium becomes greater. As a result, the saturation of blood shunted to the left side of the heart is higher, being only slightly reduced from normal.

On the other hand, in hemodynamic situations in which the resistance to flow through the lungs is increased (e.g. the neonatal period), the volume of blood flow through the lungs is nearly normal (i.e. equal to systemic blood flow). Therefore, the pulmonary and systemic venous systems contribute nearly equal volumes of blood to the right atrium, and these neonates exhibit noticeable cyanosis.

(a)

(b)

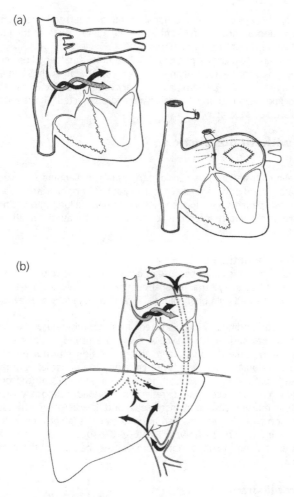

Figure 6.4 Total anomalous pulmonary venous connection. (a) Central circulation and surgical repair of unobstructed type; (b) central circulation in obstructed type.

TAPVC is an example of bidirectional shunting: a left-to-right shunt at the venous level and a right-to-left shunt at the atrial level, since all the pulmonary venous blood returns to the right atrium.

TAPVC presents two clinical pictures. One resembles atrial septal defect and has no obstruction to the venous channel (Figure 6.4a). The other shows intense cyanosis and a radiographic pattern of pulmonary venous obstruction. In this form, the connecting venous channel is narrowed and obstructed (Figure 6.4b). These two are discussed separately.

TAPVC without obstruction

History
The clinical manifestations vary considerably. Usually, the anomaly is recognized in the neonatal period or with fetal echocardiography. If not operated upon in early infancy, most patients develop congestive cardiac failure, grow slowly, and have frequent respiratory infections, but a few may be asymptomatic into later childhood.

Physical examination
The degree of cyanosis varies because of differences in the volume of pulmonary blood flow. Although systemic arterial desaturation is always present, children with greatly increased pulmonary blood flow appear acyanotic or show only slight cyanosis.

The physical findings mimic isolated atrial septal defect. Cardiomegaly, precordial bulge, and right ventricular heave are found in older unoperated infants. A grade 2/6–3/6 pulmonary systolic ejection murmur due to excess flow across the pulmonary valve is present along the upper left sternal border. Wide, fixed splitting of the second heart sound is heard and the pulmonary component may be accentuated, reflecting elevated pulmonary pressure. A mid-diastolic murmur caused by increased blood flow across the tricuspid valve is found along the lower left sternal border and is associated with greatly increased pulmonary blood flow. In TAPVC to the superior vena cava, a venous hum may exist along the upper right sternal border because of the large venous blood flow.

Electrocardiogram
The electrocardiogram reveals enlargement of the right-sided cardiac chambers with right-axis deviation, right atrial enlargement, and right ventricular enlargement/hypertrophy. Usually, the pattern reflecting volume overload is an RSR' pattern in lead V_1.

Chest X-ray

Chest X-ray findings also resemble isolated atrial septal defect. Cardiomegaly, primarily of right-sided chambers, and increased pulmonary blood flow are found. In contrast to most other admixture lesions, the left atrium is not enlarged because blood flow through this chamber is normal.

Except for TAPVC to a left superior vena cava ("vertical vein"), the contour of the heart is not characteristic. In this form, the cardiac silhouette can be described as a figure-of-eight or as a "snowman heart" (Figure 6.5a). The upper portion of the cardiac contour is formed by the enlarged left and right superior venae cavae. The lower portion of the contour is formed by the cardiac chambers.

Summary of clinical findings

The clinical, electrocardiographic, and radiographic findings resemble those of atrial septal defect because the effects on the heart are similar. Cyanosis distinguishes the conditions; although it may be minimal or not clinically evident, it is easily detectable by pulse oximetry. Unlike uncomplicated atrial septal defect, congestive cardiac failure and elevated pulmonary arterial pressure may be found in TAPVC.

Echocardiogram

Cross-sectional echocardiography reveals an atrial septal defect and enlarged right atrium, right ventricle, and pulmonary arteries. The left atrium and left ventricle appear smaller than normal. In contrast to most normal neonates, with an atrial septal defect the shunt is from the right atrium to the left atrium. Doppler demonstrates a right-to-left atrial septal defect shunt because the only blood entering the left atrium is through the atrial septal defect. The individual pulmonary veins are visualized as they join a common pulmonary vein, which then connects to the coronary sinus, the superior vena cava by way of a vertical vein (the left-sided superior vena cava), or the hepatic portal venous system after a descent into the abdomen.

Cardiac catheterization

Oxygen saturation values in each cardiac chamber and in both great vessels are virtually identical. An increase in oxygen saturation is found in the vena cava, coronary sinus, or other systemic venous sites into which the pulmonary venous blood flows. The saturation of blood in the left atrium and left ventricle is reduced because of the obligatory right-to-left atrial shunt.

(a)

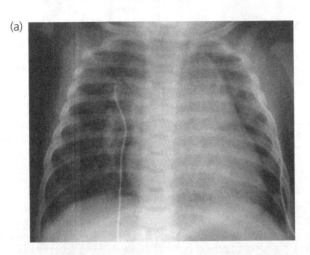

(b)

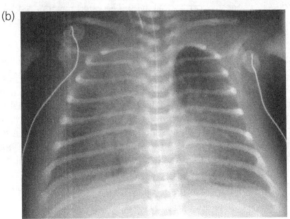

Figure 6.5 Chest X-ray in TAPVC. (a) Unobstructed (supracardiac) connection to the left superior vena cava ("snowman heart"). Upper portion of cardiac silhouette formed by dilated right and left superior venae cavae. (b) Obstructed (infradiaphragmatic) type. Pulmonary vascular congestion, a pleural effusion, and a small heart shadow.

Pulmonary hypertension may be found in infants, but some patients, particularly older ones, show near-normal levels of pulmonary arterial pressures.

Pulmonary angiography is performed, and during the later phases of the angiogram (the so-called levophase) the pulmonary veins opacify and subsequently fill the connecting venous channel, delineating the anatomic form of anomalous pulmonary venous connection.

Operative considerations

Under cardiopulmonary bypass, the confluence of pulmonary veins, which lies directly behind the left atrium, is opened and connected to it (Figure 6.4a). The atrial communication is closed, and the connecting vessel is divided. This operation can be performed with low risk, even in neonates and younger infants.

Summary

Each of the anatomic types of TAPVC is associated with cyanosis of variable extent. The physical findings are those of atrial septal defect; pulmonary hypertension may also be found. Both the electrocardiogram and the chest X-ray reveal enlargement of the right-sided cardiac chambers. Corrective operations can be performed successfully for each of the forms of TAPVC.

TAPVC with obstruction

In TAPVC, an obstruction can be present in the channel returning pulmonary venous blood to the right side of the heart (Figure 6.4b). Obstruction is always present in patients with an infradiaphragmatic connection and occasionally in patients with a supradiaphragmatic connection. In the latter, obstruction may occur intrinsically from narrowing of the channel or extrinsically if the channel passes between the bronchus and the ipsilateral branch pulmonary artery.

In infradiaphragmatic connection, four mechanisms contribute to obstruction in pulmonary venous flow: (i) the venous channel is long; (ii) the channel traverses the diaphragm through the esophageal hiatus and is compressed by either esophageal or diaphragmatic action; (iii) the channel narrows at its junction with the portal venous system; and (iv) the pulmonary venous blood must traverse the hepatic capillary system before returning to the right atrium by way of the hepatic veins.

The obstruction elevates pulmonary venous pressure. Consequently, pulmonary capillary pressure is raised, leading to pulmonary edema and a dilated pulmonary lymphatic system. Pulmonary arterial pressure is elevated because of both elevated pulmonary capillary pressure and reflex pulmonary vasoconstriction. Because of the pulmonary hypertension, the right ventricle remains thick-walled, does not undergo its normal evolution following birth, and remains relatively noncompliant. As a result, the volume of flow into the right ventricle is limited. Because of the reduced pulmonary blood flow, patients show more intense cyanosis than those with without pulmonary venous obstruction.

The clinical features of TAPVC with obstruction relate to the consequences of pulmonary venous obstruction and to the limited pulmonary blood flow.

History
Patients with obstruction present as neonates with significant cyanosis and respiratory distress. Cyanosis is often intense because of the limited volume of pulmonary flow. The cyanosis is accentuated by the pulmonary edema that interferes with oxygen transport from the alveolus to the pulmonary capillary. Respiratory symptoms of tachypnea and dyspnea result from the altered pulmonary compliance from pulmonary edema and hypertensive pulmonary arteries.

Physical examination
Cyanosis is present, and increased respiratory effort is manifested by intercostal retractions and tachypnea. On clinical examination the heart size is normal. Since the volume of flow through the right side of the heart is normal, no murmurs appear. The accentuated pulmonic component of the second heart sound reflects pulmonary hypertension. The cyanosis without cardiac findings of these neonates usually suggests a pulmonary rather than a cardiac condition.

Beyond the immediate neonatal period, the infants appear scrawny and malnourished.

Electrocardiogram
Right ventricular hypertrophy, right-axis deviation, and right atrial enlargement are found. In a normal neonate, however, the QRS axis is usually directed toward the right, the P waves may approach 3 mm in amplitude, and the R waves are tall in the right precordial leads. Therefore, the electrocardiograms of neonates with obstructed pulmonary venous connection appear similar to those of normal neonates. Such a pattern, however, is compatible with the diagnosis.

Chest X-ray
Cardiac size is normal because the volume of systemic and pulmonary blood flows is normal. The pulmonary vasculature shows a diffuse reticular pattern of pulmonary edema (Figure 6.5b). Even in young children, Kerley B lines, which are small horizontal lines at the margins of the pleura mostly in the lower lung fields, are present. The radiographic pattern, although similar to that of hyaline membrane disease, differs from it because it does not usually show air bronchograms.

Summary of clinical findings

This form of TAPVC is very difficult to distinguish from neonatal pulmonary disease because of similar clinical and laboratory findings. In both, patients present with respiratory distress and cyanosis in the neonatal period. No murmurs are present. The electrocardiogram may be normal for age and the chest X-ray shows a normal-sized heart and a diffuse, hazy pattern. Echocardiography may be misleading, so cardiac catheterization and angiography may be necessary to distinguish pulmonary disease from this form of cardiac disease.

Echocardiogram

Because the intracardiac anatomy appears normal and visualization is often limited by pulmonary hyperinflation from aggressive mechanical ventilation used in these neonates, the echocardiographic detection of this lesion is challenging. An atrial septal defect with a right-to-left shunt exists, typical of TAPVC, but this finding is also found with severe primary lung disease or persistent pulmonary hypertension. The atrial septal defect flow is much lower than in the unobstructed form because pulmonary venous obstruction results in very low pulmonary blood flow. The ductus may be large and have bidirectional or predominantly pulmonary artery-to-aorta shunt because of elevated pulmonary arteriolar resistance. Doppler shows no pulmonary venous return to the left atrium; in the most common form, the pulmonary veins return to a common pulmonary vein that courses caudad to the abdomen, usually slightly to the left of the spine.

Cardiac catheterization

As in the unobstructed form, the oxygen saturations are identical in each cardiac chamber, but with this lesion oxygen saturations are extremely low. Pulmonary hypertension is present, and also the pulmonary wedge pressure is elevated. Angiography shows the anomalous pulmonary venous connection, which is usually connected to an infradiaphragmatic site.

Operative considerations

Infants with TAPVC to an infradiaphragmatic site often die in the neonatal period. As soon as the diagnosis is made, operation is indicated, using the technique described previously. In some infants, pulmonary hypertension persists in the postoperative period for a few days and requires management with mechanical ventilation, creation of an alkalotic state, and administration of nitric oxide and other pulmonary vasodilators.

Summary

TAPVC, although of several anatomic forms, presents with one of two clinical pictures. In one, the pulmonary arterial pressures and right ventricular compliance are normal or slightly elevated. These patients' features resemble atrial septal defect but show mild cyanosis. In the other, pulmonary arterial pressure and pulmonary resistance are elevated because of pulmonary venous obstruction. Therefore, right ventricular compliance is reduced and pulmonary blood flow is limited. These patients show a radiographic pattern of pulmonary venous obstruction or severe cyanosis and major respiratory symptoms. The clinical and laboratory findings resemble neonatal respiratory distress or persistent pulmonary hypertension syndromes.

Common arterial trunk (truncus arteriosus)

In common arterial trunk or persistent truncus arteriosus (Figure 6.6), a single arterial vessel leaves the heart and gives rise to the three major circulations: pulmonary, systemic, and coronary circulations. This malformation is associated with

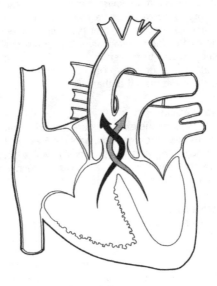

Figure 6.6 Truncus arteriosus. Central circulation.

a ventricular septal defect through which both ventricles eject into the common arterial trunk. Because the defect is large and the common trunk originates from both ventricles, the right ventricular systolic pressure is identical with that of the left ventricle.

The hemodynamics are similar to those of ventricular septal defect and patent ductus arteriosus. The volumes of systemic and pulmonary blood flow depend on the relative resistances to flow within the systemic and pulmonary circulations.

The resistance to flow through the lungs is governed by two factors: (i) the caliber of the pulmonary arterial branches arising from the common trunk and (ii) the pulmonary vascular resistance. Although differences in the size of the pulmonary arterial branches vary as they originate from the common trunk, ordinarily their size does not offer significant resistance to pulmonary blood flow, so the pulmonary arterial pressure equals that of the aorta. Therefore, the pulmonary arteriolar resistance is the primary determinant of pulmonary blood flow. In the neonatal period, when pulmonary vascular resistance is elevated, the volume of blood flow through the lungs is similar to the systemic blood flow. As the pulmonary vasculature matures, the pulmonary blood flow increases progressively.

Many of the clinical and laboratory findings of truncus arteriosus depend on the volume of pulmonary blood flow. Increased pulmonary blood flow leads to three effects: (i) the degree of cyanosis and the volume of pulmonary blood flow are inversely related, and the degree of cyanosis lessens as pulmonary blood flow increases because of the larger quantities of fully saturated pulmonary venous return mixing with the relatively fixed systemic venous return; (ii) congestive cardiac failure develops because of left ventricular volume overload; and (iii) the pulse pressure widens because the blood leaves the common trunk during diastole to enter the pulmonary arteries.

Although the truncal valve is usually tricuspid, it becomes regurgitant in some patients. Therefore, the additional volume load of regurgitation is incurred by the ventricles. Some truncal valves have four or more cusps; these are both stenotic and regurgitant, adding pressure overload to the already volume-overloaded ventricles.

Approximately 40% of truncus patients show deletion of a portion of chromosome 22 and other laboratory findings of DiGeorge syndrome, such as hypocalcemia and reduced T lymphocytes.

History

The symptoms vary with the volume of pulmonary blood flow. In the neonatal period, cyanosis is the major symptom because the elevated pulmonary vascular resistance limits the pulmonary blood flow. As pulmonary vascular resistance falls, cyanosis lessens, but congestive cardiac failure develops, usually after several weeks of age. Patients with common trunk and congestive cardiac failure mimic those with ventricular septal defect at this time because cyanosis is mild or absent. Dyspnea on exertion, easy fatigability, and frequent respiratory infections are common symptoms.

Patients whose pulmonary blood flow is limited, owing either to the development of pulmonary vascular disease or to the presence of small pulmonary arteries arising from the truncus, show predominant symptoms of cyanosis rather than congestive cardiac failure, unless significant regurgitation through the truncal valve coexists.

Physical examination
Cyanosis may or may not be clinically evident but is easily detected with pulse oximetry. Manifestations of a wide pulse pressure may appear if increased pulmonary blood flow or significant truncal valve regurgitation exists. Cardiomegaly and a precordial bulge are common. The auscultatory findings may initially resemble ventricular septal defect. The major auscultatory finding is a loud systolic murmur along the left sternal border. An apical mid-diastolic rumble present in most patients indicates large blood flow across the mitral valve from increased pulmonary blood flow.

Common arterial trunk shows three distinctive auscultatory findings: (i) the second heart sound is single since only a single semilunar valve is present; (ii) a high-pitched early diastolic decrescendo murmur is present if truncal valve regurgitation coexists; and (iii) an apical systolic ejection click that is usually heard indicates the presence of a dilated great vessel, the common trunk. The click, especially if heard at an early age, suggests that the truncal valve is stenotic to some extent.

Electrocardiogram
The electrocardiogram usually shows a normal QRS axis and biventricular enlargement/hypertrophy. The left ventricular enlargement is related to left ventricular volume overload; the right ventricular hypertrophy is related to the elevated right ventricular systolic pressure. If pulmonary vascular disease develops and reduces pulmonary blood flow, the left ventricular enlargement may disappear. Truncal regurgitation and truncal stenosis modify these findings by augmenting the ventricular volume and by increasing ventricular pressures, respectively.

Chest X-ray
The pulmonary vasculature is increased. The prominent "ascending aorta" that is usually seen represents the enlarged common trunk. Because the branch pulmonary arteries arise from the truncus arteriosus, a main pulmonary artery silhouette is absent. Most patients show cardiomegaly proportional to the volume of

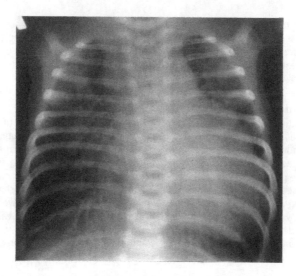

Figure 6.7 Chest X-ray in truncus arteriosus. Cardiomegaly, right aortic arch, and increased pulmonary vascularity.

pulmonary blood flow and the amount of truncal regurgitation. Left atrial enlargement is present in patients with increased pulmonary blood flow.

A right aortic arch is found in one-fourth of patients; this finding, when combined with that of increased pulmonary vascular markings and cyanosis, is virtually diagnostic of truncus arteriosus (Figure 6.7).

Summary of clinical findings

Persistent truncus arteriosus is suspected in a cyanotic patient who has a murmur suggesting ventricular septal defect and two characteristic features: a single second heart sound and a systolic ejection click. The volume of pulmonary blood flow is reflected by the degree of cyanosis and the amount of left atrial enlargement. The degree of cardiomegaly on chest X-ray or left ventricular hypertrophy on electrocardiogram is not the sole reflection of pulmonary blood flow, since coexistent truncal insufficiency can also cause these particular findings. DiGeorge syndrome is common.

Natural history

The course of common arterial trunk resembles that of ventricular septal defect but is more severe, and the development of pulmonary vascular disease, the ultimate threat to longevity and operability, is greatly accelerated. Truncal regurgitation usually progresses.

Echocardiogram

Cross-sectional echocardiography in views parallel to the long axis of the left ventricular outflow tract shows a large great vessel (the common trunk) "overriding" a large ventricular septal defect, similar to images seen in tetralogy of Fallot. A separate pulmonary artery cannot be demonstrated arising from the heart; the pulmonary arteries arise from the common trunk, and their pattern of origin is seen by echocardiography. The ductus arteriosus is usually absent unless coexisting interruption of the aortic arch is present. The truncal valve may be trileaflet, with apparent movement similar to that of a normal aortic valve, or it may be deformed, usually as a quadricuspid or multicuspid valve, with both stenosis and regurgitation. Left atrial enlargement parallels the degree of pulmonary overcirculation.

Cardiac catheterization

Usually, a venous catheter is passed through the right ventricle into the common trunk and then into the pulmonary arteries. The systolic pressures are identical in both ventricles and in the common trunk, unless truncal valve stenosis is present. In that case, ventricular systolic pressures exceed the systolic pressure in the trunk. A wide pulse pressure is often present in the trunk. An increase in oxygen saturation is found in the right ventricle with further increase in the common trunk. The blood is not fully saturated in the latter site. Truncal root injection demonstrates the origin and course of the pulmonary arteries but requires a large volume of contrast that must be administered rapidly to overcome excessive dilution from high pulmonary blood flow.

Operative considerations

For infants manifesting severe cardiac failure who do not respond to medical management, banding of the pulmonary artery or the individual branch pulmonary arteries is sometimes performed. Although the cardiac failure is improved and the infant grows, the band may complicate and increase the risk of repair. Banding surgery may also be difficult to perform when the pulmonary artery branches arise from separate origins from the truncus.

Corrective operation is almost always preferable. In this procedure, the ventricular septal defect is closed so that left ventricular blood passes into the common trunk. The pulmonary arteries are detached from the truncal wall and connected to one end of a valved conduit; its other end is inserted into the right ventricle. If severe, truncal regurgitation can be corrected simultaneously by valvuloplasty or insertion of a prosthetic valve. The risk is considerably higher for patients with truncal regurgitation, stenosis, or any element of pulmonary vascular disease. Since the conduit from the right ventricle to pulmonary arteries has a fixed diameter, reoperation is necessary as the child grows.

Summary

Common arterial trunk (persistent truncus arteriosus) is an infrequently occurring cardiac anomaly whose clinical and laboratory features resemble ventricular septal defect and patent ductus arteriosus, with similarities in hemodynamics and natural history. Early corrective operation is advised, but considerable operative risks remain, partially due to the frequent coexistence of DiGeorge syndrome.

CYANOSIS AND DIMINISHED PULMONARY BLOOD FLOW

Patients with cyanosis and roentgenographic evidence of diminished pulmonary blood flow have a cardiac malformation in which both obstruction to pulmonary blood flow and an intracardiac defect that permits a right-to-left shunt are found. The degree of cyanosis varies inversely with the volume of pulmonary blood flow. The amount by which pulmonary blood flow is reduced equals the volume of blood shunted in a right-to-left direction.

The intracardiac right-to-left shunt can occur at either the ventricular or the atrial level. In patients with a ventricular shunt, the cardiac size is usually normal, as in tetralogy of Fallot, whereas those with an atrial shunt often show cardiomegaly, as in tricuspid atresia or Ebstein's malformation.

Tetralogy of Fallot

This is probably the most widely known cardiac condition resulting in cyanosis and is the most common anomaly in this category (Figure 6.8).

Classically, tetralogy of Fallot has four components: ventricular septal defect; aorta overriding the ventricular septal defect; pulmonary stenosis, generally infundibular in location; and right ventricular hypertrophy. Because of the large ventricular septal defect, right ventricular systolic pressure is at systemic levels.

Hemodynamically, tetralogy of Fallot can be considered a combination of two lesions: a large ventricular septal defect, allowing equalization of ventricular systolic pressures, and severe pulmonary stenosis.

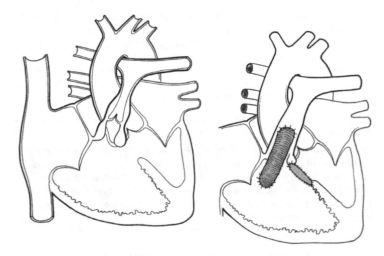

Figure 6.8 Tetralogy of Fallot. Central circulation and surgical repair.

The magnitude of the shunt through the ventricular communication depends on the relative resistances of the pulmonary stenosis and the systemic circulation. Because the pulmonary stenosis is frequently related to a narrowed infundibulum, it responds to catecholamines and other stimuli. Therefore, the amount of right-to-left shunt and the degree of cyanosis vary considerably with factors such as emotion or exercise. Many of the symptoms of tetralogy of Fallot are related to sudden changes in either of these resistance factors.

Tetralogy of Fallot with pulmonary valve atresia (Figure 6.9) has also been called pseudotruncus arteriosus. In this anomaly, blood cannot flow directly from the right ventricle into the pulmonary artery, so the entire output of both ventricles passes into the aorta. The pulmonary circulation is supplied either by multiple major aortopulmonary collateral arteries (MAPCAs) and/or through a patent ductus arteriosus. Severe hypoxic symptoms may develop in the neonatal period if the patent ductus arteriosus closes or if the MAPCAs are narrow.

Approximately 75% of patients with tetralogy of Fallot are nonsyndromic, and the other 25% have a syndrome such as trisomy 21 or DiGeorge syndrome.

History
The children often become cyanotic in the first year of life, often in the neonatal period. The time of appearance and the severity of cyanosis are directly related to the severity of pulmonary stenosis and the degree that pulmonary blood flow is reduced.

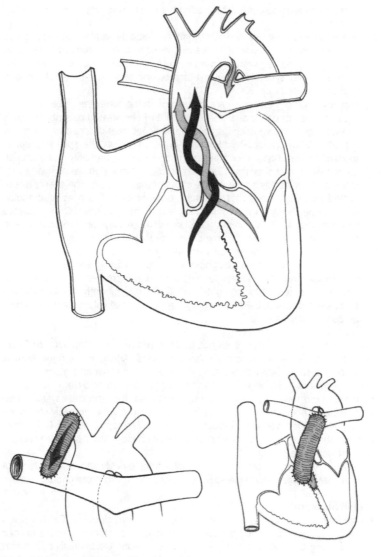

Figure 6.9 Tetralogy of Fallot with pulmonary atresia. Central circulation, showing a patent ductus. Palliative surgery and repair.

Patients with tetralogy of Fallot have three characteristic symptom complexes:

(1) The degree of cyanosis and symptoms are variable; any event that lowers systemic vascular resistance increases the right-to-left shunt and leads to symptoms associated with hypoxemia. Exercise, meals, and hot weather, for example, lower systemic vascular resistance, increase right-to-left shunt, and lead to increased cyanosis.

(2) Hypercyanotic or "tet" spells are uncommon in the current era of early operative correction or palliation with a shunt, but in unoperated patients the spells consist of episodes in which the child suddenly becomes dyspneic and intensely cyanotic. Death caused by hypoxia may result unless the spell is properly treated. The mechanism for production of tet spells is probably multifactorial. Some believe that they result from contraction of the right ventricular infundibulum, thus increasing the degree of pulmonary stenosis. This theory is supported by observations that beta-adrenergic blockers, such as propranolol, which decrease myocardial contractility, relieve the symptoms. Other evidence suggests that a fall in systemic vascular resistance plays an important role in the production of the spells; others attribute them to hyperpnea.

(3) Squatting is virtually diagnostic of tetralogy of Fallot but fortunately is now rarely seen because of early diagnosis and surgery. During exercise or exertion, the unoperated child squats to rest. Squatting increases systemic vascular resistance, thereby reducing right-to-left shunt. It also briefly increases the systemic venous return; therefore, right ventricular stroke volume and pulmonary blood flow improve.

Congestive cardiac failure does not occur in patients with tetralogy of Fallot. The left ventricle handles a normal volume of blood. Although the right ventricle develops a systemic level of pressure, it tolerates the elevated systolic pressure well, since it has been developing this level of pressure since birth. Furthermore, no matter how severe the pulmonary stenosis, the right ventricular systolic pressure cannot rise above systemic levels because the right ventricle freely communicates with the left ventricle through the ventricular septal defect. Only when another abnormality, such as anemia or bacterial endocarditis, occurs can congestive cardiac failure develop.

Children with unoperated tetralogy of Fallot fatigue easily and, as in all types of cyanotic heart disease, severe cyanosis can be associated with stroke or brain abscess.

Physical examination

The examination reveals cyanosis and, in older children, clubbing. Cardiac size is normal. The most important auscultatory finding is a systolic ejection murmur located along the middle and upper left sternal border. Occasionally a thrill may be present. The murmur is caused by the pulmonary stenosis and not by the ventricular septal defect. Although the murmur is not diagnostic of tetralogy of Fallot, the loudness of the murmur is inversely related to the severity of the stenosis. The murmur is softer in patients who have more severe stenosis because the volume of flow through the stenotic area is reduced. This useful clinical fact allows the assessment of the severity of the condition and verification that the murmur originates from the right ventricular outflow area and not from the ventricular septal defect.

> During a "tet" spell, the murmur softens and may disappear.

Patients with tetralogy of Fallot with pulmonary valvar atresia have a continuous murmur from a patent ductus arteriosus, MAPCAs, or an operative shunt; an ejection murmur is not heard.

Electrocardiogram
The electrocardiogram reveals right-axis deviation and, in more severe cases, right atrial enlargement (Figure 6.10). Right ventricular hypertrophy is always present and usually is associated with positive T waves in lead V_1.

Chest X-ray
The heart size is normal (Figure 6.11). The cardiac contour is characteristic. The heart is boot-shaped (coeur en sabot: literally, "heart like a wooden shoe"). The apex is turned upward and the pulmonary artery segment is concave because the pulmonary artery is small. Right ventricular hypertrophy and right atrial enlargement are evident. The ascending aorta is frequently enlarged and, in at least 25% of patients, a right aortic arch is present.

> *Summary of clinical findings*
>
> The history and radiographic findings are usually clearly diagnostic of tetralogy of Fallot. Once this diagnosis has been made, the loudness of the murmur, character, severity, and frequency of symptoms, pulse oximetry, and level of hemoglobin and hematocrit provide the most reliable indications of the patient's course.

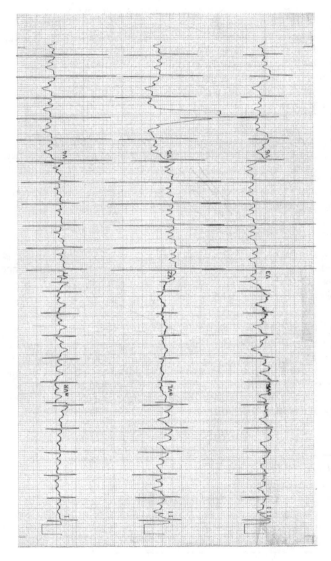

Figure 6.10 Electrocardiogram in tetralogy of Fallot. Right-axis deviation. Right ventricular hypertrophy indicated by tall R wave in V_1 and deep S wave in V_6. Tall P waves indicate right atrial enlargement.

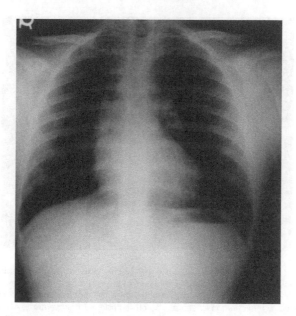

Figure 6.11 Chest X-ray in tetralogy of Fallot. Normal-sized heart and upturned apex. Decreased pulmonary vasculature and concave pulmonary artery segment.

Natural history

Symptoms progress because of increasing infundibular stenosis. Increasing frequency or severity of symptoms, rising hemoglobin, and decreasing intensity of the murmur are signs of progression. The electrocardiogram and chest X-ray show no change, however.

Echocardiogram

Cross-sectional echocardiography in views parallel to the long axis of the left ventricular outflow tract shows a large aortic root "overriding" a large ventricular septal defect, similar to the images seen in truncus arteriosus and double-outlet right ventricle (Figure 6.12). The pulmonary artery arises from the right ventricle, but the infundibulum, pulmonary valve annulus, and pulmonary arteries appear small.

Color Doppler shows accelerated, turbulent flow through the right ventricular outflow tract; a transition from laminar to disturbed color signals begins at the most proximal site of obstruction, usually the infundibulum.

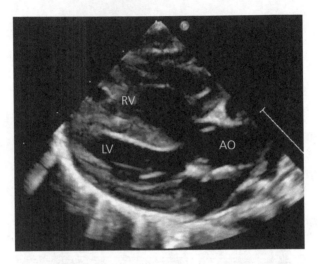

Figure 6.12 Echocardiogram in tetralogy of Fallot. A long axis parasternal view illustrates the large aorta "overriding" the VSD and the rim of the ventricular septum. Truncus arteriosus and double outlet right ventricle also show similar aortic override. The lesions are distinguished by other anatomic features. LV, left ventricle; RV, right ventricle; AO, aorta.

Cross-sectional echocardiography can define the side of the aortic arch and the anatomy and size of the proximal pulmonary artery branches. In neonates with tetralogy of Fallot, the patent ductus often appears as a long, convoluted structure, in contrast to the normal neonate's ductal course, which is shorter and more direct.

Cardiac catheterization

The oxygen values through the right side of the heart show no evidence of a left-to-right shunt. Desaturation of aortic blood is found. A pressure drop is present across the outflow area of the right ventricle; the body of the right ventricle has the same pressure as the left ventricle, and the pulmonary arterial pressure is lower than normal; however, catheter placement across the right ventricular outflow tract is avoided to minimize the risk of infundibular spasm and hypercyanotic spells ("tet" spells).

Right ventricular angiography defines the anatomic details of the right ventricular outflow area. Such studies demonstrate the site of the stenosis in the right ventricle, outline the pulmonary arterial tree, and show opacification of the aorta through the ventricular septal defect. Aortic root injection may be indicated to define anomalies of coronary artery branching that occasionally occur and that may result in operative catastrophe if unrecognized.

Ductal stenting via catheter is an alternative to palliative surgery for some neonates who are not candidates for early surgical repair.

Medical management

Most infants with tetralogy of Fallot and favorable anatomy for repair require no medical therapy before corrective operation.

As in all patients with cyanotic cardiac malformations, the development of iron-deficiency anemia must be prevented or promptly treated when it develops, because increased symptoms occur in anemic patients.

> Remember that cyanotic patients with a "normal" hemoglobin concentration (e.g. 12 g/dL) are functionally anemic: they may not have sufficient hemoglobin to counteract their level of hypoxemia.

Infants and children with tet spells should be treated by the administration of 100% oxygen (which increases systemic resistance while decreasing pulmonary resistance), by placing the child in a knee/chest position, and by having the parent console and quieten the child. Morphine or ultra-short-acting beta-blockers may be indicated. Systemic vascular resistance is increased with alpha-agonists such as phenylephrine. Administration of intravenous fluid by bolus injection may improve right ventricular performance; diuretics are contraindicated. Intractable tet spells may improve with intubation, paralysis, and ventilation to decrease oxygen consumption in preparation for performance of an emergency operation.

> *Management of hypercyanotic (tet) spells, from least to most invasive*
> - Have parent hold and calm child.
> - Knee/chest position.
> - AVOID IATROGENIC AGITATION.
>   Limit examination, venipuncture, etc.
>   NO INOTROPES (e.g. no digoxin, dopamine, or dobutamine) and
>   NO DIURETICS.
> - Oxygen (increases R_s, decreases R_p) – use least aggravating method of delivery.

- Morphine subcutaneous 0.1–0.2 mg/kg (decreases sympathetic tone, decreases oxygen consumption) *or* ketamine 1–3 mg/kg IM (sedates and increases R_s).
- Fluid bolus (warmed).
- Correct anemia.
- Convert tachyarrhythmia.
- Phenylephrine (Neo-Synephrine®; action: increases R_s).
    Bolus: 0.1 mg/kg IM or SC or IV.
    Start infusion: 0.1–0.5 µg/kg/min IV, titrate to effect (reflex bradycardia indicating raised BP; increased pulse oximeter saturation).
- β-Blockers (actions: decreases oxygen consumption; may lessen infundibular "spasm").
    Esmolol (Brevibloc®), load 500 µg/kg × 1 min, then infuse 50–950 µg/kg/min (titrate in 25–50 µg per step).
    Or propranolol (Inderal®) 0.05–0.25 mg/kg IV over five minutes.
- Sodium bicarbonate 1–2 mEq/kg/dose IV.
- Intubate/paralyze/anesthetize (reduces oxygen consumption to minimum).
- Extracorporeal membrane oxygenation (ECMO).
- Surgical shunt, emergently.

Operative and interventional considerations

Palliation. In very small infants, those with very small pulmonary arteries, or depending on the capabilities of the cardiac center, a palliative operation may be the initial surgical approach.

Several palliative procedures have been used since the first Blalock–Taussig shunt (anastomosing a subclavian artery to a branch pulmonary artery), performed in 1945. Because of early difficulties in anastomosing small subclavian arteries, the Waterston shunt (creating a communication between the right pulmonary artery and the ascending aorta) and the Potts procedure (creating a communication between the left pulmonary artery and the descending aorta) were developed. Neither the Potts nor the Waterston methods are currently used because of the tendency to create too large a communication, resulting in pulmonary vascular disease.

In a modified Blalock–Taussig shunt, a synthetic tube (polytetrafluoroethylene or Gore-Tex®), usually 4 mm in diameter, is placed between a subclavian artery and a branch pulmonary artery. This is commonly used to palliate infants with significant cyanosis. These procedures are also indicated for older children with tetralogy of Fallot whose pulmonary arteries are too small for corrective operation.

Catheterization is an alternative to palliative surgery for some neonates. A stent is inserted in the ductus arteriosus to maintain patency.

Each of these procedures allows an increased volume of pulmonary blood flow and improves arterial saturation.

Corrective repair. Tetralogy of Fallot is corrected by closing the ventricular septal defect, resecting the pulmonary stenosis, and often by inserting a right ventricular outflow tract patch. Corrective operations are usually performed in infants in lieu of performing a palliative procedure. Without complicating anatomy, such as small pulmonary arteries, the operative mortality in infants several months of age is under 1%. Early operative results are good; very few patients have congestive cardiac failure as a consequence of the right ventriculotomy or require reoperation because of residual cardiac anomalies, such as persistent outflow obstruction or ventricular septal defect.

Patients with tetralogy of Fallot with pulmonary atresia may require multiple operations to rehabilitate stenotic or disconnected pulmonary artery segments and may ultimately have a conduit placed from the right ventricle to the pulmonary artery. Reoperation is frequently necessary as these patients outgrow and/or stenose the conduit.

Patients who have a normal pulmonary annulus diameter may have resection of the infundibular stenosis without right ventriculotomy and have good pulmonary valve function postoperatively. Long-term complications in patients repaired in this way are fewer than with classical repair with its accompanying transmural right ventricular scar, marked pulmonary valve regurgitation from valve removal, and enlargement of the annulus using an outflow tract patch.

Despite highly successful corrective operations for tetralogy of Fallot that have been performed for many years, long-term risks still include right and left ventricular dysfunction, arrhythmias, and sudden death.

Summary

Tetralogy of Fallot is a frequent form of cyanotic congenital heart disease. The symptoms, physical examination, and laboratory features are characteristic. Several signs and symptoms permit evaluation of the natural progression of pulmonary stenosis. Several types of operations are available with a goal of complete correction. Long-term risks persist even for well-repaired patients.

Tetralogy "variants"

Any cardiac condition with a ventricular communication and significant pulmonary stenosis, which is not tetralogy of Fallot, can be thought of as a variant of tetralogy. Examples are single ventricle and pulmonary stenosis, and double outlet right ventricle and pulmonary stenosis. The hemodynamics and clinical and many laboratory findings are similar. Therefore, when confronted by such a patient, apply what you thought about for tetralogy of Fallot and you will understand much about the patient. Obviously, the echocardiogram and operative considerations will differ.

Tricuspid atresia

In this malformation (Figure 6.13), the tricuspid valve and the inflow portion of the right ventricle do not develop, so no direct communication exists between the right atrium and the right ventricle. Therefore, the circulation is severely altered. The systemic venous return entering the right atrium flows entirely in a right-to-left direction into the left atrium through either an atrial septal defect or a patent foramen ovale. Because the blood can take no other path, the atrial level right-to-left shunt is a form of *obligatory shunting*.

In the left atrium, the systemic venous return mixes with the pulmonary venous blood and is delivered to the left ventricle. The left ventricle ejects blood into the aorta and, in most instances, through a ventricular septal defect, into a rudimentary right ventricle and then into the pulmonary artery. Usually, the ventricular septal defect is small, the right ventricle is hypoplastic, and frequently pulmonary stenosis coexists. Therefore, a high degree of resistance to blood flow into the lungs is present. In most patients with tricuspid atresia, the pulmonary blood flow is reduced.

In one-fourth of patients with tricuspid atresia, transposition of the great vessels coexists; therefore, the pulmonary artery arises from the left ventricle and the aorta arises from the hypoplastic right ventricle. In such patients, the pulmonary blood flow is greatly increased because of the relatively low pulmonary vascular resistance and the increased resistance to systemic blood flow from the systemic vascular resistance, the small ventricular septal defect, and the hypoplastic right ventricle.

In all forms of tricuspid atresia, both the systemic and pulmonary venous returns mix in the left atrium; tricuspid atresia is an admixture lesion and the degree of cyanosis is inversely related to the volume of pulmonary blood flow. Therefore, the patient with tricuspid atresia and normally related great vessels is more cyanotic than the patient with tricuspid atresia and transposition of the great vessels. The degree of cyanosis is useful in following the course of the patient.

Two aspects of the circulation influence the clinical course of patients and direction of therapy. First is the size of the atrial communication. In most patients, an ample-sized atrial septal defect is present, but a few have only a patent foramen ovale, which causes severe obstruction.

The second aspect relates to the volume of pulmonary blood flow. Usually, pulmonary blood flow is reduced, so the resultant hypoxia and related symptoms

(a)

(b)

(c)

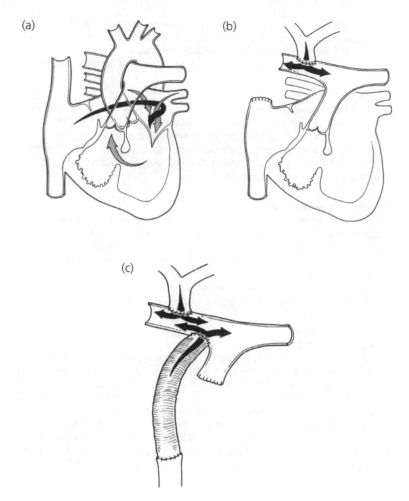

Figure 6.13 Tricuspid atresia and normally related great vessels. (a) Central circulation. Surgical options: (b) bidirectional Glenn; (c) Fontan.

require palliation. However, patients with markedly increased pulmonary blood flow, usually from coexistent transposition of the great arteries, develop congestive cardiac failure from left ventricular volume overload.

Tricuspid atresia is not usually found in association with a genetic syndrome.

History

Children with tricuspid atresia are generally symptomatic in infancy and show cyanosis. Hypoxic spells may be present, but squatting is rare. In the patient with increased pulmonary blood flow, cyanosis may be slight, and the dominant clinical features relate to congestive cardiac failure. An unusual patient with the "proper" amount of pulmonary stenosis and "balanced" pulmonary and systemic blood flow may be relatively asymptomatic for years.

Physical examination

The physical findings are not diagnostic. Cyanosis is generally evident and is frequently intense. The liver is enlarged with congestive cardiac failure or an obstructing atrial communication. In one-third of patients, either no murmur or a very soft murmur is present, indicating marked reduction in pulmonary blood flow. In patients with a large ventricular septal defect or with coexistent transposition of the great vessels, a grade 3/6–4/6 murmur is present along the left sternal border; in these patients, an apical mid-diastolic murmur may also be found. The second heart sound is single.

Electrocardiogram

The electrocardiogram is usually diagnostic of tricuspid atresia (Figure 6.14). Left-axis deviation is almost uniformly present and is typically between 0 and −60°. Tall, peaked P waves of right atrial enlargement and a short PR interval are common. Because the right ventricle is rudimentary, it contributes little to the total electrical forces forming the QRS complex. Therefore, the precordial leads show a pattern of left ventricular hypertrophy with an rS complex in lead V_1 and a tall R wave in V_6. This precordial pattern is particularly striking in infancy because of the marked difference from the normal infantile pattern of tall R waves in the right precordium. In older patients, the T waves may become inverted in the left precordial leads.

Chest X-ray

The pulmonary vasculature is decreased in most patients; but in those with transposition of the great vessels or large ventricular septal defect, it is of course increased. Cardiac size is increased. The cardiac contour is highly suggestive of tricuspid atresia because of the prominent right heart border (enlarged right atrium) and the prominent left heart border (enlarged left ventricle).

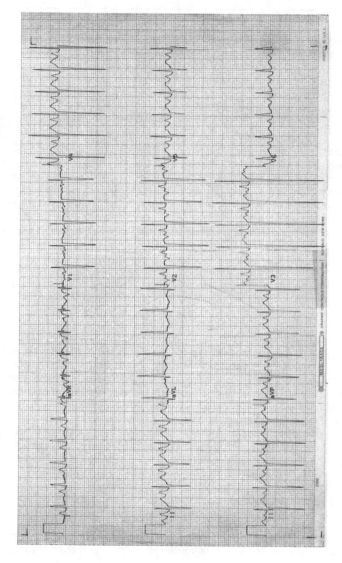

Figure 6.14 Electrocardiogram in tricuspid atresia. Left-axis deviation (−45°). Right atrial enlargement.

Summary of clinical findings

In patients with cyanosis, the electrocardiogram presents the most important diagnostic clue. The combination of left-axis deviation and pattern of left ventricular enlargement/hypertrophy is highly suggestive of tricuspid atresia. The chest X-ray findings also help if the pulmonary vasculature is decreased. The auscultatory findings and history are not diagnostic but are useful for providing clues about the condition's severity.

Echocardiogram

The diagnosis is easily confirmed by demonstrating that the tricuspid valve is absent using the four-chamber cross-sectional view obtained from the apex. An atrial septal defect is seen, and an obligatory right-to-left atrial shunt is demonstrated by Doppler. If the great vessels are normally related, Doppler is used to define the degree of obstruction to pulmonary blood flow (at the ventricular septal defect, right ventricular infundibulum, and/or the pulmonary valve). If the great vessels are malposed, Doppler is used to estimate the degree of obstruction to aortic outflow. Doppler estimates of obstruction performed in neonates with tricuspid atresia may mislead the physician because the gradient is minimal in the presence of the large patent ductus and relatively high pulmonary vascular resistance at this stage of life and because narrowing of the muscular portions of the outflow pathway (ventricular septal defect and infundibulum) increases with age and hypertrophy.

Cardiac catheterization

Oximetry data reveal a right-to-left shunt at the atrial level. The oxygen values in the left ventricle, aorta, and pulmonary artery are similar; they are inversely related to pulmonary blood flow. In some patients, the right atrial pressure is elevated, indicating a restricted interatrial communication. Patients who are candidates for a cavopulmonary connection should have normal left ventricular end-diastolic pressure and pulmonary vascular resistance.

Left ventriculography shows simultaneous opacification of both great vessels and permits the identification of the level of obstruction to pulmonary blood flow.

If cardiac catheterization is carried out in infancy, a balloon atrial septostomy may be performed to reduce obstruction to flow into the left atrium.

Operative considerations

Various palliative procedures are available for patients with tricuspid atresia.

Pulmonary artery banding. This procedure is indicated in infants with increased pulmonary blood flow and is often performed by one to three months of age. It is an essential step to protect the pulmonary vascular bed from high flow and pressure, in consideration for future palliative surgery.

Modified Blalock–Taussig (Gore-Tex® interposition) shunt. This, or a similar shunt, is performed in neonates with markedly reduced pulmonary blood flow. Ductal stenting may be employed in lieu of surgery in some neonates.

After several weeks to months of age, when pulmonary resistance has fallen sufficiently, a cavopulmonary anastomosis (connecting systemic venous return directly into the pulmonary arteries without an intervening pump) is considered.

"Bidirectional" Glenn procedure or "hemi-Fontan". In this procedure (Figure 6.13b), the superior vena cava is anastomosed to the roof of the right pulmonary artery, allowing systemic venous blood to pass into both pulmonary arteries. It is the first part of a staged cavopulmonary anastomosis.

Complete cavopulmonary anastomosis (Fontan procedure). This is available for older patients with tricuspid atresia and normally related great vessels after a previous bidirectional Glenn procedure. With this operation (Figure 6.13c), the inferior vena caval return is conducted to the pulmonary arteries, usually by way of a conduit coursing through or external to the right atrium. This effectively separates the pulmonary venous and systemic venous returns, as in a normal heart; but unlike normal, a ventricle does not pump blood from the systemic veins to the pulmonary arteries. Therefore, the Fontan procedure is considered palliative but not corrective.

The long-term results of the Fontan procedure vary. Some patients develop complications from chronically elevated systemic venous pressure, including pleural, pericardial, and ascitic effusions, liver dysfunction, and protein-losing enteropathy. Stroke and arrhythmia are long-term risks. Many patients who appear well palliated for years after the Fontan procedure develop left ventricular dysfunction of unknown cause and heart failure. It is probably independent of the type of palliation, since ventricular dysfunction develops in patients with Blalock–Taussig and other aorticopulmonary shunts. Some speculate that the myocardium is congenitally myopathic in tricuspid atresia patients.

Summary

Children with tricuspid atresia present with cyanosis and cardiac failure. A murmur may or may not be present. The electrocardiogram reveals left-axis deviation, right atrial enlargement, and left ventricular enlargement/hypertrophy. Chest X-rays show right atrial and left ventricular enlargement. Palliative, but not corrective, operations are available.

Pulmonary atresia with intact ventricular septum

In this malformation (Figure 6.15), the pulmonary valve is atretic, no blood flows directly from the right ventricle to the pulmonary artery, and the right ventricle is usually hypoplastic. In a few neonates, significant tricuspid regurgitation is present; in these patients, the right ventricle is enlarged. An atrial communication, either foramen ovale or atrial septal defect, allows a right-to-left shunt. Pulmonary blood flow depends entirely upon a patent ductus arteriosus. As the ductus arteriosus closes in the neonatal period, the infant's hypoxia progresses.

The right ventricle frequently communicates with the coronary artery system through myocardial sinusoids. During systole, blood flows from the high-pressure right ventricle into the major coronary artery branches and even as far as the aortic root. During the first year of life, these progressively enlarge and form a way for the right ventricle to decompress.

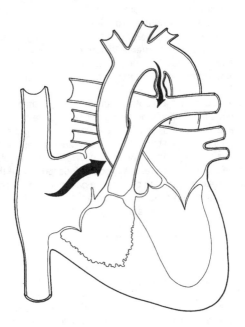

Figure 6.15 Pulmonary atresia with intact ventricular septum.

History

Patients present in the neonatal period with progressive cyanosis and its complications. Features of congestive cardiac failure may appear if the atrial communication is small or if left ventricular dysfunction is present.

Physical examination

The infant presents with intense cyanosis and dyspnea. No murmur is usually present; however, in some a soft, continuous murmur of patent ductus arteriosus is found. In neonates with tricuspid regurgitation, a holosystolic murmur is heard along the lower left and right sternal border. The second heart sound is single. Hepatomegaly is present if the atrial septal defect is restrictive.

Electrocardiogram

The electrocardiogram usually shows a normal QRS axis. Peaked P waves of right atrial enlargement usually appear. Since the right ventricle is hypoplastic, the precordial leads show an rS complex in lead V_1 and an R wave in lead V_6. This pattern resembles left ventricular hypertrophy and contrasts strikingly with the normal pattern for a newborn. The T waves are usually normal. If tricuspid regurgitation and an enlarged right ventricle are present, a pattern of right ventricular hypertrophy is found.

Chest X-ray

The pulmonary vasculature is reduced. The cardiac contour resembles tricuspid atresia by showing prominent right atrial and left ventricular borders. The cardiac size is enlarged.

Summary of clinical findings

In a cyanotic infant, the combination of X-ray findings of cardiomegaly and reduced pulmonary vascular markings and left ventricular enlargement/ hypertrophy on the electrocardiogram suggests the diagnosis of pulmonary atresia. This condition may be distinguished from tricuspid atresia by the difference in the QRS axis, but this distinction is not always reliable.

Echocardiogram

Cross-sectional echocardiography shows a small, hypertrophied, poorly contracting right ventricle and no motion at the location of the pulmonary valve, which appears plate-like. The tricuspid valve motion may appear so limited by poor flow into the blindly ending right ventricle that, echocardiographically, the diagnosis may be confused with tricuspid atresia. In contrast to tricuspid atresia, Doppler usually demonstrates some tricuspid regurgitation. If marked tricuspid valve regurgitation is present, the right ventricle is enlarged. The right ventricular systolic pressure (which can be estimated from the tricuspid regurgitation velocity) is often suprasystemic (i.e. greater than that of the left ventricle).

An atrial septal defect with right-to-left atrial shunt is present.

The patent ductus, which shows a continuous aorta-to-pulmonary artery shunt, appears long and convoluted, similar to that in tricuspid atresia and tetralogy of Fallot with pulmonary atresia.

Left ventricular function may be subnormal, especially if abnormal right ventricle-to-coronary artery connections (sinusoids) are present. These connections are often demonstrated with color Doppler.

Cardiac catheterization

The oxygen saturation shows a right-to-left atrial shunt and marked systemic arterial oxygen desaturation because of severe limitation of pulmonary blood flow. The right atrial pressure is often elevated by a narrowed atrial communication. The hypoplastic right ventricle, entered with a catheter via the tricuspid valve, reveals high (often suprasystemic) pressure.

Right atrial angiography shows a right-to-left shunt at the atrial level and resembles tricuspid atresia. Left ventriculography usually distinguishes this anomaly because the ventricular septal defect and right ventricular outflow areas are not visualized in pulmonary atresia; instead, the aorta is opacified and, subsequently, the pulmonary artery opacifies by a patent ductus arteriosus. The right ventricle may be very cautiously injected by hand with a small volume. This allows the determination of the distance between the right ventricle cavity and the main pulmonary artery (filled from the ductus with a separate injection). Abnormal connections, called sinusoids, between the right ventricular cavity and coronary arteries may fill from the right ventricle. They represent a poor prognostic sign, since myocardial function may depend on retrograde perfusion and limit operative efforts to return the right ventricular pressure to normal.

Placement of a stent in the ductus arteriosus to maintain long-term patency may be an option for some neonates.

Operative considerations

Neonates require emergency palliation with prostaglandin to maintain ductal patency. A pulmonary valvotomy, usually surgical (or using various transcatheter methods to puncture and then balloon dilate the valve), is performed so that the hypoplastic right ventricle will grow in size and compliance. Even if adequate pulmonary valvotomy is achieved, a large right-to-left-atrial shunt persists because of the small, poorly compliant right ventricle. A modified Blalock–Taussig shunt is then performed to take the place of the ductus. Pulmonary valvotomy may be contraindicated in infants with retrograde coronary artery flow through sinusoids, the so-called RV-dependent coronary circulation.

Summary

Pulmonary atresia resembles tricuspid atresia with normally related great vessels in hemodynamics, clinical and laboratory findings, and operative considerations. In both conditions, the severity of symptoms is related to the adequacy of the communication between the atria and to the volume of pulmonary blood flow. The conditions are distinguished by the difference in the QRS axis.

Ebstein's malformation of the tricuspid valve

In Ebstein's malformation (Figure 6.16), the leaflets of the tricuspid valve attach to the right ventricular wall rather than to the tricuspid valve annulus. The tricuspid valve is displaced into the right ventricle, so a part of the right ventricle between the tricuspid annulus and the displaced tricuspid valve (the "atrialized" portion) is functionally part of the right atrial chamber. An atrial septal defect is usually present.

The malformation has two hemodynamic consequences. First, the tricuspid valve frequently permits tricuspid regurgitation. Second, the portion of the right ventricle between the tricuspid and pulmonary valves is small and noncompliant. As a result, right ventricular inflow is impeded so that a right-to-left shunt exists at the atrial level so the pulmonary blood flow is decreased.

No particular genetic condition has been associated with Ebstein's anomaly, although familial forms, often with noncompaction cardiomyopathy, can occur.

History

Patients frequently have a history of variable cyanosis, being cyanotic in the first week of life, then acyanotic or minimally cyanotic for a variable period, only to become increasingly cyanotic later in life. Mild forms are not infrequently first diagnosed in adults. As pulmonary vascular resistance decreases in the neonatal period, a symptomatic neonate improves as pulmonary blood flow increases. In those with a more deformed and significantly displaced valve, cyanosis is greater and survival less likely. Congestive cardiac failure is present in those with more severe forms but, transiently, in neonates with less abnormal anatomy. Supraventricular tachycardia

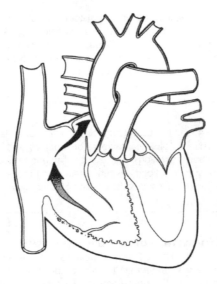

Figure 6.16 Ebstein's malformation. Central circulation.

or atrial flutter, related to the right atrial dilation, and in one-fifth of patients, to pre-excitation (Wolff–Parkinson–White syndrome), may coexist.

Physical examination

Cyanosis may be minimal or absent. A precordial bulge may be found. The auscultatory findings are characteristic. A quadruple rhythm is often present. Both the first and second heart sounds are split, and a fourth heart sound may be present. Usually, a holosystolic murmur of variable intensity that indicates tricuspid regurgitation is found. In addition, a rough mid-diastolic murmur is often heard in the tricuspid area.

Electrocardiogram

The electrocardiographic features are characteristic (Figure 6.17). Right atrial enlargement is evident and the P wave may be 8–9 mm in height. The QRS duration is prolonged because of complete right bundle branch block or Wolff–Parkinson–White syndrome, which is present in 20% of patients. The precordial leads show a pattern of ventricular hypertrophy and the R wave in lead V_1 rarely exceeds 10 mm in height.

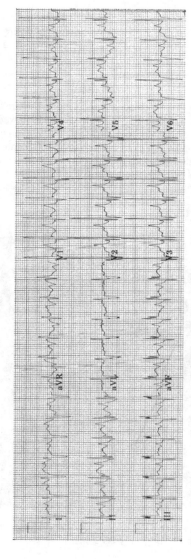

Figure 6.17 Electrocardiogram in Ebstein's malformation. Indeterminate frontal-plane QRS axis. Tall P waves indicate right atrial enlargement. Right bundle branch block with an RSR' pattern in V_1.

Chest X-ray

The heart is enlarged, possibly having a box-like configuration. The right atrium is enlarged. In neonates with severe right atrial enlargement, cardiomegaly may be massive (Figure 6.18). The pulmonary vascular markings are diminished.

Echocardiogram

Cross-sectional four-chamber views demonstrate the apical displacement of the tricuspid valve into the right ventricle. The right atrium is markedly dilated. The cross-sectional area of the right atrium and the atrialized portion of the right ventricle, when compared with the area of the remaining right ventricle, left atrium, and left ventricle, correlates with survival. Patients with the most displaced tricuspid valves and the largest right atria do less well. Doppler shows tricuspid regurgitation that varies in severity among patients. A right-to-left atrial shunt is generally present.

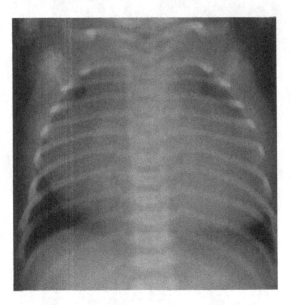

Figure 6.18 Chest X-ray in Ebstein's malformation. Massive cardiomegaly (so-called wall-to-wall heart) and decreased pulmonary vascularity.

Cardiac catheterization

The oximetry data show a right-to-left shunt at the atrial level. Right ventricular systolic pressure is normal, whereas right atrial pressure is elevated. Angiography may be diagnostic in showing the abnormal position of the tricuspid valve, reduced right ventricular size, enlarged right atrium, and right-to-left atrial shunt. Arrhythmias are common during catheterization, so the patient must be monitored carefully and treated promptly.

Operative considerations

The preferred approach is avoidance of operation. Shunt procedures should be avoided, since within the first few days of life, cyanosis improves as pulmonary vascular resistance falls and right ventricular compliance improves somewhat. A shunt procedure is indicated only for patients with persistent and markedly reduced pulmonary blood flow. In some older patients, particularly those with congestive failure, an operation to reconstruct the tricuspid valve may be possible; otherwise a prosthetic valve is placed in the tricuspid annulus; the huge right atrium is reduced in size by resection of part of its wall.

Summary

The diagnosis of Ebstein's malformation can usually be made clinically because of the history and auscultatory and electrocardiographic findings. Palliative procedures are available.

Summary of cyanotic lesions

Cardiac conditions with cyanosis generally present in the neonatal period or are recognized before birth by fetal echocardiography. Although many are complex conditions, in most a corrective or palliative procedure can be performed. With prompt recognition of the neonate, correct diagnosis, and medical management (usually including prostaglandin), an operation can be performed with relatively low risk and good results considering the size and condition of the neonate.

Chapter 7
Unusual forms of congenital heart disease in children

CONGENITALLY CORRECTED TRANSPOSITION OF THE GREAT VESSELS/ARTERIES

As mentioned in Chapter 6, the term *transposition* means a reversal of anteroposterior anatomic relationships. Therefore, in transposition of the great vessels/arteries (I-TGV, I-TGA), the aorta arises anteriorly and the pulmonary artery arises posteriorly. Normally, the anterior blood vessel arises from the infundibulum, which is the outflow portion of the morphologic right ventricle.

Moller's Essentials of Pediatric Cardiology, Fourth Edition.
Walter H. Johnson, Jr. and Camden L. Hebson.
© 2023 John Wiley & Sons Ltd. Published 2023 by John Wiley & Sons Ltd.

In congenitally corrected transposition of the great arteries, these anatomic relationships are present and the circulation is physiologically correct (i.e. systemic venous return is delivered to the pulmonary arteries; pulmonary venous return is delivered to the aorta).

The anatomy of congenitally corrected transposition of the great arteries differs from complete dextrotransposition of the great arteries (d-TGA) because ventricular inversion coexists. The term *inversion* indicates an anatomic change in the left–right relationships. Therefore, inversion of the ventricles indicates that the morphologic right ventricle lies on the left side and that the morphologic left ventricle lies on the right side. The inversion of the ventricles in corrected transposition of the great arteries allows the circulation to flow in a normal pattern (Figure 7.1).

The systemic venous return from the inferior and superior venae cavae passes into the normally positioned right atrium. This blood then flows across a *mitral* valve into a ventricle that has the morphologic features of a left ventricle: it is a finely trabeculated chamber, and fibrous continuity exists between the atrioventricular (AV) (mitral) and semilunar valves (pulmonary). This ventricle is located to the right of

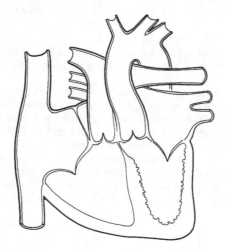

Figure 7.1 Congenitally corrected transposition of the great vessels/arteries (l-TGV, l-TGA). In addition to levo-transposed great vessels, ventricular inversion is found. The morphologic right ventricle (trabeculated) is left-sided and is located between the left atrium (fully oxygenated blood) and the aorta. The morphologic left ventricle is right-sided and is positioned between the right atrium (deoxygenated blood) and the pulmonary artery. Therefore, the circulation is physiologically correct.

the other ventricle. This anatomic left ventricle ejects blood into a posteriorly and medially placed pulmonary artery.

The pulmonary venous blood returns into the normally placed left atrium. The flow then crosses a *tricuspid* valve into a ventricle having the morphologic features of a right ventricle: it is coarsely trabeculated and the AV (tricuspid) and semilunar valves (aortic) are separated by an infundibulum. The aorta arises from the infundibulum and lies anteriorly and left of the pulmonary artery.

The flow of blood, therefore, is normal and the anatomic relationship of the great vessels fulfills the definition of transposition of the great arteries. This type of transposition has also been termed levo-transposition because the aorta lies to the left of the pulmonary artery.

This condition alone would lead to no cardiovascular symptoms or murmurs (although there are concerns of the ability of the systemic right ventricle to sustain the systemic circulation). Virtually all patients with congenitally corrected transposition, however, have coexisting cardiac anomalies. Ventricular septal defect, pulmonary stenosis, and insufficiency of the left-sided AV valve are the most common associated cardiac anomalies.

These coexistent anomalies lead to clinical and laboratory findings similar to those found in patients with the same anomaly but with normal relationships between the ventricles and the great vessels.

Three clinical findings, however, allow the detection of congenitally corrected transposition of the great arteries as the underlying cardiac malformation:

(1) The second heart sound is loud, single, and best heard along the upper left sternal border (in the so-called pulmonary area). Because the aorta is located anteriorly and leftward, the aortic valve lies immediately beneath this area. The second sound appears single because the pulmonary valve is distant (posteriorly positioned), so its component is inaudible.

(2) On chest X-ray, the left cardiac border is straight or shows only two rounded contours (the upper being the leftward-positioned ascending aorta and the lower the inverted right ventricle). This is in contrast to patients with normally related great vessels who have three contours – the aortic knob, pulmonary trunk, and left ventricular border.

(3) Electrocardiographic findings are distinctive and related to ventricular inversion. The bundle of His is also inverted, so the ventricular septum depolarizes from right to left, the opposite of normal. This leads to a Q wave in lead V_1, and an initial positive deflection in lead V_6 (the opposite of the normal pattern of an initial R wave in lead V_1, and a Q wave in lead V_6). Such a pattern is present in almost all patients with congenitally corrected transposition of the great arteries. A word of caution: patients with severe right ventricular hypertrophy may also show such a pattern, so this electrocardiographic finding alone is not diagnostic.

Patients with congenitally corrected transposition of the great arteries often spontaneously develop partial or complete heart block.

While the basic anatomic anomaly in congenitally corrected transposition of the great arteries does not require treatment, hemodynamically significant coexistent conditions do, generally by operation.

Operative treatment

The associated anomalies are corrected using the same general techniques as in those with normally related ventricles and great arteries, although the risk of operative heart block is higher. The treatment of the regurgitant systemic AV valve, the morphologic tricuspid valve (often described as Ebstein's anomaly), is challenging because the basic approach to the operation on the valvar condition varies with the anatomy of the valve. Additionally, as in any patient with left AV valve regurgitation, it is critical that the operation reduces the degree of regurgitation. Because of the concern about the ability of the inverted right ventricle to function adequately for a long period at systemic levels of pressure, this has prompted some centers to perform a "double switch" procedure. This involves performing an arterial switch so that the aorta is connected to the left ventricle and the pulmonary artery is connected to the right ventricle. This creates the circulatory pattern of complete transposition. To address this, an atrial switch is carried out during the same operation so that systemic venous blood flows to the right ventricle and then to the pulmonary artery. Pulmonary venous blood is directed to the left ventricle and then the aorta.

Natural history

The natural history is affected by three issues. The first determinate is the nature and severity of the coexistent cardiac conditions. If the conditions are significant, they will require correction or palliation early in life. Second, there is a 2% annual development of heart block which requires treatment. Third, systemic right ventricular dysfunction develops often by the third decade and requires anticongestive measures.

MALPOSITION OF THE HEART

The heart may assume an abnormal position in either the left or the right side of the chest. Various classifications of cardiac malposition have been developed, but the authors favor the one presented here, although the terminology may differ from that of other authors.

Certain anatomic features are important in understanding cardiac malpositions. In normal patients and virtually all those with cardiac malposition, certain fundamental anatomic relations are constant.

The inferior vena cava (at the diaphragm), the anatomic right atrium, and the major lobe of the liver are located on one side of the body, whereas the aorta (at the diaphragm), the anatomic left atrium, and the stomach are located on the opposite side of the body.

The inferior vena cava is crucial in our considerations, as it is an important link between the abdominal and thoracic contents.

Situs solitus

Situs solitus (Figure 7.2) describes the anatomic relationships in a normal individual wherein the liver, inferior vena cava, and right atrium are present on the right side of the body and the stomach, aorta, and left atrium are present on the left side.

Dextrocardia

This general term indicates that the cardiac apex is located in the right side of the chest.

Three anatomic variations associated with dextrocardia are presented here.

Situs inversus totalis (mirror image dextrocardia)

This condition is the opposite of the usual situs solitus (Figure 7.2). The inferior vena cava, major lobe of the liver, and anatomic right atrium are located on the left side of the body, and the stomach, anatomic left atrium, and aorta (at the diaphragm) on the right side. This has also been termed mirror image dextrocardia because the anatomic relationships are exactly the reverse of normal. Other anatomic findings include the presence of two lobes in the right lung, of three lobes in the left lung, and of the appendix in the left lower quadrant.

Situs inversus is probably associated with an increased incidence of cardiac anomalies, but the type and distribution of the anomalies parallel those of patients with situs solitus.

About 40% of patients have ciliary dyskinesia, usually Kartagener syndrome, characterized by chronic sinusitis, bronchitis/bronchiectasis, and sterility.

Dextroversion with situs solitus

In this condition, the fundamental anatomic relationships of situs solitus are present, but the cardiac apex is directed toward the right (Figure 7.2). The atria are anchored by the venae cavae, but the ventricles can rotate on the long axis of the heart and lie in the midline or right chest.

In dextroversion, the heart may show one of two anatomic forms. In one, the ventricles and great arteries are normally related; and ventricular septal defect and pulmonary stenosis are common. In the other form, corrected transposition of the

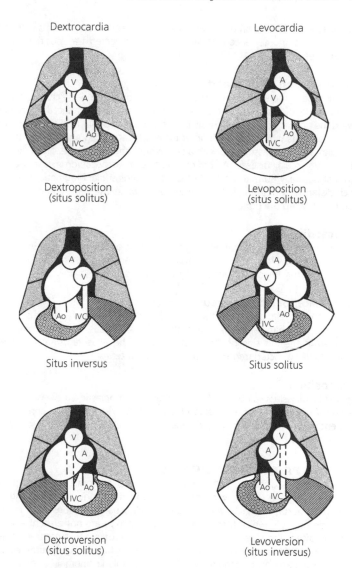

Figure 7.2 Malposition of the heart. Ao, aorta; IVC, inferior vena cava; V, venous atrium; A, arterial atrium.

great arteries and inversion of the ventricles are present. These patients show the type of cardiac anomalies commonly found with corrected transposition of the great arteries.

Dextroposition of the heart

This is another condition with the situs solitus relationship and the cardiac apex in the right side of the chest (Figure 7.2). In this instance, cardiac displacement toward the right is caused by extrinsic factors, such as hypoplasia of the right lung. In many patients with dextroposition of the heart, cardiac anomalies coexist. The anomalies are often associated with a left-to-right shunt; patients often develop pulmonary vascular disease. A common cause of dextroposition in the neonate with a structurally normal heart is left-sided congenital diaphragmatic hernia, in which distended gut in the left side of the chest forces the heart and mediastinal structures toward the right.

Levocardia

Levocardia is a general term indicating that the cardiac apex is located in the left side of the chest. Situs solitus is one form of levocardia; in other conditions, the cardiac apex may be located abnormally in the left side of the chest.

Levoversion of situs inversus

This anatomic relationship is the opposite of dextroversion of situs solitus (Figure 7.2). The basic anatomic relationship is situs inversus, but the cardiac apex is located in the left side of the chest. As might be expected, many of these patients have corrected transposition of the great arteries.

Levoposition

In patients with situs solitus, the left lung may be hypoplastic, so the heart is displaced further into the left hemithorax than normal. When this condition exists in a patient with a cardiac anomaly, a tendency to develop pulmonary vascular disease exists.

HETEROTAXY SYNDROMES

In the conditions discussed above, the fundamental anatomic relationships are present among the inferior vena cava, liver, and right atrium and among the descending aorta, stomach, and left atrium. Unusual conditions with cardiac malposition exist in which these anatomic relationships are not present and the spleen is often abnormal. There is often symmetry of organ structures. These conditions have been given various names, such as heterotaxy syndromes and isomerism syndromes, or named after the type of splenic anomaly or pattern of symmetry, and they have been classed as either right or left atrial appendage isomerism.

Asplenia syndrome (bilateral right-sidedness, right atrial isomerism, right atrial appendage isomerism)

In this syndrome, the heart may be located in either the left or right side of the chest, the spleen is absent, and numerous visceral and cardiac anomalies are found. The atrial appendages each appear like those of a right atrium, being broad and pyramidal. The visceral anomalies reflect a tendency toward symmetrical organ development, with paired organs each having the form of the right-sided organ; left-sided structures are absent. Thus, each lung has three lobes (like a right lung); the spleen, a left-sided structure, is absent; and the liver is symmetrical. Malrotation of the bowel is often present.

Cardiac anomalies are complex, including atrial and ventricular septal defects, often in the form of AV septal defect, severe pulmonary stenosis or atresia, transposition of the great arteries, and, in about 75% of instances, total anomalous pulmonary venous connection. This combination of anomalies leads to clinical and radiographic features that resemble severe tetralogy of Fallot. Despite palliative procedures, the outlook for these patients is often bleak.

Because of the symmetry of the liver, malrotation of the bowel, and midline position of the inferior vena cava, the important anatomic relationships that allow the definition of situs are disrupted, so classifying the type of cardiac malposition in patients with asplenia is difficult.

Polysplenia syndrome (bilateral left-sidedness, left atrial isomerism, left atrial appendage isomerism)

In this syndrome, as in asplenia, the heart may be located in either the left or right side of the chest. Both atrial appendages are long and finger-like as in a left atrium. The spleen is present but is divided into multiple masses. A tendency for symmetrical organ development also exists, in this case bilateral left-sidedness, in which both lungs appear as the left lung, the gallbladder may be absent, and there are multiple spleens. Malrotation of the bowel often occurs.

Cardiac anomalies include atrial and/or ventricular septal defect, partial anomalous pulmonary venous connection, and interrupted inferior vena cava with azygous continuation.

The clinical picture resembles that of left-to-right shunt. The prognosis is good and many patients undergo corrective operation.

As in asplenia, difficulty is encountered in determining situs because of the malrotation of the bowel and the fact that in about two-thirds of patients the inferior vena cava is interrupted at the level of the diaphragm.

VASCULAR RING

Normally, no vascular structure passes behind the esophagus, but in a vascular ring the aortic arch or a major arch vessel lies behind the esophagus. Radiographic barium swallow and echocardiography are the most useful noninvasive means of confirming the diagnosis. Computed tomography angiography (CTA), magnetic resonance imaging (MRI)/magnetic resonance angiography (MRA), or catheterization with aortography are often used to provide detailed anatomic information prior to surgical intervention.

An understanding of the anatomic variations of the vascular ring is gained by studying the development of the fourth and sixth aortic arches (Figure 7.3). Early in embryonic development, the ascending aorta gives rise to both a right and a left fourth aortic arch. These paired arches encircle the trachea and the esophagus and join to form the descending aorta. In addition, both a left and a right ductus arteriosus (sixth aortic arches) are found.

In the normal development of the fourth arch, the right arch is interrupted beyond the right subclavian artery, and the right ductus arteriosus regresses. This leads to the normal left aortic arch (fourth arch). The proximal portion of the primitive right arch becomes the innominate artery, which in turn gives rise to the right carotid and right subclavian arteries. The left carotid and left subclavian arteries arise directly from the left aortic arch. The left sixth arch persists as the left ductus arteriosus and connects the left pulmonary artery to the proximal descending aorta beyond the left subclavian artery.

Right aortic arch

If the left aortic arch is interrupted beyond the left subclavian artery, a right aortic arch with mirror-image branching is formed (Figure 7.3). The ascending aorta arises; the first branch is an innominate artery representing the proximal portion of the left aortic arch. From this arise the left subclavian and left carotid arteries. The aortic arch passes toward the right and gives rise to the right carotid and right subclavian arteries. The ductus arteriosus may be on either the left or right side. The aorta descends in the thorax and crosses into the abdomen to the left of the spine.

Double aortic arch

Rarely, neither aortic arch is interrupted during embryonic development. The resultant anomaly is one form of vascular ring – a double aortic arch. The ascending aorta divides into two aortic arches. One of the aortic arches passes anteriorly to the trachea and the other passes posteriorly to the esophagus. They join to form the descending aorta that then courses in either the left or right side of the thorax. Thus, the trachea and esophagus are encircled by vascular structures and can be compressed, leading to respiratory symptoms and difficulty in swallowing.

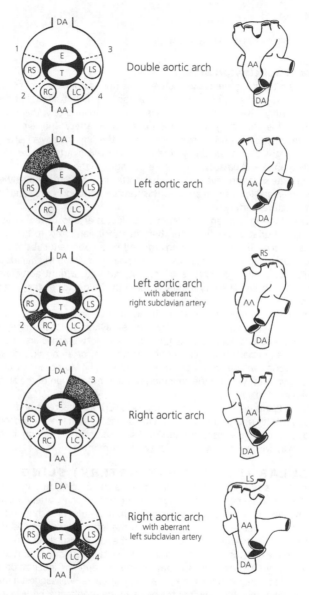

Double aortic arch

Left aortic arch

Left aortic arch
with aberrant
right subclavian artery

Right aortic arch

Right aortic arch
with aberrant
left subclavian artery

Figure 7.3 Development of aortic arch anomalies based on the concept of primitive double aortic arch and the resultant aortic arch patterns. The primitive double aortic arch may be uninterrupted developmentally, and a double arch results. It may also be interrupted at any of four locations (1–4). These result, respectively, in a normal left aortic arch, left aortic arch with aberrant right subclavian artery, right aortic arch, and right aortic arch with aberrant left subclavian artery. AA, ascending aorta; DA, descending aorta; LC, left carotid artery; LS, left subclavian artery; RC, right carotid artery; RS, right subclavian artery; E, esophagus; T, trachea.

Aberrant subclavian artery

If the right aortic arch is interrupted between the right carotid and right subclavian arteries instead of the usual location, the aortic arch is left-sided, but the right subclavian artery arises aberrantly. There is no innominate artery; the first branch arising from the ascending aorta is the right carotid artery. The remaining arch vessels are, respectively, the left carotid artery, the left subclavian artery, and, finally, the right subclavian artery. The right subclavian artery arises from the descending aorta and passes behind the esophagus to the right arm.

The opposite situation develops if the left aortic arch is interrupted between the left subclavian and left carotid arteries. This forms a right aortic arch and an aberrant left subclavian artery.

The vascular ring is often completed by a ductus arteriosus, either ligamentous or patent, that passes from the aberrant subclavian artery to the ipsilateral pulmonary artery. These vascular rings formed by an aberrant subclavian artery can also cause symptoms that are usually relieved by dividing the ductus arteriosus, which is usually ligamentous. Many patients with a right aortic arch and aberrant left subclavian artery require division of the ductus as they are usually symptomatic.

In summary, a number of variations in aortic arch anatomy exist, depending on the site(s) of interruption of the developmental aortic arches. If they are not interrupted, a double aortic arch is formed. If the aortic arches are interrupted at one site, a normal aortic arch, a right aortic arch, or an aortic arch with an aberrant subclavian artery can be formed. Rarely, the aortic arches are interrupted at two sites, yielding the condition termed interruption of the aortic arch (see Chapter 8).

In many patients with vascular ring, symptoms such as wheeze or stridor suggest respiratory infection, bronchiolitis, or airway disease, and tracheobronchomalacia may indeed accompany vascular ring. After surgical relief of the ring, respiratory and/or airway symptoms may persist for weeks or months.

VASCULAR (PULMONARY ARTERY) SLING

This condition is not an anomaly of the aortic arch complex, but an anomalous origin of the left pulmonary artery from the right pulmonary artery (Figure 7.4). The left pulmonary artery passes above the right mainstem bronchus and courses between the trachea and esophagus toward the left lung, creating tension and compression of the tracheobronchial tree near the carina. Usually, one lung is overinflated and the other is underinflated, which results in respiratory symptoms.

It is the only vascular anomaly that creates an anterior indentation on the barium-filled esophagus. Sometimes, a lateral chest X-ray will suggest a mass (the left pulmonary artery) between the trachea and the esophagus, particularly if the position of the esophagus is outlined by a feeding tube.

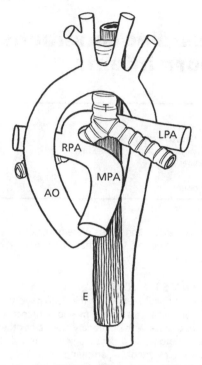

Figure 7.4 Pulmonary artery sling. The left pulmonary artery (LPA) arises anomalously from the right pulmonary artery (RPA) and courses between the trachea (T) and esophagus (E). MPA, main pulmonary artery; AO, aorta. Illustration courtesy of David C. Mayer, MD.

Surgical reimplantation of the anomalous left pulmonary artery into the main pulmonary artery can relieve the sling effect, but tracheobronchomalacia and symptoms often persist, and in many children, the left pulmonary artery is hypoplastic. Pulmonary artery sling has been associated with various genetic conditions, including Mowat–Wilson syndrome.

Chapter 8
Unique cardiac conditions in newborn infants

As indicated previously, several conditions present in neonates, but they are not exclusively seen in that age period. In this chapter, we present conditions that are symptomatic in neonates.

NEONATAL PHYSIOLOGY

The distinctive and transitional features of the neonatal circulation may lead to cardiopulmonary abnormalities not only in newborn infants with cardiac malformations but also among those with pulmonary disease or other serious illnesses.

Understanding the anatomic and physiologic features of the transition from fetal to adult circulation aids the physician caring for critically ill neonates.

Normal fetal circulation

Normal fetal circulation differs from that of the postnatal state. In the fetus, the pulmonary and systemic circulations are parallel, rather than occurring in series as in the normal circulation. In the fetal circulation, both ventricles eject blood into the aorta and receive systemic venous return. The right ventricle ejects a greater volume than the left ventricle. Postnatally, the circulation differs because the ventricles and the circulation are in series. The right ventricle receives the systemic venous return and ejects it into the pulmonary artery. The pulmonary venous return passes through the left atrium and the left ventricle alone ejects blood

Moller's Essentials of Pediatric Cardiology, Fourth Edition.
Walter H. Johnson, Jr. and Camden L. Hebson.
© 2023 John Wiley & Sons Ltd. Published 2023 by John Wiley & Sons Ltd.

into the aorta. Left ventricular and right ventricular outputs are equal. The transition from a parallel to a series circulation normally occurs soon after birth; however, in a distressed neonate, the parallel circulation may persist, delaying the evolution to series circulation.

The fetal circulation also has three distinctive anatomic structures: the placenta, the patent ductus arteriosus, and the patent foramen ovale. The blood returning to the fetus from the placenta enters the right atrium and flows predominantly from the right to the left atrium through the patent foramen ovale (Figure 8.1). This stream passes to the left ventricle and the ascending aorta, supplying the head with the proper level of oxygenated blood. The blood that leaves the head returns to the heart in the superior vena cava and flows principally into the right ventricle. Right ventricular output passes into the pulmonary artery, and the major portion (90%) flows through the ductus into the descending aorta, while a smaller amount (10%) flows into the lungs.

The major factor influencing the pattern and distribution of fetal blood flow is the relative vascular resistances of the pulmonary and systemic circuits. In contrast to the adult circulation, the pulmonary vascular resistance in the fetus is very elevated and the systemic vascular resistance is low. Prenatally, the lungs are airless, and the pulmonary arterioles possess thick media and a narrowed lumen.

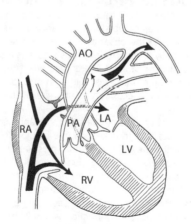

Figure 8.1 Central circulation in the fetus. Predominant flow from the inferior vena cava is through the patent foramen ovale into the left atrium. The major portion of right ventricular flow is through the patent ductus arteriosus. AO, aorta; LA, left atrium; LV, left ventricle; PA, pulmonary artery; RA, right atrium; RV, right ventricle.

These anatomic features of the pulmonary arterioles are accentuated by the relative hypoxic environment of the fetus, as hypoxia is a potent stimulus for pulmonary vasoconstriction. The systemic vascular resistance is unusually low, primarily because of the large flow through the placenta, which has low resistance. In the fetus, the pulmonary vascular resistance is perhaps five times greater than the systemic vascular resistance, the reverse of the adult circulation.

Because the systolic pressures in both ventricles and great vessels are identical, the distribution of blood flow depends upon the relative vascular resistances. As a result, a relatively small volume of blood flows through the lungs and a large volume passes through the ductus from right to left into the descending aorta. A considerable proportion (about 40%) of the combined ventricular output flows through the placenta.

The right-to-left shunt at the atrial level in the fetus depends in part upon the streaming effect caused by the position of the valve of the foramen ovale. This ridge tends to divert blood from the inferior vena cava into the left atrium through the fossa ovalis. Since the atrial pressures are identical, the shunt also depends on the relative compliances of the ventricles. Approximately one-third of the total flow returning to the right atrium crosses the foramen ovale.

Transition to postnatal circulatory physiology

At birth, the distinctive features of fetal circulation and the vascular resistances are suddenly changed. A major reversal of resistance occurs because of the separation of the placenta and the onset of respiration. The loss of the placenta, which has acted essentially as an arteriovenous fistula, is associated with a doubling of systemic vascular resistance. The expansion of the lungs is associated with a sevenfold drop in pulmonary vascular resistance, principally from vasodilation of pulmonary arterioles secondary to an increase in inspired oxygen level to normal.

Coinciding with the fall in pulmonary vascular resistance, the volume of pulmonary blood flow increases and thus the volume of blood returning to the left atrium increases proportionately. The left atrial pressure rises, exceeds the right atrial pressure, and closes the foramen ovale functionally. In most infants, for up to several months, a small left-to-right shunt occurs via the incompetent flap of the foramen ovale. Anatomically, the atrial septum ultimately seals in 75% of children and remains either patent or "probe-patent" in 25%.

The ductus narrows by muscular contraction within 24 hours of birth, although anatomic closure may take several days. The closure of the ductus is associated with a lowering of pulmonary arterial pressure to normal levels. When the ductus and foramen ovale close, the pulmonary blood flow equals systemic blood flow and the circulations are in series.

In the neonatal period, the changes that occur in the ductus, foramen ovale, and pulmonary arterioles are reversible. The pulmonary arterioles and the ductus arteriosus are responsive to oxygen levels and acidosis. An increase in the vascular resistance occurs in conditions associated with hypoxia. Although minor changes occur at a PaO_2 of 50 mmHg, large increases in pulmonary vascular resistance occur at PaO_2 levels less than 25 mmHg. If acidosis coexists with hypoxia, the increase in pulmonary resistance is far greater than at comparable levels of PaO_2 occurring at normal pH.

Persistent pulmonary hypertension of the newborn

Neonates with pulmonary parenchymal disease, such as respiratory distress syndrome, develop increased pulmonary vascular resistance and increased pulmonary arterial pressure because of hypoxia. If acidosis complicates the illness, the changes are even greater. This condition has been called persistent fetal circulation (PFC), or by the more physiologically descriptive term persistent pulmonary hypertension of the newborn (PPHN).

Because of the elevation of right ventricular systolic pressure, right atrial pressure increases, causing a right-to-left shunt at the foramen ovale. In a similar way, the ductus arteriosus of a neonate is also responsive to oxygen. With hypoxia, the ductus may reopen and, should the pulmonary resistance be simultaneously elevated, a right-to-left shunt could occur through the ductus arteriosus. Clinically, this is recognized by a lower PaO_2 (or pulse oximetry saturation) in the legs than arms.

Thus, cyanosis in the neonate with pulmonary parenchymal disease can result from right-to-left shunting of blood, as well as from intrapulmonary shunting and diffusion defects. Administration of 100% oxygen improves both of these abnormalities, but often the improvement is not great enough to exclude cyanotic cardiac malformations. Administration of oxygen to cyanotic patients with a cardiac anomaly generally also lessens the degree of cyanosis. With the development of echocardiography, the ability to distinguish these has been greatly enhanced.

CARDIAC DISEASE IN NEONATES

Most cardiac malformations cause no problems in utero or in the immediate postnatal state. However, during the transition to the normal circulatory pattern, particularly as the ductus arteriosus is closing and then closes, certain malformations become evident. These malformations have one of three circulatory patterns in which the ductus played an important role during fetal life, and as it closes postnatally the neonatal circulatory pattern is disrupted.

The three types of malformations dependent upon ductal blood flow following birth are as follows:

(1) Transposition of the great arteries. In this condition, the blood flow from the aorta through the ductus into the pulmonary artery provides an important pathway for mixing of blood.
(2) Anomalies with pulmonary atresia or severe stenosis and an intracardiac shunt. In these conditions, the ductus provides the sole or major flow into the lung and therefore the pulmonary circulation. As the ductus closes in the first two days of life, the neonate becomes increasingly cyanotic.
(3) Anomalies with major aortic obstructive lesions. In hypoplastic left heart syndrome (HLHS), the blood flow through the ductus from right to left provides the entire systemic circulation and in interruption of the aortic arch it provides the entire blood flow to the descending aorta. Thus, closure of the ductus is a major disruption of the circulation. In neonates with a coarctation, the aortic obstruction does not become evident until the ductus closes completely. Prior to closure, blood can pass from the ascending to descending aorta through the aortic orifice of the ductus as it closes from the pulmonary artery toward the descending aorta.

Because of cardiovascular problems that result from ductal closure, the severity of the neonatal condition, and the potential for correction or palliation in the first days of life, guidelines for screening of all neonates by peripheral oximetry are being incorporated in newborn nurseries as a method of identifying such neonates.

The guidelines are presented in the form of an algorithm (Figure 8.2). Pulse oximetry is used to measure oxygen saturations of the right hand and one lower extremity to detect the presence of hypoxia or a clinically important difference between upper and lower extremity saturations. When done after 24 hours of age, the specificity of the test is maximized (false-positive readings are minimized). The test is highly sensitive for detecting most cyanotic malformations and some left heart obstructive lesions with a right-to-left ductal shunt. However, the test has limitations as many obstructive lesions may not exhibit detectable levels of right-to-left ductal shunt, and some cyanotic lesions (such as truncus arteriosus and unobstructed total anomalous pulmonary venous return [TAPVR]) may have relatively high oxygen saturation levels. Also, left-to-right shunt lesions are not detected.

Cardiac malformations may lead to severe cardiac symptoms and death in the neonatal period. The types of cardiac malformations causing symptoms in this age group generally differ from those leading to symptoms later in infancy. Among the latter group, symptoms usually derive from a large volume of pulmonary blood flow, such as in ventricular septal defect (VSD), in which congestive failure develops at about six weeks of age. Other conditions, such as tetralogy of Fallot, await the

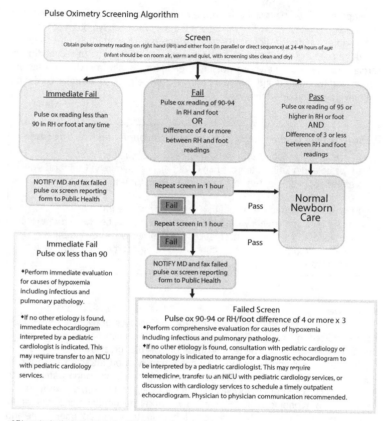

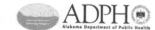

Figure 8.2 Pulse oximetry screening algorithm. Reprinted with the kind permission of the Alabama Department of Public Health (www.adph.org).

development of sufficient stenosis before becoming symptomatic. In the neonate, hypoxia and congestive cardiac failure are the major cardiac symptom complexes.

An aggressive diagnostic and therapeutic approach is warranted in neonates. If not diagnosed in fetal life, this approach begins with the prompt recognition of cardiac disease in the newborn nursery. Treatment, usually involving prostaglandin, should be initiated and the infant immediately referred to a cardiac center for definitive diagnosis and therapy.

Management of the cyanotic neonate with congenital heart disease

(1) Assess and manage ABCs (Airway/Breathing/Circulation) *first.*
(2) Prostaglandin E (PGE, alprostadil) 0.025–0.1 µg/kg/min IV: Common side effects: apnea, hypotension, fever, rash. Monitor respiratory status continuously.
(3) Consider endotracheal intubation, especially before transport.
(4) If PGE is not immediately available: intubate, ventilate, begin neuromuscular blockade, *and* sedate or anesthetize to minimize oxygen consumption.
(5) Arrange prompt transfer to a congenital cardiac center for definitive diagnosis and therapy.

Hypoxia

Severe cardiac symptoms also occur in neonates because of hypoxia from conditions discussed in Chapter 6. Two circulatory patterns can be the cause: inadequate mixing as in complete transposition of the great arteries, or severe obstruction to pulmonary blood flow coexisting with an intracardiac shunt. In neonates, tetralogy of Fallot, often with pulmonary atresia, pulmonary atresia with intact ventricular septum (hypoplastic right ventricle), and tricuspid atresia are the most common conditions in this category. Critical pulmonary stenosis is valvar pulmonary stenosis with a large right-to-left shunt through a foramen ovale and with various degrees of right ventricular hypoplasia and abnormal compliance; the physiology is similar to that of pulmonary atresia with intact ventricular septum.

Neonates with hypoxia show extreme cyanosis. Rapid, difficult respiration occurs from metabolic acidosis, which can develop quickly because of the hypoxia; cardiac failure is usually not a major problem. Administration of oxygen is usually of little benefit. Malformations with inadequate pulmonary blood flow are improved by prostaglandin administration followed by a corrective operation if possible, an aorticopulmonary shunt to improve oxygenation, or catheter intervention. Neonates with complete transposition of the great arteries require prostaglandins to keep the ductus patent and a Rashkind atrial septostomy to improve intracardiac mixing.

Thus, a diverse group of cardiac conditions cause symptoms in the neonatal period. Because of the potential for correction or palliation, any neonate with severe cardiac symptoms should be stabilized. Then echocardiography and, in many neonates, cardiac catheterization and angiocardiography are used to define the anatomic and physiologic details of the cardiac malformation. Although there is some risk (1% mortality) when performing a cardiac catheterization in neonates, it is outweighed by the benefits of the data obtained or the therapeutic interventions performed. Following definition of the malformation, appropriate decisions are made concerning an operation; and in some malformations (e.g. critical aortic stenosis, critical pulmonary stenosis), balloon dilation of the obstruction is successful.

Congestive cardiac failure

In the neonatal period, congestive cardiac failure results most commonly from (i) anomalies that cause severe outflow obstruction, particularly to the left side of the heart, and often associated with a hypoplastic left ventricle, (ii) volume overload from an insufficient cardiac valve or systemic arteriovenous fistula, and (iii) cardiomyopathy or myocarditis.

Cardiac conditions with a left-to-right shunt (e.g. VSD) almost never place large volume loads upon the ventricles and cause symptoms in the neonatal period. Occasionally, in prematurely born infants, a patent ductus arteriosus may lead to signs of cardiac failure. Presumably, the pulmonary vasculature approaches normal levels more quickly than in full-term infants. The resultant large volume of pulmonary blood flow causes overload of the left ventricle.

Left heart obstruction

Hypoplastic left heart syndrome (HLHS). HLHS is the most frequent cause of cardiac failure in neonates (Figure 8.3a). The term encompasses several cardiac malformations, each associated with a diminutive left ventricle and similar clinical and physiologic features, and includes aortic atresia, mitral atresia, and severe ("critical") aortic stenosis. In each, severe obstruction to both left ventricular inflow and outflow is present.

Whether from an atretic mitral valve or from a small left ventricle, filling of the left ventricle is impeded or impossible. The foramen ovale is often small and restrictive, permitting only a small amount of blood to flow from the left to the right atrium. The volume of shunt is not sufficient to decompress the left atrium, so its pressure rises, elevating pulmonary capillary pressure and ultimately causing pulmonary edema. Left ventricular outflow is either severely obstructed or totally occluded.

Patent ductus arteriosus is a major component of all forms of HLHS. The flow through the ductus is from right to left and represents the sole or major source of systemic arterial blood flow. The left ventricular output may be absent or is so

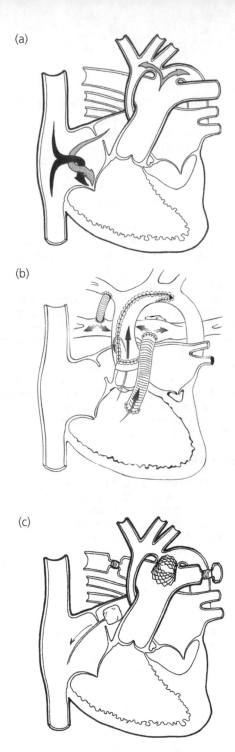

Figure 8.3 Hypoplastic left heart syndrome (HLHS). Aortic atresia. (a) Central circulation; (b) Norwood procedure (stage 1). Both a modified Blalock–Taussig shunt and a Sano shunt are shown. (c) Hybrid procedure.

small that the flow in the ascending aorta and to the coronary arteries is retrograde through the arch from the ductus arteriosus. Coarctation of the aorta may complicate the anatomic features.

History. These patients show severe congestive cardiac failure and/or low cardiac output, usually in the first week of life, with a clinical presentation similar to coarctation of the aorta.

Physical examination. The peripheral pulses are weak and the skin is mottled because of poor tissue perfusion. A soft, nonspecific murmur may be heard, but often no murmur is found. Rarely, systolic clicks may be heard; they likely result from a dilated main pulmonary artery.

Electrocardiogram. The electrocardiogram may appear normal for age. The absence of a Q wave in V_6 is common, but normal infants may lack this if the electrode for V_6 is not placed properly.

Chest X-ray. Chest X-rays show an enlarged heart and accentuated pulmonary arterial and venous markings. The condition has been said to cause the largest heart the earliest.

Natural history. Death usually occurs in the first week of life as the ductus closes, although rarely infants are not recognized with this condition until later in the first month of life.

Echocardiogram. Echocardiography demonstrates a hypoplastic ascending aorta and diminutive left ventricle, although in some patients a left ventricular cavity is not seen. Doppler displays the typical pattern of the pulmonary artery to aorta flow and retrograde blood flow in the aortic arch and ascending aorta.

Cardiac catheterization. Cardiac catheterization is usually unnecessary unless a restrictive atrial septum is found that requires blade atrial septectomy or balloon septostomy. Some infants awaiting cardiac transplantation require balloon dilation of the ductus or a ductal stent to maintain adequate ductal size. See the hybrid procedure (under 'Operative considerations').

Medical management. Prostaglandin should be administered to maintain ductal patency and thus systemic blood flow. Because the systemic and pulmonary circulations are connected at the great vessel level, systemic blood flow may fall with a decrease in pulmonary vascular resistance; therefore, oxygen administration is avoided once the diagnosis has been made because of its effect on lowering pulmonary vascular resistance.

Operative considerations. Corrective operations are not available for infants with HLHS. Palliative operations include the Norwood procedure, which essentially converts the physiology from aortic atresia to pulmonary atresia by using the native pulmonary trunk as a neoaorta (Figure 8.3b). Controlled pulmonary blood flow is supplied to the disconnected branch pulmonary arteries from a systemic artery through a prosthetic, usually Gore-Tex®, shunt. An alternative (Sano shunt) inserts a valveless prosthetic tube between the right ventricle and pulmonary artery to maintain pulmonary blood flow.

A hybrid procedure, sometimes employed for infants of very low birth weight or with multiple noncardiac anomalies, may allow for delay of the cardiopulmonary bypass the Norwood procedure entails; the hybrid approach involves catheterization for ductal stenting and atrial septostomy, and surgical banding of the individual branch pulmonary arteries (Figure 8.3c). Physiologically, this limits excess pulmonary blood flow, protects the pulmonary arterioles, allows pulmonary venous blood to reach the right ventricle, and maintains systemic blood flow which is supplied from the right ventricle.

Infants palliated with a Norwood procedure have a univentricular heart and later may be candidates for cavopulmonary anastomosis (Glenn and Fontan) operations.

Because results of these palliations vary, many infants with HLHS may become candidates for cardiac transplantation. The long-term prognosis for children who have survived either of these two operative approaches is unknown. Neonates not considered for intervention die in early infancy; controversy exists as to the most suitable management for HLHS.

Summary

HLHS is a common cause of shock and congestive heart failure in the neonate. Although palliative options, including Norwood operation and transplantation, exist, mortality is higher than for most other cardiac malformations.

Coarctation of the aorta. Coarctation of the aorta (see Chapter 5), either isolated or coexisting with other cardiac malformations, is another common cause of congestive cardiac failure in neonates.

Clinical diagnosis is difficult because the low cardiac output from congestive failure minimizes the blood pressure difference between the arms and legs. Following treatment with inotropes, a blood pressure differential may develop as the cardiac output increases. Prostaglandin also helps widen the juxtaductal area of the descending aorta. Cardiomegaly and an electrocardiographic pattern of right ventricular hypertrophy and inverted ST segment and T waves in the left precordium are found. Much less frequently, aortic and pulmonary stenosis may lead to congestive cardiac failure early in life.

Interrupted aortic arch. Interrupted aortic arch (Figure 8.4), a complex anomaly resulting from the absence of a segment of the aortic arch, is associated with various degrees of hypoplasia of the left ventricular outflow tract and aortic valve; a VSD is virtually always present. The aortic arch may be interrupted distal to the left subclavian artery origin (type A) or between the left carotid artery and the left subclavian artery (type B). Many patients, particularly those with type B, have DiGeorge syndrome. Blood flow to the descending aorta is only by way of the ductus arteriosus. As the ductus undergoes normal closure, flow to the lower body is markedly reduced.

History. All patients with interrupted aortic arch as neonates have a clinical presentation similar to coarctation of the aorta, characterized by signs and symptoms of low cardiac output and shock.

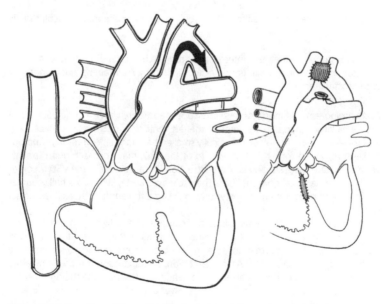

Figure 8.4 Interruption of the aortic arch. Central circulation and surgical repair.

Physical examination. Neonates have a difference in oxygen saturation between the upper (normal saturation) and lower (lower saturation) extremities because the right ventricle supplies all the lower body cardiac output via the ductus.

As the ductus arteriosus narrows, decreased lower extremity pulses become apparent, a finding similar to that in neonates with coarctation. With interruption occurring between the origin of the left carotid artery and the left subclavian artery (type B), only the right-upper extremity pulses may be palpable, whereas in neonates with interruption distal to the left subclavian artery (type A), pulses in both upper extremities may feel equal.

Ventricular function becomes reduced and all pulses may be difficult to palpate. This stage is characterized by nonspecific signs of shock, including poor perfusion, cyanosis, listlessness, and marked tachypnea. A murmur and systolic click are not usually apparent.

Electrocardiogram. The electrocardiogram shows findings similar to those of coarctation, including right ventricular enlargement/hypertrophy.

Chest X-ray. The cardiac silhouette is enlarged and pulmonary vasculature is increased.

Natural history. If untreated, interrupted aortic arch is fatal in neonates. As with coarctation, temporary palliation is accomplished by maintaining ductal patency with prostaglandin.

Echocardiogram. All neonates with interrupted aortic arch have a large VSD, often 1.5 times larger than the diameter of the left ventricular outflow tract because it and the aortic valve annulus are typically smaller than normal. A spur of infundibular septum, which forms part of the rim of the VSD, may encroach upon the left ventricular outflow tract and cause obstruction. Because of this, the VSD is sometimes termed a malalignment VSD. The ascending aorta, which is small, courses cephalad and does not curve posteriorly to become the aortic arch, as in a normal neonate.

The ductus arteriosus, which is large, curves posteriorly to join the thoracic descending aorta so seamlessly that the ductus itself may be mistaken for the aortic arch. Unlike a normal aortic arch, the brachiocephalic arteries cannot be seen arising from the ductus. As in coarctation, the ductal shunt is predominantly right to left (from pulmonary artery to descending aorta) because the right ventricle is the sole source of blood flow to the lower body.

Cardiac catheterization. Oxygen data show a left-to-right shunt at ventricular level and a right-to-left shunt via the ductus arteriosus, with normal saturation in the ascending aorta and its branches and decreased saturation in the descending aorta, corresponding to the level of right ventricular saturation.

Left ventriculography demonstrates the location of the arch interruption, the origin and courses of the aortic branches, and the degree of left ventricular outflow tract hypoplasia; the last effect is better demonstrated by echocardiography.

Operative considerations. Operation is designed to create an unobstructed connection from ascending to descending aorta and to either close or limit the flow through the VSD.

Two options exist: (i) primary repair of the arch and closure of the VSD, or (ii) repair of the arch and pulmonary artery banding, with later de-banding and VSD closure.

The latter approach may have less overall mortality risk, especially in neonates who have a hypoplastic left ventricular outflow tract that could grow in the interval between pulmonary artery banding and operative closure of the VSD. If the left ventricular outflow tract is of an inadequate size or is severely obstructed, a palliative operation, similar to a Norwood operation, can be done.

Summary

Interrupted aortic arch is a form of left heart obstruction that presents in neonates in a manner similar to coarctation of the aorta; it is highly associated with DiGeorge syndrome. The success of operative repair depends on the degree of left ventricular outflow tract hypoplasia and on whether associated noncardiac anomalies are present.

Volume overload

Volume overload placed on either ventricle may lead to neonatal cardiac failure, and may result from rare lesions such as valvular insufficiency, or arteriovenous malformations.

Systemic arteriovenous fistula or malformation (AVM). AVM (e.g. in the great vein of Galen or in the liver) results in a high-output cardiac failure and is the most common noncardiac cause. The arteriovenous fistula is associated with low systemic arterial resistance and an increased volume of blood flow through the shunt. The increased flow through the right side of the heart leads to profound cardiac symptoms early in life.

Prior to birth, cardiac failure is absent because of the normally low systemic vascular resistance prenatally. With the loss of the placenta, systemic resistance increases and so does the volume shunted through the fistula. However, systemic resistance does not rise to normal postnatal levels because of the malformation, a circumstance that contributes to clinical findings of "persistent fetal circulation." An arteriovenous fistula may be recognized by auscultation for a continuous murmur over the head, liver, or other peripheral sites and by increased pulse pressure, similar to that seen in large patent ductus arteriosus. Operative or transcatheter obliteration of the fistula, if possible, is curative, although, in some, pulmonary hypertension persists.

Chapter 9
The cardiac conditions acquired during childhood

Moller's Essentials of Pediatric Cardiology, Fourth Edition.
Walter H. Johnson, Jr. and Camden L. Hebson.
© 2023 John Wiley & Sons Ltd. Published 2023 by John Wiley & Sons Ltd.

In pediatric cardiology, congenital heart disease, arrhythmias, and murmurs have been emphasized. An important wide spectrum of other conditions affect the structure and/or function of the cardiovascular system in pediatric-aged patients. These include genetic, infectious, and inflammatory diseases and in many instances the etiology is unknown. In some patients, a cardiac condition can be suspected because of a known association between the primary disease with a specific cardiovascular abnormality. In other instances, the family history may indicate the possibility of a genetic cardiac condition. Finally, the patient may present with cardiac symptoms or signs and the underlying cardiac condition can be diagnosed.

KAWASAKI DISEASE

Kawasaki disease (mucocutaneous lymph node syndrome) is a systemic vasculitis of unknown etiology. First described in Japan in 1967 by Dr. Tomisaku Kawasaki, it is a common cause of acquired cardiac disease among children in the United States, affecting at least 5000 children yearly. It is exclusively a childhood disease, with 80% of cases occurring by the age of five years. Occasionally, adolescents and older teenagers are diagnosed with this disease. Adults may present with coronary artery aneurysms thought to be the result of undiagnosed and untreated childhood Kawasaki disease.

Coronary artery aneurysms are the most common and potentially dangerous sequelae of Kawasaki disease, occurring in one in four untreated patients. Mortality is less than 0.1%, usually from myocardial infarct, although severe myocarditis can occur. The greatest risk of death occurs in the first 45 days, often from coronary artery thrombosis, but myocardial infarction can occur years later. Other systemic arteries can be affected, and clinical overlap exists with a disseminated vasculitis, infantile polyarteritis nodosa.

Diagnosis

Clinical features
The illness is characterized by the following features: (i) bilateral conjunctivitis without discharge; (ii) erythematous mouth and dry, fissured lips; (iii) a generalized erythematous rash; (iv) nonpitting, painful induration of the hands and feet, often with marked erythema of the palms and soles; and (v) lymphadenopathy (Table 9.1). Initially, these occur with a high persistent fever without obvious origin. Patients with five days or more of high fever and at least four of these five features have Kawasaki disease, analogous to the use of the Jones criteria for the diagnosis of rheumatic fever. Kawasaki disease is much more pleomorphic than rheumatic fever, and many cases of "atypical" Kawasaki disease occur. The diagnosis remains based on clinical and laboratory findings, as no definitive laboratory test exists.

Natural history
If untreated, Kawasaki disease is self-limited, with a mean duration of 12 days for fever, although irritability and anorexia, both prominent during the febrile acute phase, often persist for two to three weeks after the fever ends. During the subacute or convalescent phase, usually from day 10 to 20 after onset of fever, most patients have a highly specific pattern of desquamation of the hands and feet that begins periungual and proceeds proximally to involve the palms and soles. Occasionally, the perineal skin desquamates. The trunk and face do not peel, in contrast to scarlet fever.

Laboratory studies
Laboratory tests are supportive but not diagnostic. The erythrocyte sedimentation rate (ESR), C-reactive protein (CRP), and other acute-phase reactants are often very elevated. The platelet count is often normal throughout the acute phase (the first 10–14 days), so it cannot be used to exclude the diagnosis. An echocardiogram (or, if unavailable, a chest radiograph to screen for cardiomegaly) and 12-lead

Table 9.1 Clinical features of Kawasaki disease.

Fever
Conjunctivitis, nonexudative, and bilateral
Erythematous and fissured oral changes
Erythematous rash
Painful hand and foot induration
Lymphadenopathy

electrocardiogram are advisable at the time of diagnosis. Echocardiography during the acute phase usually does not show aneurysms; however, diffusely enlarged coronary arteries and other nonspecific signs of mild carditis may be present. Therefore, echocardiography cannot be used to "rule out" Kawasaki disease. The echocardiogram should be repeated at about one to two weeks after diagnosis, to evaluate for possible rapidly expanding aneurysms. Echocardiogram should be repeated four to six weeks after onset of illness, since coronary artery changes may have occurred by then. Patients with carditis or aneurysms detected early require more frequent follow-up.

Treatment

Aspirin

Aspirin does not decrease the incidence of aneurysm formation, even in anti-inflammatory doses (100 mg/kg/day), although it is indicated in low dose (3–5 mg/kg/day) for inhibition of platelet aggregation.

Intravenous gamma (immune) globulin (IVGG or IVIG)

Intravenous immune globulin (IVIG) is a preparation from human plasma containing mostly nonspecific polyclonal immunoglobulin G (IgG) from several thousand donors. Treatment with IVIG (2 g/kg as a single dose) within the first 10 days after onset of fever reduces the incidence of coronary artery aneurysm from 25% to 5% or less. Treatment should be given as soon as possible after the diagnosis, and can be given even after the 10th day if inflammation is still present. Many patients show prompt and impressive resolution of fever and other acute-phase symptoms within hours after IVIG. About 10% of patients require a second treatment because of failure to improve following the initial dose.

The mechanism of action is unknown but probably involves attenuation of an autoimmune response that may be the prime pathophysiologic factor in Kawasaki arteritis.

Adverse effects of IVIG treatment are rare, but hepatitis C infection was associated with some preparations decades ago. Continuing concern over the possibility of unknown transmissible agents and the high cost of IVIG have led to its overly conservative use in atypical Kawasaki disease. As a result, many patients not treated early enough in their illness ultimately manifest aneurysms. Interestingly, only a small percentage of childhood IVIG doses are given for Kawasaki disease; most IVIG use in the United States is for other conditions.

Current guidelines also stress that infants are more likely to have an incomplete clinical picture and that empiric treatment should be considered.

The authors recommend timely treatment with IVIG whenever a reasonable suspicion of Kawasaki disease exists, even if less than five of the classic criteria are not met.

Corticosteroids and other immune mediators

Steroids in high intravenous doses over several days have been successful in up to 10% of patients who fail to respond to IVIG. Oral steroids are not a substitute for IVIG, as data from the pre-IVIG era suggest that the risk of aneurysms was unchanged or possibly higher than with aspirin alone.

Other agents, including monoclonal antibodies, infliximab, and related drugs, often relieve signs of inflammation in children who appear to fail IVIG treatment, yet prevention of aneurysms is unproven.

Follow-up care

Echocardiography

Because the peak time to detect an aneurysm by echocardiography or angiography is 30 days after onset and resolution of fever, a normal echocardiogram during the febrile period does not exclude this vascular complication. Echocardiography should be repeated within one to two weeks after treatment and at four to six weeks after the onset of illness.

Laboratory

A striking finding during the convalescent phase, thrombocytosis (often >1 000 000/mm^3) does not peak until the second week after onset of fever. Therefore, a normal platelet count during the acute phase cannot be used as evidence against a diagnosis of Kawasaki disease. The ESR slowly falls to normal over several weeks.

Low-dose aspirin

Low-dose aspirin should be started for its antiplatelet effect, although some have advocated high-dose aspirin for a variable period to aid resolution of inflammation before commencing low-dose aspirin.

Children with persistent dilation, and those with small aneurysms, may need to continue aspirin indefinitely, and those with large or rapidly dilating aneurysms may require more aggressive antithrombotic therapy early in the disease. But, usually, if coronary arteries are normal at the time of the four- to six-week echocardiogram, aspirin is discontinued.

Low-dose aspirin may confer a small risk during certain viral illnesses; it should be temporarily suspended during acute varicella or influenza and perhaps after varicella vaccination.

Recurrent disease

As in rheumatic fever, recurrent disease can develop, requiring retreatment with IVIG and aspirin and resetting of follow-up echocardiography. The risk is approximately 1 : 50, with most cases recurring within the first few months of the initial episode.

Coronary aneurysm

The natural history of patients who develop coronary artery aneurysms varies. In 90% of patients the aneurysms resolve on echocardiogram, although some have continued narrowing of the coronary artery lumen leading to stenotic lesions. Coronary artery stenoses may be impossible to image by echocardiography, and catheterization or computed tomography angiography (CTA) may be indicated.

In children with anginal symptoms or electrocardiogram abnormalities who have fully recovered from acute Kawasaki disease and who have no echocardiographically apparent lesions, nuclear myocardial perfusion scans at rest and with exercise may help in differentiating benign chest pain from true ischemia and/or infarct.

The effect of childhood Kawasaki disease (without aneurysms) on the risk of coronary atherosclerosis in adulthood is unknown.

RHEUMATIC FEVER

Rheumatic fever is a systemic disease affecting several organ systems, including the heart. It is a sequela of group A beta-hemolytic streptococcal infections, usually tonsillopharyngitis, and develops in <1% of infected patients, yet different populations may show differing susceptibilities. Rheumatic fever usually develops 10 days to 2 weeks following a streptococcal pharyngitis that almost always is associated with fever greater than 101°F (38.3°C), sore throat, and cervical adenitis. The pathogenesis of the systemic manifestations is unknown. Despite a minor resurgence in the 1980s, the incidence of rheumatic fever in North America decreased markedly in the last half of the twentieth century. Worldwide, however, rheumatic fever remains the most common cause of acquired heart disease in the young.

Rheumatic fever is diagnosed by use of the modified Jones criteria (Table 9.2). These criteria comprise the various combinations of clinical and laboratory manifestations reflecting the multiple sites of disease involvement. The original (1944) intent of the Jones criteria was to minimize overdiagnosis. Several modifications have been made to attempt to improve the balance between under- and overdiagnosis. There must be two major criteria or one major and two minor criteria, plus evidence of a preceding streptococcal infection, to diagnose acute rheumatic fever, except in recurrent cases in which three minor criteria suffice.

The proof of a prior streptococcal infection can be established by either of three methods. The first is the recovery of beta-hemolytic streptococcus by throat culture. This finding must be interpreted with care because streptococcal carrier states exist and are not considered a streptococcal infection. The second is the history of positive rapid antigen test to streptococcal group A carbohydrate. The third finding is an increase in streptococcal antibodies. Following a streptococcal infection, antibodies to various streptococcal components, such as antistreptolysin-O (ASO) and

Table 9.2 Modified Jones criteria for the diagnosis of acute rheumatic fever.

Major criteria:
  Carditis[a]
  Arthritis
  Chorea[a]
  Erythema marginatum
  Subcutaneous nodules
Minor criteria:
  Arthralgia
  Prolongation of the PR interval
  Elevated acute phase reactants (ESR and CRP)
  Fever
Other:
  Previous history of rheumatic fever[a]

[a]See "Exceptions to the Jones Criteria" noted in the text.
Evidence of prior streptococcal infection is necessary before these criteria are considered.

antideoxyribonuclease B (ant-DNase B), rise significantly. Titers for several antibodies should be measured because an individual may not form antibodies to each streptococcal product. Significant antibody rise indicates a recent streptococcal infection and is more meaningful than statically elevated titers.

Diagnosis

Jones criteria

Five major and four minor criteria (Table 9.2) can be used to fulfill the Jones criteria.

Major criteria

Carditis. Carditis can involve any layer of the heart, but valvulitis is the most consistent manifestation of rheumatic fever.

Pericarditis can occur in this disease and can be suspected by the occurrence of chest pain that may be referred to the abdomen or shoulders. It is diagnosed by finding a pericardial friction rub, ST segment elevation/depression on the electrocardiogram, or thickened pericardium or effusion by echocardiogram.

Cardiac enlargement or cardiac failure without evidence of valvar anomalies is evidence of myocardial involvement. Rarely, cardiac failure occurs from myocardial involvement itself. Various degrees of heart block, gallop rhythm, and muffled heart sounds are other manifestations of myocarditis. Prolonged PR interval in itself is not a criterion for carditis.

Valvulitis is the most serious manifestation of carditis because it can lead to permanent cardiac sequelae. Both the aortic and mitral valves may be involved acutely. Three types of murmurs may be present that suggest acute rheumatic fever. (i) An apical holosystolic murmur of mitral regurgitation is the most frequently occurring murmur. (ii) At times a mid-diastolic murmur may also be heard at the apex. The origin of this murmur is unknown, but it is perhaps related to turbulence from either valvulitis or blood flow into a dilated left ventricle. (iii) An early diastolic murmur of aortic regurgitation may be found during the acute episode but is more frequently a late manifestation. Aortic stenosis does not occur during the acute episode of rheumatic fever.

These valvar abnormalities, particularly aortic and mitral regurgitation, may be demonstrated by echocardiography and color Doppler.

The role of echocardiography in diagnosing subclinical valvar changes is now considered an essential component of diagnosis. Subclinical carditis refers to echocardiographic evidence of valvulitis in the absence of the typical murmurs noted above.

Arthritis. Typically, arthritis is migratory and several joints may be involved, often sequentially, but at a given time there may be involvement of only one joint. Usually the large joints are involved. Diagnosis of arthritis rests on finding warm and tender joints that are painful on movement. The changes are not permanent.

Chorea. Chorea is a late manifestation of rheumatic fever and often develops several months after the streptococcal infection. At that time, other manifestations of rheumatic fever may not be found. It is often said that fortunately for the patient, painful arthritis, usually an early finding, never occurs at the same time as chorea. The presence of chorea alone is sufficient for the diagnosis of rheumatic fever, as there are virtually no other causes in childhood, although lupus must be excluded. Chorea is more common in females and prior to puberty.

Chorea is characterized by involuntary, nonrepetitive, purposeless motions, often associated with emotional instability. The parents may complain that their child is clumsy, is fidgety, cries easily, or has difficulty in writing or reading.

Classic physical findings of chorea exist. The milkmaid (or grip) sign describes the fibrillatory nature of a hand grasp. Other findings are related to exaggerated muscle movements, such as the hyperextension of the hands or apposition of the backs of the hands when the arms are extended above the head. Although lasting for months in some children, it is not usually permanent.

Erythema marginatum. Erythema marginatum is a fleeting, characteristic cutaneous finding. It is characterized by pink macules with distinct sharp margins; these change rapidly in contour. Warmth tends to bring out these lesions. With time the center fades, whereas the margin persists as a circular or serpentine border. While not as common as the first three major criteria, erythema marginatum is highly specific.

Subcutaneous nodules. Subcutaneous nodules are a rare manifestation of rheumatic fever, occurring late in the course of the disease. These are non-tender, firm, pea-like nodules over the extensor surfaces, particularly over the knees, elbows, and spine. They have a strong association with chronic carditis.

Minor criteria

Arthralgia. The symptom of painful joints without subjective evidence of arthritis may be used as a minor criterion, if arthritis has not been used as a major one.

Prolongation of the PR interval. This can be used as a minor criterion, if carditis has not been used as a major one.

Elevated acute-phase reactants. Laboratory evidence of acute inflammation, such as elevated ESR or CRP, meets requirements for a minor criterion.

Fever. The temperature is usually in the range 101–102°F (38.3–38.9°C).

Exceptions to the Jones criteria

A presumptive diagnosis of rheumatic fever may be made without strict adherence to the criteria in at least three circumstances:

(1) Chorea, which may be the only manifestation.
(2) Carditis and its sequelae in patients presenting long after an episode of acute rheumatic fever.
(3) Previous history of rheumatic fever and a recent streptococcal infection, but care must be taken that the diagnosis of the previous episode of rheumatic fever was carefully made according to the Jones criteria.

In any of these situations, other etiologies must be excluded by appropriate testing. As with other diagnostic criteria, strict adherence to the Jones criteria may lead to underdiagnosis of acute rheumatic fever.

Treatment

Bedrest and activity
Bedrest was traditionally prescribed for the duration of the acute febrile period of the illness, with gradual increases in activity, provided that there was no

recurrence of signs or symptoms. Serial determination of ESR is helpful in reaching decisions concerning activity levels. The return to full activity may be achieved by six weeks in patients with arthritis as the only major criterion; but in those with carditis, three months may be advisable. There is little evidence to guide such decisions and virtually no consensus on the timing and degree of activity restriction, yet experience suggests that children do not suffer greater long-term effects from pursuing activities of daily living during their recovery.

Salicylates

Salicylates are preferred to reduce the inflammatory response, and arthritis promptly improves. Aspirin does not improve the natural history of carditis or valvulitis. Temperature associated with rheumatic fever returns to normal within a few days. Aspirin is administered in a dose sufficient to achieve a blood salicylate level of approximately 20 mg/dL (1.45 mmol/L); usually this dosage is about 75–100 mg/kg/day. Salicylates are continued until the ESR is normal, and then tapered.

Corticosteroids

Steroids have been used to treat acute rheumatic fever, but there is no evidence that they are better than aspirin in preventing cardiac valvar damage. Steroids may, however, lead to a more prompt reduction in symptoms than aspirin. Since steroids are more hazardous, their use should be reserved for patients with severe pancarditis.

A patient with acute rheumatic fever should be treated for streptococcal infection even if streptococcal cultures are negative, as described later, in the section "Prevention of Acute Rheumatic Fever".

Rheumatic fever prophylaxis ("secondary" prophylaxis)

Once patients have had an episode of rheumatic fever, the risk of developing a second episode is higher, particularly within the first five years. A slight added risk continues throughout life. Since rheumatic fever develops following a streptococcal infection, preventive measures are directed at eliminating such infections in susceptible individuals.

The American Heart Association has recommended that all patients with a history of rheumatic fever be placed on long-term penicillin prophylaxis. The duration of prophylaxis is partly determined by the presence or absence of carditis, but for children it is a minimum of 5 years or until 21 years of age, whichever is longer; some authorities recommend lifelong prophylaxis in all patients.

> *Secondary rheumatic fever prophylaxis*
>
> Penicillin can be administered in two forms: (i) penicillin V, 250 mg orally twice per day; or (ii) benzathine penicillin G, 1.2 million units, intramuscularly monthly. Some advocate a reduced dosage for children weighing ≤60 lb (27.3 kg) and ≤5 years of age (see "Additional reading"). If the patient is allergic to penicillin, sulfonamides should be given. Although sulfa drugs are not bactericidal and should not be used for the treatment of a streptococcal infection, they are bacteriostatic for streptococcus and prevent colonization of the nasopharynx. Patients allergic to penicillin and sulfonamides may receive erythromycin or another macrolide antibiotic, or an azalide.

Prevention of acute rheumatic fever ("primary" prophylaxis)

Physicians should prevent the initial episode of rheumatic fever by recognition and proper treatment of group A beta-hemolytic streptococcal infections. Only by adequate treatment of such infections can rheumatic fever be prevented. The throat of any child with the symptoms and findings of tonsillopharyngitis should be tested, because the absolute clinical differentiation of streptococcal versus viral infection is not possible.

Two types of tests are available: culture and rapid screening tests. Rapid streptococcal tests that detect the group A carbohydrate antigen are highly specific, so positive results do not demand additional culture. However, the rapid tests vary in sensitivity, so a negative result should be backed up with culture. If beta-hemolytic streptococcus is present, the throat culture becomes positive within 24 hours. The child with a positive culture may be treated; to initiate treatment at the time of culturing the child is unnecessary, since antibiotic treatment does not alter the early course of acute streptococcal tonsillopharyngitis. The aim of treatment of this infection is the eradication of the streptococcus.

> *Primary rheumatic fever prophylaxis*
>
> This is done by administering either:
>
> (1) penicillin V, 250 mg (400 000 U) orally twice or three times daily for 10 days for children, and 500 mg (800 000 U) for adolescents and adults; or
> (2) benzathine penicillin, 600 000 U for children weighing less than 60 lb (27.3 kg) and 1.2 million U for larger children and adults, intramuscularly in a single dose.

The intramuscular route is associated with a slightly better rate of eradication and is better for patients in whom compliance may be a factor. Mixtures containing procaine penicillin are often used to minimize the pain of injection.

Penicillin-allergic patients may receive erythromycin or other macrolides, but resistance is a problem in some parts of the world. First-generation cephalosporins may be used, but tetracyclines and sulfonamides are not advisable for acute streptococcal eradication.

Long-term care

After the acute episode of rheumatic fever, the patient should be seen periodically. The purposes of these visits are to (i) emphasize the continuing need for penicillin prophylaxis for rheumatic fever and (ii) to observe for the development of valvar rheumatic heart disease.

In half of patients with evidence of valvar abnormality during the acute episode, the murmurs disappear, but over a period of years the other half may develop more severe cardiac manifestations, such as mitral stenosis, mitral regurgitation, or aortic regurgitation. These patients may ultimately require a cardiac operation or intervention.

MYOCARDIAL DISEASES

The term *myocardial disease* includes a variety of conditions affecting principally the myocardium that lead to similar clinical and physiologic states. It excludes obvious valvar heart disease, cardiac malformations, hypertension, and coronary arterial disease.

Despite the various etiologic factors of myocardial disease, the major signs and symptoms are similar. Because of the myocardial involvement, there is failure of the heart to (i) act as a pump, (ii) initiate and maintain its rhythm, and (iii) maintain its architecture. Each of these three effects of myocardial involvement has clinical and laboratory findings in common.

The inability of the myocardium to act efficiently as a pump is shown clinically by features of congestion and inadequate forward flow of blood. Symptoms of fatigue, angina, dizziness, and exercise intolerance indicate inadequate systemic output. Signs of congestive cardiac failure are found: pulmonary edema, dyspnea, hepatomegaly, peripheral edema, and gallop rhythm.

Cardiac arrhythmias are common. Two types of arrhythmias can be present. Slowing of conduction, particularly through the atrioventricular node, may occur, leading to first-degree, or more advanced, heart block. Ectopic pacemaker sites may develop, leading to atrial or ventricular tachycardias. Low-voltage QRS complexes and abnormalities of repolarization are also common.

Finally, a group of signs and symptoms relate to the inability of the heart to maintain its normal muscular architecture. The most obvious finding on clinical examination is the displacement of the cardiac apex. Cardiomegaly is found on the chest X-ray and may be so extensive as to interfere with the left-sided bronchi, resulting in atelectasis of the left lower lobe. Mitral regurgitation may develop from either dilation of the mitral ring or papillary muscle dysfunction. Prominent third and fourth heart sounds develop and are related to increased left ventricular filling pressure.

Typically, infants present with congestive cardiac failure, cardiomegaly (particularly involving the left side of the heart), absence of a cardiac murmur, and faint heart sounds. In older children, the features develop more gradually.

The myocardial diseases may be divided into three broad categories: myocarditis, myocardial disease of obscure origin (idiopathic dilated, hypertrophic, and restrictive cardiomyopathies), and myocardial involvement with systemic disease.

Myocarditis

The myocardium may be involved in an inflammatory process related to infectious agents, autoimmune (collagen-vascular) disease, or unknown causes. Although many instances are considered to be of viral origin, this relationship is often difficult to prove, even using molecular biologic techniques to evaluate for viral genome. Within diseased myocytes, echo, coxsackie, and rubella viruses have been associated with myocarditis in childhood. Severe acute respiratory syndrome coronavirus 2 (SARS CoV-2) and coronavirus (COVID-19) have been associated both with acute myocarditis during infection and as a feature of multisystem inflammatory syndrome in children (MIS-C) several weeks following acute infection. A mild and usually self-limited form of carditis has been associated with COVID vaccine.

Idiopathic myocarditis is generally a disease of the neonatal period or early infancy, but occurs sporadically thereafter. Onset may be abrupt, with sudden cardiovascular collapse and death within hours, or the development of congestive cardiac failure may be more gradual. The cardiac failure may respond well to treatment. The infant is mottled and has weak peripheral pulses. Evidence of cardiomegaly is found clinically and the heart sounds are muffled. Sinus tachycardia is a regular feature and episodic tachyarrhythmias are common. The electrocardiogram shows normal or reduced QRS voltages. ST-segment depression and T-wave inversion are usually found in the left precordial leads. Cardiomegaly and pulmonary congestion are seen on chest X-ray. The echocardiogram shows a dilated left atrium and left ventricle with a global decrease in contractility. Mitral regurgitation is almost always present, even without a murmur. Frequently, a mitral regurgitation murmur is noted only after treatment results in improved cardiac output.

The prognosis varies. Corticosteroids and other immunosuppressants may be indicated when autoimmune disease is the etiology of myocardial dysfunction, but they are not beneficial in apparent myocarditis. IVIG has been used to attenuate the inflammatory response in myocarditis. Some patients spontaneously improve to normal cardiac structure and function without treatment or with only symptomatic therapy. Treatment with anticongestive heart failure drugs (see Chapter 11) usually improves the patient's status, although the course may be chronic with long-standing evidence of cardiomegaly. Many patients progress slowly over several months or years to irreversible severe myocardial dysfunction and death; cardiac transplant may be the only option for survival.

Myocardial disease of obscure origin

Dilated cardiomyopathy. This diffuse group of diseases, usually of unknown etiology, shows no evidence of myocardial inflammation. Most pediatric conditions in this category are clinically and pathologically indistinguishable, with the following notable exceptions.

Anomalous origin of the left coronary artery. In the differential diagnosis of infants with manifestations of primary myocardial disease, anomalous origin of the left coronary artery from the pulmonary artery leads to similar findings but differs from the others in being a congenital anomaly and one that may be improved by operation.

In this condition, the left coronary artery arises from the pulmonary artery, whereas the right coronary artery arises normally from the aorta. As a result, the left ventricular myocardium is poorly perfused because of the low pulmonary artery pressure, so that ischemia and infarction occur. Subsequently, collaterals develop between the high-pressure right and the low-pressure left coronary arterial systems. In this situation, blood flows from the right into the left coronary arterial system. The left ventricular myocardium is poorly perfused because blood flows in a retrograde direction into the pulmonary artery.

History. Neonates are usually asymptomatic. Around the age of six weeks, they typically develop episodes described as angina. The infant suddenly cries as if in pain, becomes pale, and perspires profusely. These episodes are short and are believed to represent transient myocardial ischemia. Other children may show no symptoms, but many of the patients develop signs and symptoms of congestive cardiac failure. The lesion is sometimes recognized only at postmortem examination (e.g. in the adolescent patient who dies suddenly during a sports activity).

Physical examination. The child usually appears normal. No abnormal auscultatory findings may exist, or a soft, apical holosystolic murmur of mitral regurgitation may be found.

Electrocardiogram. The electrocardiogram is usually diagnostic, showing a pattern of anterolateral myocardial infarction, manifested by deep Q waves and inverted T waves in leads I, aVL, V_5, and V_6. In a few patients, it shows only left ventricular hypertrophy and strain or a pattern of complete left bundle branch block.

Chest X-ray. The chest X-ray reveals cardiomegaly and a left ventricular contour.

Echocardiography. Echocardiography shows nonspecific cardiac dilation and left ventricular dysfunction. Only the right coronary artery, which is enlarged, can be identified arising from the aorta. Using color Doppler, the origin of the anomalous coronary artery may be seen as a jet of flow from the left coronary artery into the pulmonary artery.

Management. Patients with cardiac failure should receive anticongestive therapy and should undergo cardiac catheterization or CTA to precisely define the anatomy. Surgical options include reimplantation of the left coronary artery to the aorta, or surgical creation of a tunnel within the pulmonary artery to establish continuity between the coronary artery and the aorta. Cardiac transplantation may be indicated in patients with severe irreversible left ventricular damage.

Anthracycline cardiotoxicity. Anthracycline chemotherapeutic agents, such as doxorubicin (Adriamycin®), through unclear mechanisms possibly involving excessive oxygen radical formation, can cause a cardiomyopathy. Most chemotherapeutic protocols limit the cumulative dose of these agents to 400 mg/m², because the incidence of cardiac dysfunction rises sharply with larger doses. A small number of patients, however, develop cardiac failure at levels below that considered the threshold for toxicity, suggesting that the toxic effect occurs at a low dose but only manifests clinically in certain patients. Patients may develop chronic congestive heart failure years after the conclusion of therapy.

Treatment is nonspecific, as with other dilated cardiomyopathies. Various drugs are being investigated that may prevent cardiac injury during chemotherapy.

Endocardial fibroelastosis. Endocardial fibroelastosis (EFE) was a common cause of dilated cardiomyopathy in the 1950s and 1960s but since then has virtually disappeared. Some believe it resulted from a viral infection, possibly mumps. The endocardium could be 2 mm thick, whereas in the normal individual it is only a few cells thick. The myocardium showed minimal change.

The disease usually presented in infancy as congestive cardiac failure. Electrocardiograms showed left ventricular hypertrophy and inverted T waves in the left precordial leads. Gross cardiomegaly, particularly of the left atrium and left ventricle, was seen on chest X-ray.

The echocardiogram showed a strikingly echogenic endocardium, left ventricular enlargement, decreased systolic function, and mitral regurgitation. (A similar echocardiographic picture, from subendocardial ischemia accompanying severe aortic stenosis, is often called EFE.)

Tachycardia-induced cardiomyopathy. Tachycardia-induced cardiomyopathy is a rare but curable type of dilated cardiomyopathy. It is caused by an incessant tachyarrhythmia, either ventricular or "supraventricular" (see Chapter 10). Certain rare types of supraventricular tachyarrhythmias, automatic (ectopic) atrial tachycardia (AET or EAT), and the permanent form of junctional reciprocating tachycardia (PJRT) are particularly likely to cause myocardial dysfunction. Although PJRT has a distinctive electrocardiographic appearance – deep negative P waves in leads II, III, and aVF – other chronic tachyarrhythmias may be difficult to diagnose because they masquerade as sinus tachycardia, a common, nonspecific feature of dilated cardiomyopathy.

Following elimination of the tachyarrhythmia, normal cardiac function usually recovers, although some degree of left ventricular dilation may persist.

Hypertrophic cardiomyopathy (idiopathic hypertrophic subaortic stenosis). In hypertrophic cardiomyopathy (HCM), also known as idiopathic hypertrophic subaortic stenosis (IHSS), the myocardium is greatly thickened, but not in response to pressure overload. The hypertrophy may be concentric, involving the ventricular walls diffusely, or asymmetric, unevenly affecting portions of the wall, usually the ventricular septum.

In contrast to dilated cardiomyopathy, the left ventricular cavity has a normal or decreased size. During systole, the hypertrophied myocardium bulges into the left ventricular outflow tract and may result in subaortic obstruction. Other names for this condition are hypertrophic obstructive cardiomyopathy and asymmetric septal hypertrophy.

HCM has pleomorphic clinical features and course, with some patients progressing to obstruction, others to malignant arrhythmia, and still others to predominant diastolic dysfunction. The disease may be caused by mutations of genes coding for various contractile proteins, and less commonly, as the result of certain storage diseases. This condition frequently occurs as an autosomal dominant or sex-linked condition (occurring in males). Multiple generations may be involved. The natural history and prognosis are variable; sudden death is not uncommon, even in patients who have no important obstruction or sentinel arrhythmia.

History. Syncope may be present, but congestive cardiac failure is rare unless significant diastolic dysfunction is present. Chest pain and palpitations, common benign symptoms in children, may result from myocardial ischemia and/or obstruction and ventricular tachycardia associated with HCM. The family history may reveal other members with similar diagnosis or a history of sudden death.

Physical examination. The peripheral pulses are brisk, and palpation of the apex may reveal a double impulse. A long systolic ejection murmur is present along the left sternal border and faintly radiates to the base. The murmur varies in intensity with change in the patient's body position; it is usually loudest with the patient standing, in contrast to functional flow murmurs. Third and fourth sounds may be present.

Electrocardiogram. The electrocardiogram shows a normal QRS axis, left ventricular hypertrophy, and occasionally left atrial enlargement. ST-segment and T-wave changes are common. Deep Q waves may be found in the left precordial leads. Conduction abnormalities of a nonspecific nature may alter the QRS complex.

Chest X-ray. Chest X-ray does not usually show cardiac enlargement related to the left ventricle and left atrium because hypertrophy alone may not alter the external silhouette. In contrast to other forms of aortic stenosis, the ascending aorta (AAO) is usually of normal size.

Echocardiogram. The echocardiogram shows striking thickening of the left ventricular walls, particularly the interventricular septum, which may be 2–3 cm thick, compared with the normal 1 cm.

Systolic anterior motion (SAM) of the mitral valve anterior leaflet is a classic two-dimensional (2D) echocardiographic finding. SAM results from the high-velocity flow occurring in the left ventricular outflow tract. This creates low pressure that "pulls" the valve leaflet toward the interventricular septum during systole.

Color Doppler reveals disturbed flow within the left ventricular outflow tract, beginning proximal to the aortic valve. Spectral Doppler allows estimation of the systolic gradient by measurement of the maximum velocity; this may change from beat to beat because of the dynamic nature of the muscular obstruction.

Management. Because the subsequent therapies increase the gradient, the use of digoxin or other inotropes is contraindicated in these patients. Beta-blockers, calcium channel blockers, and other "negative inotropes" have been advocated for these patients but do not necessarily prevent sudden death.

Implantable cardioverter/defibrillator (ICD) devices may abort potentially lethal arrhythmia in some patients.

Surgical excision of portions of the septal myocardium (myomectomy) has been helpful in some patients with obstruction. Alcohol injected via a coronary artery catheter can achieve a form of nonsurgical myomectomy by selectively destroying obstructing myocardium. Ventricular pacing via a transvenous right ventricular electrode may reduce the gradient in some patients, presumably by altering the activation sequence of the left ventricular myocardium, but the response varies.

Restrictive cardiomyopathy. This, the rarest of the three general types of cardiomyopathy, is characterized by poor ventricular compliance and limited filling. Some patients have a mutation of myocardial regulatory proteins, such as troponin, but most forms are idiopathic.

Symptoms are nonspecific and similar to those of congestive heart failure seen with dilated cardiomyopathy. In contrast to dilated cardiomyopathy, the left ventricle is of normal size and may have normal systolic function. Unlike HCM, the left ventricular walls are normal in thickness. This condition alters diastolic ventricular function, so the clinical manifestations are those of elevated left and right atrial pressures.

Examination reveals hepatic and splenic enlargement and jugular venous distension. Electrocardiographic abnormalities are usually limited to atrial enlargement. Chest X-ray shows pulmonary vascular congestion with a relatively normal cardiac silhouette.

The echocardiogram reveals striking dilation of the atria and great veins but normal or small ventricles. Physiologically, the condition is similar to restrictive pericarditis; differentiating the two can be difficult.

The prognosis is poor, as clinical decline is often rapid and mortality high. Cardiac transplantation is the only effective treatment.

Myocardial involvement with systemic disease

The myocardium of children with certain generalized diseases may be altered by the particular disease process. Children may present clinically with features of dilated, hypertrophic, or restrictive pathophysiology. Inflammatory changes may occur in conditions such as lupus erythematosus. Abnormal substances may accumulate in the heart, as in glycogen storage disease type II (Hurler syndrome). Myocardial fibrosis may develop in neuromuscular disease such as Friedreich's ataxia or muscular dystrophy.

Glycogen storage disease, type II (Pompe disease)

Deficiency of the enzyme acid maltase (acid alpha-glucosidase or α-1,4-glucosidase) leads to accumulation of glycogen in the myocardium, which becomes thickened to more than twice normal.

The infants present within the first three months with congestive cardiac failure because of the cardiac involvement. Generalized skeletal muscular weakness is prominent clinically because of its involvement. The liver, which may contain increased glycogen content, is enlarged out of proportion to the degree of cardiac failure.

Cardiac examination is unrevealing except for evidence of cardiomegaly. The electrocardiogram is diagnostic, showing greatly increased QRS voltages, often a shortened PR interval, and a delta wave consistent with Wolff–Parkinson–White (WPW) syndrome. Cardiomegaly, particularly left ventricular enlargement, is found.

The prognosis is poor; death occurs in the first year of life without therapy. Bone marrow transplantation and enzyme replacement therapy have been employed with generally increased survival but with variable response.

Hurler syndrome, Hunter syndrome, and other mucopolysaccharidoses

These storage diseases affect the heart to variable degrees, but less severely than in Pompe disease. Valves may become thick and regurgitant. Coronary artery changes occur prematurely.

Neuromuscular diseases

These include Friedreich's ataxia, a neurodegenerative disease, with an abnormal electrocardiogram (most commonly nonspecific ST–T changes) and variable expression of both hypertrophic and dilated cardiomyopathy. The cardiac findings may precede the onset of neurologic symptoms.

Duchenne muscular dystrophy and similar diseases frequently show electrocardiographic abnormalities (including ST–T changes, right bundle branch block (RBBB), and abnormalities of the QRS axis), some of which may relate to the chronic hypoventilation that accompanies the patient's progressive skeletal muscle weakness.

Both disorders may manifest dilated, hypertrophic, and/or restrictive type cardiomyopathy. The severity of the cardiac dysfunction may be masked by the limitations to physical activity imposed by the skeletal muscle disease. Although heart failure and arrhythmias can occur, these patients almost always succumb to progressive muscular weakness leading to respiratory failure.

Tuberous sclerosis

Tuberous sclerosis is a phacomatosis manifesting with seizures and skin findings, such as hypopigmented macules ("ash leaf spots"), facial angiomas, and a typical facial lesion, adenoma sebaceum.

The myocardium often contains benign tumors, rhabdomyomas, which can be extremely large, especially in neonates. These tend to dwindle in size with age and may even disappear. Although, rarely, obstruction or an arrhythmia from cardiac rhabdomyoma may occur, myocardial performance is normal in most; the diagnosis is often made from incidental echocardiogram findings in a child being evaluated for other complaints, such as murmur.

Considerations in the differential diagnosis of cardiomyopathy

In infancy, the underlying cause of cardiomyopathy is often indicated by the electrocardiographic and echocardiographic findings. Although most causes of cardiomyopathy are associated with ST-segment and T-wave changes, the QRS patterns may differ.

Myocarditis shows normal or reduced QRS voltages; glycogen storage disease, with greatly increased voltages; EFE, with left ventricular hypertrophy and strain; and anomalous left coronary artery, with a pattern of anterolateral myocardial infarction. Infants with incessant tachycardia, especially with an abnormal or frequently changing P-wave axis, may have tachycardia-induced cardiomyopathy.

The echocardiogram can visualize the size and function of the ventricles, particularly the left, whether the wall is thickened or the chamber is dilated or normal in size. Abnormalities of the coronary arteries or the presence of rhabdomyomas are examples of precise echocardiographic diagnoses.

In the older child, other clinical signs and symptoms are related to the underlying disease, such as the characteristic facies and habitus of Hurler syndrome or the presence of the recurrent fever and antinuclear antibodies in a patient with myocardial involvement in lupus erythematosus. Often, however, no findings exist that allow an etiologic diagnosis because many cases are of unknown origin.

Management of myocardial diseases

Management of myocardial disease is directed at the cardiovascular problems developing from the myocardial involvement. Specific treatment is rarely available for the underlying condition. The major therapeutic efforts address cardiac failure and diminished cardiac output. Mainstays of drug therapy include inotropes (e.g. digoxin) to improve myocardial contraction, diuretics, such as furosemide, to control pulmonary congestion, and afterload reduction (see Chapter 11).

Cardiomyopathies may lead to mitral regurgitation, probably not so much from dilation of the mitral annulus as from papillary muscle dysfunction. The regurgitation may be from infarction of the papillary muscle or subjacent ventricular wall or ventricular dilation leading to abnormal position of papillary muscles. Regardless of the cause, if major mitral regurgitation results, the left ventricular volume load is further increased; and congestive cardiac failure worsens. Annuloplasty (plication of the mitral ring) or replacement of the mitral valve may have a strikingly beneficial effect, but surgical mortality is high.

Cardiac arrhythmias, both heart block and tachyarrhythmias, occur and may require treatment. Heart block may not require treatment if the patient is asymptomatic. Should syncope occur or congestive cardiac failure worsen, pacemaker implantation may be indicated.

Tachyarrhythmias, such as premature contractions, are usually ventricular in origin and may be harbingers of ventricular tachycardia. Supraventricular tachyarrhythmias, such as atrial flutter or fibrillation, may develop secondary to atrial dilation and require treatment, as they often worsen the cardiac status. Except for treatment of incessant tachyarrhythmias which cause cardiomyopathy, treatment of secondary arrhythmias is controversial. Aggressive drug therapy of secondary rhythm abnormalities may increase mortality, perhaps because of their proarrhythmic effect on the abnormal myocardium or by worsening of myocardial function, because most of these drugs are negative inotropes. Implantation of automatic defibrillators may slightly prolong survival in some patients but may not improve the quality of life.

The overall prognosis of primary myocardial disease is unknown and variable, since a number of diseases cause this symptom complex. Without specific etiologic diagnosis, it is difficult to give a precise prognosis. Some conditions, such as idiopathic myocardial hypertrophy, progress and lead to death, whereas others, such as myocarditis, improve but may cause residual cardiac abnormalities.

Cardiac transplantation (see Chapter 11) is reserved for patients who are severely ill and have a poor prognosis for recovery because of a deteriorating clinical course. Transplantation is often a difficult choice in a severely ill child near death but who (rarely) might recover good cardiac function without transplantation. Recipients must have suitable pulmonary vascular resistance determined by pretransplantation catheterization; otherwise, the right ventricle of the donor heart fails acutely and the patient dies. Donor organs for children are scarce, so many succumb to their disease before a suitable organ is available. Side effects of antirejection medication can be considerable and are a major factor in post-transplant mortality. Children who have been bedridden for months or years with severe cardiac failure often become asymptomatic and return to normal activity within days of successful cardiac transplantation. Because rejection cannot be controlled completely, surveillance for its effects, particularly myocardial dysfunction and a unique form of coronary artery occlusive disease, is necessary over the long term.

INFECTIVE ENDOCARDITIS
Infective endocarditis involves bacterial or fungal invasion of the endocardium or endothelium of the great vessels.

This condition usually occurs in a patient with congenital or rheumatic heart disease but occasionally develops without pre-existing heart disease.

Infective endocarditis has been divided into subacute and acute forms – the latter is of shorter duration, is more commonly caused by a staphylococcus, and more frequently occurs without pre-existing heart disease. This classification has limited use clinically because considerable overlap exists between acute and subacute types.

Streptococcus viridans is the most common causative agent; *Streptococcus faecalis* and *Staphylococcus aureus* occur less frequently. Rarely, other bacteria or fungi are involved. Fungal endocarditis occurs more commonly in immunocompromised patients and in those with an indwelling line or a prosthetic valve.

Infective endocarditis usually occurs in cardiac conditions with a large pressure difference. A high-velocity jet results and creates an endocardial lesion susceptible to blood-borne bacteria. The cardiac malformations most often associated with endocarditis are ventricular septal defect, patent ductus arteriosus, aortic stenosis, and tetralogy of Fallot. Endocarditis also occurs in patients with an aorticopulmonary shunt, such as a Blalock–Taussig shunt. It can involve the mitral or aortic valves in patients with rheumatic heart disease. Endocarditis is extremely rare in patients with atrial septal defect.

The lesion of endocarditis is a vegetation consisting of fibrin, leukocytes, platelets, and bacteria. Many clinical manifestations are related to destructive aspects of the infection or to embolization of portions of the vegetation. Endocarditis, particularly from staphylococcus, may cause valvar damage, including perforation of aortic cusps or ruptured chordae tendinae of the mitral valve. Embolization may occur into either the pulmonary or the systemic circulations and cause infarction, abscess, or inflammation of various tissues. Emboli to the lungs, kidneys, spleen, or brain are reported most frequently because of their major clinical or laboratory findings.

Efforts should be made to prevent the development of bacterial endocarditis in children with cardiac anomalies (see Chapter 12).

History

Endocarditis rarely occurs before the age of five years. Fever, weight loss, anemia, and elevation of the ESR and CRP are common but nonspecific clinical findings of bacterial endocarditis. The diagnosis should be suspected in any child with a significant cardiac murmur and a prolonged fever. An age exception is premature infants with an indwelling catheter who can become infected with a fungus.

Physical examination

The appearance of a new murmur may indicate endocarditis. A change in murmur intensity is not necessarily an indication of endocarditis, since cardiac output and murmur loudness increase normally with fever.

Congestive cardiac failure may develop, especially if aortic or mitral valve regurgitation is created by the infection. Half of patients with endocarditis have signs or symptoms of embolic phenomenon. Signs of recurrent pneumonia or a pleuritic type of pain may indicate embolization of infected material to the lungs. Signs of systemic embolization, such as splenomegaly, hematuria, splinter hemorrhages, and central nervous system signs, should be sought in any febrile patient with a cardiac anomaly.

Laboratory findings

The diagnosis is confirmed by obtaining the organisms from a blood culture. At least six blood cultures should be taken within the first 12 or 24 hours that endocarditis is suspected.

It is not necessary to wait for a fever spike, since the chance of obtaining a positive culture depends primarily upon the volume of blood drawn.

It is important that blood cultures of ample volume be obtained prior to antibiotics; otherwise the chance of recovering an organism is reduced by an estimated 40%.

Nonspecific acute-phase reactants such as ESR, CRP, and rheumatoid factor are usually very elevated; the tests are useful in following the progress of therapy.

Echocardiography is not usually helpful in making a diagnosis, because the absence of valve changes or vegetations does not exclude endocarditis. Echocardiography can be helpful by confirming acute changes in valve function suspected clinically. When vegetations are seen, they may persist long after successful antibiotic treatment is concluded. Endocarditis is a clinical and a laboratory diagnosis, not necessarily an echocardiographic diagnosis.

Treatment

If the patient is very ill or if the clinical findings are typical, antibiotic treatment can be initiated immediately after the cultures have been obtained and before the results of cultures are available. If the diagnosis is questionable, initiation of therapy should await the results of the blood cultures.

The general principles of treatment are that antibiotics must be parenteral (usually intravenously administered, although some limited use of oral antibiotics after initial parenteral treatment is currently being used in some adults) and bactericidal, and that treatment must be prolonged. The exact treatment depends on the organism isolated and its antibiotic sensitivities.

Initial empiric treatment varies according to the clinical situation: for example, whether the patient has been treated with antibiotics prior to cultures, whether prosthetic valves, material, or devices such as pacing leads are present, and whether the presentation is acute (and more likely to be staphylococcal) or subacute. Other considerations are patient allergy to particular drugs and the knowledge of local antibiotic resistance patterns. Several regimens have been proposed. Usually, a penicillin (e.g. ampicillin, amoxicillin) or vancomycin (until *S. aureus* has been excluded) are the preferred initial antibiotics and are given in large dosages parenterally. Antibiotics may need to be changed if antibiotic sensitivities so indicate. Low-dose gentamicin, rifampin, or other antibiotics are often added for synergistic effect. Intravenous therapy is continued for four to six weeks.

During and following completion of therapy, blood cultures should be obtained to verify eradication of the infection.

Despite the availability of antimicrobials, endocarditis can lead to major complications, such as valvar damage or permanent sequelae resulting from embolization; occasionally, the disease is fatal.

MARFAN SYNDROME

Marfan syndrome is an autosomal dominant disease affecting connective tissue and leading to characteristic physical findings and cardiac lesions. A mutation of the gene *FBN1*, on chromosome 15, coding for the structural protein fibrillin is usually the cause. Marfan syndrome patients are typically tall and thin, showing a high incidence of kyphoscoliosis, pectus carinatum or excavatum, arachnodactyly, high-arched palate, and loose joints. Dislocation of the lens is common.

Cardiac anomalies occur in almost all patients and lead to premature death, although death rarely occurs in childhood. Aneurysmal dilation of the AAO and aortic sinuses occurs and leads to aortic regurgitation, which may become severe. Dissecting aneurysms can develop in the AAO and lead to death. Mitral valve prolapse and regurgitation are common, resulting from elongated chordae tendinae and redundant valve leaflets.

Genetic testing may be helpful, especially for the family members of patients known to have an *FBN1* mutation or deletion. The differential diagnosis includes other conditions from which patients may be at risk for aortopathy, such as Loeys–Dietz syndrome, some forms of Ehlers–Danlos syndrome, and disorders associated with other rarer gene mutations affecting the integrity of the aorta and other arteries.

Criteria for diagnosis are available, most recently published as the article "The revised Ghent nosology for the Marfan syndrome" (see "Additional reading").

Physical examination

General physical findings have been described earlier. Cardiac auscultation may be normal, or a systolic ejection click may result from aortic root dilation. If aortic regurgitation is present, an early diastolic murmur may or may not be audible. Mitral valve prolapse, if present, creates sounds as described in the next main section "Mitral valve prolapse".

Electrocardiogram

The electrocardiogram is usually normal, unless the heart is displaced by severe pectus excavatum or unless chamber enlargement from associated aortic or mitral regurgitation exists.

Chest X-ray

The chest X-ray may be normal or can show dilation of the AAO. Pectus excavatum, scoliosis, and other skeletal anomalies may be evident.

Echocardiogram

An echocardiogram is useful for the screening and diagnosis of patients suspected of Marfan syndrome (Figure 9.1). For patients diagnosed with a connective tissue

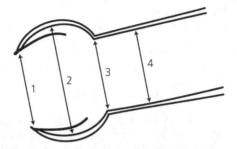

Figure 9.1 Two-dimensional echocardiographic assessment of the aortic root in Marfan syndrome. A parasternal long axis view of the aortic root in systole is used to measure diameter at four levels (1–4), denoted annulus (ANN), sinuses of Valsalva (SOV), sinoaortic ridge (SAR), and ascending aorta (AAO), respectively. These dimensions are usually referenced to the individual patient's body size (traditionally, body surface area; BSA) and compared against normal persons of similar size; however, there are many ways to accomplish this and there is no single agreed-upon standard normal data set for the calculation of a z-score. Additional references for health professionals and diagnostic aids, including z-score calculators, are available from the Marfan Foundation at www.marfan.org.

disorder, periodic echocardiography is indicated to detect progressive aortic dilation and valve regurgitation.

Treatment
Many children with Marfan syndrome are asymptomatic, but treatment with beta-blockers (e.g. atenolol and propranolol) or other drugs (angiotensin receptor blockers) has been recommended to reduce or slow aortic dilation.

Aortic surgery is performed prophylactically to reduce the risk of sudden death by aortic dissection.

The timing of aortic surgery depends on family history and individual patient findings, such as the presence of aortic dissection, important valvar regurgitation, rapid enlargement of the aortic root, and absolute size of the aorta. Guidelines that have been proposed include the following:

- In children, enlargement of the AAO diameter by >10 mm/year.
- In adolescents and adults, enlargement of the AAO diameter by >5 mm/year or absolute aortic diameter of >45–50 mm (the lower number advised for patients with a family history of dissection).

Severe aortic or mitral regurgitation requires valve replacement. Replacement of the aortic valve is often combined with replacement of the AAO with a prosthetic graft or homograft to prevent dissecting aneurysm. In some patients, the aortic root is replaced with prosthetic material, leaving the native aortic valve in place. The long-term prognosis following these operations is good, but other segments of the aorta may remain at risk for aneurysm and dissection.

MITRAL VALVE PROLAPSE

Mitral valve prolapse, originally thought to occur predominantly in females, may be equally prevalent in males. Usually first recognized in adolescence, it is rare in childhood; thus, it may represent an acquired condition or a congenital condition with late presentation, analogous to connective tissue disorders.

When a child is diagnosed with mitral valve prolapse, subtle congenital anomalies, such as mitral cleft or anomalous coronary artery, must be ruled out, in addition to acquired disorders such as hyperthyroidism or cardiac inflammatory diseases, genetic conditions including Marfan syndrome, and certain storage diseases including mucopolysaccharidoses.

A positive family history may exist, but the etiology and pathology are largely unknown. Because of its seeming ubiquitous nature in young adults and the lack of consensus about what constitutes prolapse, controversy persists about the true incidence.

Various symptoms are often attributed to mitral valve prolapse, including chest pain, palpitations, near-syncope, syncope, and "panic attacks." Controlled studies have failed to show a strong correlation between patients with these symptoms and those with mitral prolapse. The symptoms may represent a mild form of autonomic nervous system dysfunction, for which mitral prolapse is a weak marker.

Physical examination

The auscultatory findings are diagnostic. At the apex a mid- or late-systolic murmur exists that often begins with one or multiple mid-systolic to late-systolic clicks. The characteristics of the murmur vary. Any maneuver that decreases left ventricular diastolic volume, such as a Valsalva maneuver, standing, or inhalation of amyl nitrate, causes the murmur to begin earlier and last longer. The increase in murmur intensity with the patient standing is similar to that in HCM and is unlike innocent flow murmurs. The click occurs earlier with standing and later with squatting or in the supine position.

Laboratory findings

The electrocardiogram and chest X-ray are usually normal in the absence of significant regurgitation.

Echocardiography may show either one or both mitral valve leaflets prolapsing into the left atrium. The prolapse occurs maximally in mid-systole and may be associated with mitral regurgitation beginning in mid or late systole. Mitral regurgitation is easily demonstrated by color Doppler. Current equipment is sufficiently sensitive that "physiologic" trace mitral regurgitation is commonly seen in normal individuals without prolapse.

Treatment
The prognosis is good for patients with mitral valve prolapse. There is very little risk of sudden death, provided that mitral regurgitation is not severe and that mitral prolapse is not related to another condition, such as intrinsic cardiomyopathy, systemic disorder, or myocardial ischemic problem. Embolic stroke is so rare that the association with mitral prolapse remains controversial. Endocarditis is rare in individuals with mitral valve prolapse, and the indications for prophylactic antibiotics are controversial; the American Heart Association no longer recommends routine prophylaxis. Some with marked mitral regurgitation and/or myxomatous valve leaflets may be at greater risk and the decision to provide prophylaxis is individualized.

PERICARDITIS
Pericarditis can result from a variety of diseases. The most common in our experience are (i) idiopathic, presumed viral; (ii) purulent; (iii) juvenile rheumatoid arthritis or systemic lupus erythematosus; (iv) uremia; (v) neoplastic diseases; and (vi) postoperative (postpericardiotomy syndrome).

In these conditions, both the pericardial sac and the visceral pericardium are involved. As a result of the inflammation, fluid may accumulate within the sac. The symptoms that result from pericardial fluid depend on the status of the myocardium and the volume and the speed at which the fluid accumulates. A slow accumulation of a large volume is better tolerated than the rapid accumulation of a small volume.

Cardiac tamponade can develop because of fluid accumulation within the pericardial sac. The pericardial fluid can compress the heart and interfere with ventricular filling. Three mechanisms compensate for the tamponade: (i) elevation of atrial and ventricular end-diastolic pressures; (ii) tachycardia to compensate for lowered stroke volume; and (iii) increased diastolic blood pressure from peripheral vasoconstriction to compensate for diminished cardiac output. These compensatory mechanisms must be considered in selecting medical treatment.

Clinical and laboratory findings are related to (i) inflammation of the pericardium, (ii) cardiac tamponade, and (iii) etiologic factors.

History and physical examination

Pericarditis is accompanied by pain in about half of patients. This pain may be dull, sharp, or stabbing. It is located in the left thorax, neck, or shoulder and is improved when the patient is sitting.

A pericardial friction rub, a rough scratchy sound, may be present over the precordium. It is louder when the patient is sitting, or when the stethoscope is pressed firmly against the chest wall. The rub is evanescent, so repeated examinations may be needed to identify it. No relationship between the amount of pericardial fluid and the presence of a rub has been found, but with a large effusion a rub is often not heard.

Cardiac tamponade is reflected by several physical findings. The patient may appear to be in distress and more comfortable when sitting. The neck veins are distended and, in contrast to normal, increase on inspiration. The heart sounds may be muffled. Hepatomegaly may be present. Tachycardia develops and is a valuable means of following the patient. As the stroke volume falls because of the tamponade and limited ventricular filling, the heart rate increases to maintain cardiac output. The pulse pressure also narrows, and this can be measured accurately and serially to follow the patient's course. Peripheral pulses diminish as systemic vasoconstriction heightens and the pulse pressure narrows. Central pulses diminish because of the narrow pulse pressure and decreased stroke volume.

Excess pulsus paradoxus, a decrease in pulse pressure of more than 20 mmHg with inspiration (normal is less than 10 mmHg), is also highly diagnostic of tamponade and can often be identified by palpation of the radial pulse. It is not absolutely specific for tamponade – it often occurs in a severe asthmatic episode, for example.

Historical and physical findings may suggest an etiology of the pericardial effusion, such as a history of neoplasm or uremia.

In many patients, no etiology is found for the episode of acute pericarditis. Certain viral agents, such as Coxsackie B, have been identified as causative agents for pericarditis. In these patients, frequently a history of a preceding respiratory infection is found. Among patients with purulent pericarditis, *Hemophilus influenzae*, pneumococcus, and staphylococcus are the most common organisms. Purulent pericarditis usually occurs in infancy and may follow or be associated with infection at another site, such as pneumonia or osteomyelitis. The infants often show a high leukocyte count and appear to be very septic. An important clue in some infants and toddlers may be grunting respirations in the absence of auscultatory or radiographic evidence of pneumonia.

Pericarditis can develop secondary to juvenile rheumatoid arthritis and may occur before other manifestations of this disease. Usually, children show high fever, leukocytosis, and other systemic signs. Tamponade is rare.

Electrocardiogram

The electrocardiogram (Figure 9.2) usually shows ST-segment and T-wave changes. Early in the course of the disease, the ST segment is elevated and the T wave is upright. Subsequently, the ST segments return to the isoelectric line and the T waves become diffusely inverted. Reciprocal ST–T changes (elevation in one group of leads and depression in the opposite leads) are common early. Later, both ST segments and T waves return to normal. The QRS voltage may be reduced, particularly with a large fluid accumulation.

Chest X-ray

The chest X-ray may be normal, but the cardiac silhouette enlarges proportionately with accumulation of pericardial fluid.

Echocardiogram

Pericardial effusion can be recognized fairly accurately by echocardiography, and this technique may be helpful in diagnosing suspicious cases. Often the fluid can be characterized as purulent rather than serous because leukocytes are more echogenic (giving an echo-bright cloudy or smoky appearance) than fluid alone (which appears black by 2D echocardiography). Left ventricular diastolic diameter may be reduced because of inability of the ventricle to fill properly. The systolic function of the left ventricle is normal or even hyperdynamic. Tamponade is accompanied by dilation of the hepatic veins, vena cavae, and early diastolic "collapse" of the right atrium and right ventricle.

Treatment

Pericardiocentesis is indicated in many patients to confirm the diagnosis, identify the etiology, or treat tamponade. In patients with purulent pericarditis, pericardiocentesis is indicated, since reaching an etiologic diagnosis is imperative so that appropriate antibiotic therapy can be initiated. Other than in patients with neoplasm and purulent pericarditis, the analysis of the fluid rarely yields a diagnosis.

Pericardiocentesis is often indicated as an emergency procedure to treat the significant cardiac tamponade by removing fluid, thereby allowing adequate cardiac filling.

At times, particularly with recurrent tamponade, a thoracotomy with creation of a pericardial window is indicated to decompress the pericardial sac. Pericardiectomy, removal of a large panel of the parietal pericardium, is sometimes performed, especially in purulent pericarditis, in the hopes of avoiding late restrictive pericarditis as the sac scars and contracts.

Symptomatic relief of pain is indicated. Digoxin and diuretics are contraindicated because they slow the heart rate and reduce the filling pressure, contrary to the normal compensatory mechanisms for tamponade.

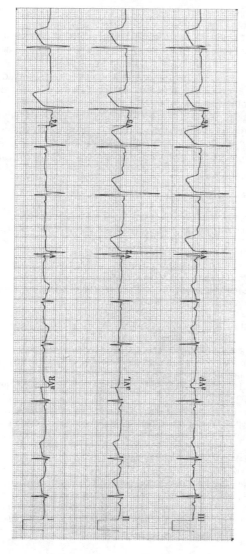

Figure 9.2 Electrocardiogram in acute pericarditis. Marked ST-segment and T-wave elevation in multiple leads, which are unlike the ST–T changes seen with acute myocardial ischemia or with coronary artery anomalies.

High doses of antibiotics are indicated in purulent pericarditis, the type to be determined by antibiotic sensitivities, and open or closed drainage may be necessary. Appropriate cultures for mycobacteria and fungus should be performed, especially in immunocompromised patients. Tests for mycobacterial and fungus infection may be helpful, especially if cultures prove negative.

In children and adolescents with noninfectious pericarditis, including some with postoperative pericardial effusion (postpericardiotomy syndrome), the use of aspirin or other nonsteroidal anti-inflammatory drugs (NSAIDs) or colchicine can be useful. These are administered in anti-inflammatory doses. In patients with a primary inflammatory disorder, such as lupus, effective treatment of the underlying disorder with appropriate agents, such as steroids and other immunosuppressants, usually results in resolution of the pericarditis and effusion.

ADDITIONAL READING

Baddour, L.M., Wilson, W.R., Bayer, A.S., et al. (2015) Infective endocarditis in adults: diagnosis, antimicrobial therapy, and management of complications: a scientific statement for healthcare professionals from the American Heart Association [published corrections appear in *Circulation* 2015; **132** (17):e215; *Circulation* 2016; **134** (8):e113; *Circulation* 2018; **138** (5):e78–e79]. *Circulation* **132** (15):1435–1486. https://doi.org/10.1161/CIR.0000000000000296.

Baltimore, R.S., Gewitz, M., Baddour, L.M. et al. (2015). Infective endocarditis in childhood: 2015 update: a scientific statement from the American Heart Association. *Circulation* **132** (15): 1487–1515. https://doi.org/10.1161/CIR.0000000000000298.

Gerber, M.A., Baltimore, R.S., Eaton, C.B. et al. (2009). Prevention of rheumatic fever and diagnosis and treatment of acute streptococcal pharyngitis: a scientific statement from the American Heart Association. *Circulation* **119**: 1541–1551.

Gewitz, M.H., Baltimore, R.S., Tani, L.Y. et al. (2015). Revision of the Jones criteria for the diagnosis of acute rheumatic fever in the era of Doppler echocardiography: a scientific statement from the American Heart Association [published correction appears in *Circulation* 2020; **142** (4):e65]. *Circulation* **131** (20): 1806–1818. https://doi.org/10.1161/CIR.0000000000000205.

Habib, G., Lancellotti, P., Antunes, M.J. et al. (2015). 2015 ESC guidelines for the management of infective endocarditis: the task force for the management of infective endocarditis of the European Society of Cardiology (ESC). Endorsed by European Association for Cardio-Thoracic Surgery (EACTS), the European Association of Nuclear Medicine (EANM). *Eur. Heart J.* **36** (44): 3075–3128. https://doi.org/10.1093/eurheartj/ehv319.

Kimberlin, D.W. (ed.) (2021). *Red Book: 2021–2024 Report of the Committee on Infectious Diseases*. Elk Grove Village, IL: American Academy of Pediatrics.

Kumar, R.K., Antunes, M.J., Beaton, A. et al. (2020). Contemporary diagnosis and management of rheumatic heart disease: implications for closing the gap: a scientific statement from the American Heart Association [published correction appears in *Circulation* 2021;**143** (23):e1025–e1026]. *Circulation* **142** (20): e337–e357. https://doi.org/10.1161/CIR.0000000000000921.

Loeys, B.L., Dietz, H.C., Braverman, A.C. et al. (2010). The revised Ghent nosology for the Marfan syndrome. *J. Med. Genet.* **47**: 476–485. www.marfan.org.

McCrindle, B.W., Rowley, A.H., Newburger, J.W., et al. (2017) Diagnosis, treatment, and long-term management of Kawasaki disease: a scientific statement for health professionals from the American Heart Association [published correction appears in *Circulation* 2019;**140** (5):e181–e184]. *Circulation* **135** (17):e927–e999. https://doi.org/10.1161/CIR.0000000000000484, www.heart.org.

Roy, C.L., Minor, M.A., Brookhart, M.A., and Choudhry, N.K. (2007). Does this patient with a pericardial effusion have cardiac tamponade? *JAMA* **297**: 1810–1818.

Wilson, W., Taubert, K.A., Gewitz, M., et al. (2007) Prevention of infective endocarditis: guidelines from the American Heart Association [published erratum appears in *Circulation* 116:e376–e377]. *Circulation* **116**: 1736–1754. www.heart.org.

Chapter 10
Abnormalities of heart rate and conduction in children

Disturbance of cardiac rate and conduction occur in children with no history of preceding cardiac disease, as a manifestation of congenital or acquired cardiac disease, as a complication of drug therapy, particularly digoxin therapy, or as a manifestation of metabolic, particularly electrolyte, abnormalities.

Cardiac arrhythmias can be generally classified as (i) alterations in cardiac rate or (ii) abnormalities of cardiac conduction.

ALTERATIONS IN CARDIAC RATE
Cardiac arrhythmias result from either of two mechanisms: (i) automatic tachy-cardias – alterations in the rate of discharge of pacemakers at the atrial, junctional, or ventricular level; or (ii) re-entry mechanisms, occurring solely within the atria (primary atrial tachyarrhythmias) or the ventricles (some types of ventricular tachycardia [VT]), or from re-entry circuits involving atria, ventricles, junctional tissue, and abnormal atrial-to-ventricular connections (atrioventricu-lar (AV) tachyarrhythmias).

Moller's Essentials of Pediatric Cardiology, Fourth Edition.
Walter H. Johnson, Jr. and Camden L. Hebson.
© 2023 John Wiley & Sons Ltd. Published 2023 by John Wiley & Sons Ltd.

Atrial and atrioventricular arrhythmias

Sinus arrhythmia

Sinus arrhythmia is a normal variation of sinus rhythm (SR) (Figure 10.1). It describes the normal increase in cardiac rate with inspiration and the slowing with expiration. Sometimes with expiration, nodal escape occurs.

Premature atrial systoles

Premature atrial systoles (or contractions, PACs) (Figure 10.2) occur commonly in the fetus and young infant less than two months of age but uncommonly in older children; they arise from ectopic (and automatic) atrial foci. On the electrocardiogram (ECG) this condition is recognized by a P wave with an abnormal shape which differs in contour from the patient's usual P waves. The P waves occur earlier than normal, so prematurely, in fact, that the AV node is completely refractory and a QRS complex does not occur. PACs that occur during partial AV node refractoriness may be conducted aberrantly, mimicking multiform premature ventricular contractions (PVCs). PACs occurring after the AV node has ceased to be refractory are conducted normally, resulting in a narrow QRS complex. No treatment is required.

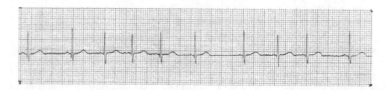

Figure 10.1 Electrocardiogram of sinus arrhythmia. Each QRS complex is preceded by a P wave, but the interval between each P wave is variable, usually changing with the respiratory cycle.

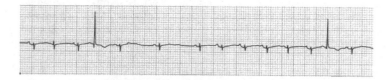

Figure 10.2 Electrocardiogram of premature atrial contractions.

Sinus tachycardia

The normal sinoatrial node (SAN) can discharge at a rapid rate of up to 210 beats per minute (bpm) in response to some stimuli such as fever, shock, atropine, or epinephrine. The increased heart rate does not require treatment, but the tachycardia should be considered a clinical finding that requires diagnosis and perhaps treatment of the root cause.

Distinguishing sinus tachycardia from a tachyarrhythmia

In infants and children, the cardiac rate varies considerably and may reach 210bpm during physical activity or with a high fever. Thus, it may be difficult to distinguish this from various types of tachyarrhythmia.

In both sinus and tachyarrhythmia, the QRS complex is almost always narrow, but in the latter the cardiac rate usually exceeds 210bpm.

There are other clues to identify an ectopic tachycardia. One relates to the P-wave axis. In sinus tachycardia, the P-wave axis is normal (0–90°), whereas in a tachyarrhythmia a normal P-wave axis is found in only 20%, or the P waves may not be visible at all.

Second, the clinical situation should be considered. Tachycardia in the presence of sepsis, dehydration, or fever is almost always of sinus origin. Improvement following treatment of the underlying condition leads to slowing of the cardiac rate in sinus tachycardia.

The history of onset and disappearance of the tachycardia differs between the two. Sinus tachycardia does not instantly increase or disappear but changes gradually. When an effort is made to intervene by a vagal maneuver, if the tachycardia rate changes abruptly, its origin is tachyarrhythmia. In contrast, the heart rate of a sinus rhythm decreases gradually. However, the rate may not change in either situation with this maneuver.

Paroxysmal supraventricular tachycardia

Paroxysmal supraventricular tachycardia (SVT, PSVT, PAT), often occurring with minimal or no symptoms, rarely leads to death if untreated. Typically, a previously healthy infant develops poor feeding, sweating, irritability, and rapid respiration. If the arrhythmia is unrecognized and untreated, congestive cardiac failure may progress to death in 24–48 hours. Recognition of arrhythmia is not difficult when examining the heart. The measured heart rate of 250–350bpm (Figure 10.3) is remarkably regular, showing no variation when the child breathes, cries, or becomes quiet.

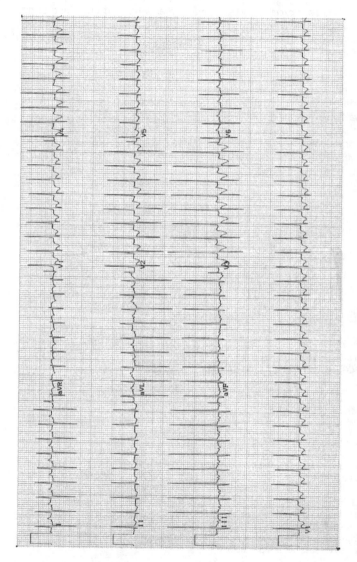

Figure 10.3 Electrocardiogram of supraventricular tachycardia. A regular narrow-QRS tachycardia without easily seen P waves. Heart rate 220 bpm.

The prognosis is excellent because many infants have no underlying cardiac malformation and recurrent episodes are rare or infrequent and are well tolerated, if of short duration. Patients with coexistent Ebstein's malformation and/or Wolff–Parkinson–White (WPW) syndrome, however, may have repeated episodes of SVT.

Orthodromic reciprocating AV tachycardia (ORT). The mechanism of this type of tachycardia is virtually always re-entry via an accessory pathway between the atria and ventricles (Figure 10.4). Normally, only one electrically conductive pathway, the penetrating bundle of His, exists between the atria and ventricles. In more than 95% of fetuses, infants, and young children with SVT, an abnormal accessory connection exists between the atria or ventricles, a possible vestige of the multiple connections that exist in the embryonic cardiac tube before separate cardiac chambers are formed.

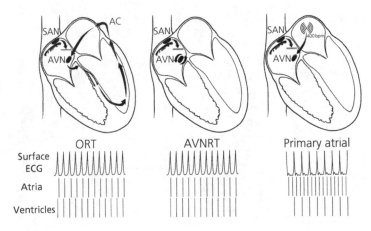

Figure 10.4 Mechanisms of supraventricular tachycardia. ORT is the most common in children. An abnormal accessory connection (AC) with the atrioventricular node (AVN) and the atria and ventricles constitutes a re-entrant circuit. In atrioventricular node re-entry tachycardia (AVNRT), the circuit includes two pathways within the AVN and also the atria and ventricles. Both types result in a regular narrow-QRS tachycardia without discernible P waves. Primary atrial tachycardia (e.g. atrial flutter) originates in the atria (true SVT) and conducts via the AVN to the ventricles – in this case, in a 2 : 1 ratio. P waves may or may not be seen. The lower panel allows simultaneous comparison of the surface ECG with electrograms recorded in the atria and ventricles. In each type, the sinoatrial node (SAN) is suppressed because of the more rapid SVT.

This accessory connection together with the AV node, the atria, and the ventricles may create a large re-entrant circuit (Figure 10.4). Impulses may conduct normally via the AV node (orthodromic conduction) but pass retrograde to the atria via the accessory connection when the AV node is refractory. Then the impulse passes from the atria through the AV node, to the ventricles, then to the atria via the accessory connection, as the sequence is repeated. This creates ORT, the most common mechanism for childhood SVT. Because the tachycardia is not truly supraventricular but actually atrioventricular and is dependent on four components – atria, AV node, ventricles, and accessory connection – any of these components can be altered slightly to terminate the tachycardia. In practical terms, the AV node is the component most amenable to intervention by vagal stimulation or medication such as adenosine.

Since conduction is antegrade at all times, the QRS complex appears normal during the tachycardia. The tachycardia rate slows with age, being up to 300 bpm in neonates and 200 bpm in adolescents. Because of the length of the re-entrant circuit, the P wave may be more clearly seen *following* the QRS complex often best in lead V_1.

Atrioventricular nodal re-entry tachycardia (AVNRT). The second most common tachycardia mechanism involves a small re-entrant circuit within or near the AV node itself (Figure 10.4). It can be thought of as an acquired form of SVT, since it has never been reported in children less than four years of age but does occur in half of adults with SVT. As in ORT, the tachycardia depends on the atria, ventricles, and a fast and a slow pathway within the AV node. This AV tachycardia is called AVNRT. The ECG shows a regular, narrow-QRS tachycardia similar in appearance to ORT. Conversion is best accomplished by altering AV node conduction via vagal stimulation or medication.

Differentiation of AV re-entrant tachyarrhythmias. ORT must be distinguished from AVNRT at the time of catheter ablation, but clinically and by noninvasive means this can be challenging. In a practical sense, the medical treatments of ORT and AVNRT are often the same or very similar. The location of the P wave in relation to the QRS complex is a valuable diagnostic sign, being close in AVNRT and further removed in ORT. In most children, visualization of the retrograde P wave is difficult if not impossible by a standard surface ECG. (Other than by electrophysiologic catheterization, techniques such as transesophageal electrocardiography, i.e. recording of an atrial electrogram by positioning an electrode catheter within the esophagus behind the left atrium, can allow good visualization of the P wave and the R–P interval.) Clinically, AVNRT may be more frequent, occurring several times per day, and the tachycardia rate varies between episodes by a greater degree than with ORT.

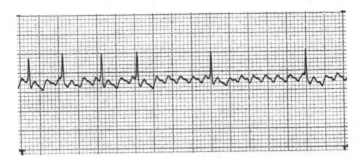

Figure 10.5 Electrocardiogram of atrial flutter. Regular P waves with less than 1 : 1 AV conduction. Atrial rate >300 bpm.

Atrial flutter

In atrial flutter, the atrial rate may be between 280 and 400 bpm, with a 2 to 1 or greater, degree of AV block, so that the ventricular rate is slower than the atrial rate (Figure 10.4). On the ECG, the atrial activity does not appear as distinct P waves; instead, it has a sawtooth appearance (Figure 10.5).

This arrhythmia can occur in infants without an underlying condition or in children with conditions such as dilated cardiomyopathy, Ebstein's malformation, or rheumatic mitral valvar disease that leads to a greatly enlarged left atrium.

Medication usually slows the ventricular rate by slowing the AV node, but rarely does it result in conversion. Cardioversion (synchronized with the R wave to avoid induction of dangerous ventricular rhythms) with very low energy (usually 0.25 J/kg) converts the rhythm to a sinus mechanism.

Atrial fibrillation

Atrial fibrillation is associated with chaotic atrial activity at a rate of more than 400 bpm. Distinct P waves are not seen, but atrial activity is evident as small, irregular wave forms on the ECG (Figure 10.6). The ventricular response is irregular. This arrhythmia results from conditions that chronically dilate the atria.

Hyperthyroidism is a rare cause in childhood. Medications such as digoxin, beta-blockers, or calcium channel blockers are indicated to slow the ventricular response. Cardioversion may require high energy (1–2 J/kg), although biphasic shocks are often successful at lower energy compared with monophasic shocks.

Reinitiation of atrial fibrillation is common, especially with underlying structural heart disease or cardiomyopathy. Antithrombotic therapy, usually with a

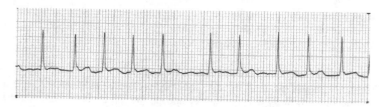

Figure 10.6 Electrocardiogram of atrial fibrillation. The wavy isoelectric line reflects the irregular and rapid atrial activity. Typically, the ventricular rate is "irregularly irregular."

vitamin K antagonist (warfarin), is often used to minimize the risk of embolic stroke. In some patients, particularly those with complex postoperative problems, atrial fibrillation may be refractory to antiarrhythmic medication. Such patients may be candidates for a surgical or catheter (radiofrequency [RF] ablation) procedure to create multiple linear scars within the atria to prevent atrial fibrillation from becoming sustained (Maze procedure). In other patients, tolerance of chronic atrial fibrillation may be achieved by control of ventricular rate, using a variety of techniques, including medication or AV node ablation plus pacemaker implantation.

Other primary atrial tachyarrhythmias

Primary atrial tachycardia arises from a specific automatic (not re-entrant) atrial focus and does not involve the SA or AV nodes or ventricles in maintaining the abnormal rhythm. Various types may involve one or more foci and have been termed atrial ectopic tachycardia, ectopic atrial tachycardia, or chaotic atrial tachycardia. Occurring at any age during childhood, atrial tachycardia is an incessant or frequently occurring tachycardia and often presents as a tachycardia-induced cardiomyopathy. The heart rate varies, being as high as 300 bpm in infants and ranging from 150 to 250 bpm in children. The rate can vary abruptly. P-wave morphology is usually abnormal and depends on the location of the ectopic focus. P waves are generally observed and the PR interval can be normal, short, or prolonged. Sinus tachycardia is the major condition from which this tachyarrhythmia must be distinguished.

Because of the natural history, treatment depends on age. In infants and young children, the tachycardia often resolves, so these patients are treated with medications. After a few years, medications can be withdrawn if the tachycardia has resolved. For older children, ablation of the ectopic focus is successful and may need to be performed acutely if the child is ill and has poor ventricular function.

Junctional arrhythmias

These ectopic (automatic) arrhythmias arise from the AV node; they are called nodal or junctional premature beats or tachycardia.

Premature junctional contractions (PJCs)

The QRS complex is normal because the impulses propagate along the normal conduction pathway. The P waves may appear with an abnormal form shortly before the QRS complex, may be buried within the QRS complex, or may follow the QRS complex.

Junctional ectopic tachycardia (JET)

Junctional ectopic tachycardia (JET) occurs almost exclusively following a cardiac operation. This ectopic (automatic) tachycardia arises from the area around the AV node and bundle of His because of edema, hemorrhage, or trauma around the node. The maximum heart rate of JET varies with age, ranging from up to 300 bpm in infants to 200 bpm in adolescents.

The atria and ventricles are dissociated, with the ventricular rate being faster than the atrial rate. The QRS complex may be either normal or altered as a result of the cardiac operation (e.g. RBBB).

In a postoperative patient, the tachycardia usually resolves within two to three days of the operation, but JET can result in severe hemodynamic compromise and may be difficult to control. Treatment is directed at stabilizing the patient's hemodynamics and minimizing inotropic medications that may be proarrhythmic. If the tachycardia persists, the body temperature is reduced, patient sedation is optimized, and medications (amiodarone, procainamide) can be infused.

Permanent junctional reciprocating tachycardia (PJRT)

This rare form of incessant tachycardia is frequently associated with reversible myocardial dysfunction (tachycardia-induced cardiomyopathy), although the heart rate is usually only 150–200 bpm. The P-wave axis is always abnormal, with negative P waves in leads II, III, and aVF. Permanent junctional reciprocating tachycardia (PJRT) is actually an AV tachycardia caused by an accessory atrioventricular connection (AC) located near the os of the coronary sinus. Although an occasional child may have spontaneous disappearance of PJRT, medication or radiofrequency ablation is usually required.

Ventricular arrhythmias

Ventricular arrhythmias are characterized by widened QRS complexes and large abnormal T waves generally with opposite polarity to the QRS complex. They arise from ectopic foci in the bundles of His, re-entrant pathways within the ventricular myocardium, or automatic foci in the myocardium.

Premature ventricular contractions (PVCs)

In children, PVCs are usually benign. They are recognized by bizarre QRS complexes falling irregularly in the normal cardiac rhythm (Figure 10.7). This widened QRS has a different configuration from the normal QRS complex, does not follow a P wave, and is associated with a large T wave. Following the ectopic beat, a compensatory pause occurs. Generally, PVCs are unifocal, meaning that each of the aberrant QRS complexes has an identical configuration. PVCs occur more frequently at slow sinus rhythm rates, happening as often as every other beat (bigeminy), and decrease in frequency or disappear at fast sinus rates, as occurs with exercise. They do not usually occur in pairs (couplets).

A useful office diagnostic technique to evaluate PVCs is as follows. Have the child perform mild exercise; then determine if the PVCs disappear with increased heart rate. Continue to listen or monitor with ECG following exercise, while the heart rate is returning to normal. The PVCs tend to return as the heart rate slows.

PVCs in children usually require no treatment, as the prognosis is excellent. Patients with a benign history (including family history) and normal physical examination should have an ECG to exclude the presence of multifocal PVCs and of abnormalities such as hypertrophic cardiomyopathy, WPW, or long QT syndrome. Patients with PVCs who otherwise have a normal evaluation are said to have benign PVCs of childhood.

In some patients, PVCs with QRS complexes of varying contours are present. These multifocal PVCs are often related to myocardial disease. They tend to increase

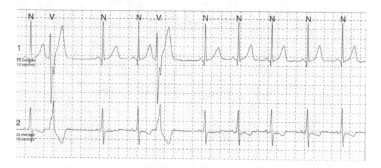

Figure 10.7 Electrocardiogram of PVCs. These ectopic beats occur as wide-QRS premature complexes associated with abnormal T waves.

with exercise. A cause should be sought by history, physical examination, electrolytes, and echocardiography, as indicated. PVCs may develop as a sign of a metabolic abnormality (e.g. hyperkalemia) or drug toxicity (especially digoxin) and require treatment of the metabolic abnormality or discontinuance of the medication, followed by careful monitoring. Occasionally, multifocal PVCs result from a right atrial central venous catheter tip intermittently entering the right ventricle in diastole.

Ventricular tachycardia (VT)

Ventricular tachycardia (VT) arises as a rapidly discharging ventricular focus at a rate of 150–250 bpm. These arrhythmias are usually serious and associated with symptoms of chest pain, palpitations, or syncope. This rhythm may occur in normal children as a manifestation of digoxin or other drug toxicity, in myocarditis, or as a terminal event after a catastrophic injury or metabolic derangement.

The ECG shows regular wide-QRS complexes (Figure 10.8a) and often P waves that occur at a slower rate (AV dissociation). Patients with antiarrhythmic drug toxicity (particularly procainamide) and those with the long QT syndrome may have a distinctive type of VT called torsades de pointes (literally, "twisting of the points" or axis) (Figure 10.8b).

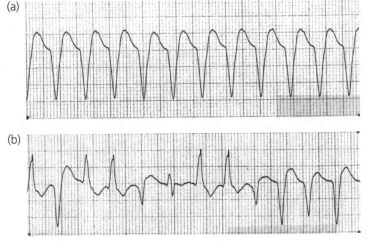

Figure 10.8 Electrocardiogram of VT. Wide-QRS complexes occurring at regular intervals without evidence of atrial activity. (a) Monomorphic VT, the most commonly seen. (b) Torsades de pointes.

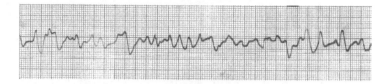

Figure 10.9 Electrocardiogram of ventricular fibrillation. Irregular disorganized ventricular activity.

Rare patients, usually infants, have a self-limited, apparently benign, monomorphic VT that usually requires no treatment. In almost all other patients, VT requires cardioversion, either by external direct current (DC) shock, intracardiac pacing in the catheterization laboratory, or drug therapy; the immediacy and type of cardioversion depend on whether or not the child is hemodynamically stable and, if stable, upon the degree of symptoms.

Ventricular fibrillation
The electrocardiographic finding of ventricular fibrillation often represents a terminal event and appears as wide, bizarre, irregularly occurring wave forms of various amplitudes (Figure 10.9). Cardiac output is markedly decreased. VT may degenerate into ventricular fibrillation. It is treated by the methods used for management of cardiopulmonary arrest and by external nonsynchronized DC shock.

CONDUCTION DISTURBANCES
Most major conduction disturbances occur between the atrium and the ventricles at the level of the AV node.

Shortened AV conduction (pre-excitation syndromes)
In pre-excitation syndromes, conduction through or around the AV node is accelerated; such patients tend to develop episodes of paroxysmal SVT.

One of these conditions, WPW syndrome, has three electrocardiographic features: (i) a shortened PR interval; (ii) a widened QRS complex; and (iii) a delta wave, a slurred broadened initial portion of the QRS complex (Figure 10.10).

WPW syndrome results from a microscopic accessory AC (Figure 10.11), consisting of working myocardium (i.e. lacking the electrical properties of the AV nodal tissue that allow for normal delay in atrial to ventricular impulse transmission). Such a delay, called the PR interval, is necessary for efficient movement of blood from the atria to ventricles before ventricular systole.

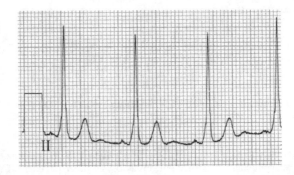

Figure 10.10 Electrocardiogram in WPW syndrome. Short PR interval and wide-QRS complex with a delta wave, indicated by slurred initial portion of QRS complex.

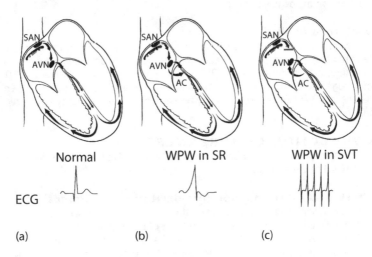

Figure 10.11 Mechanism of WPW syndrome. (a) Normal is shown for comparison. (b) During sinus rhythm (SR), WPW patients have early activation (pre-excitation) of a portion of the ventricular myocardium via an abnormal accessory connection (AC) that conducts more rapidly from the atrium to the ventricle than the atrioventricular node (AVN). (c) If a WPW patient has "supraventricular tachycardia" (SVT), the AC conducts from the ventricle to the atrium; therefore, a delta wave is not present, and the QRS is narrow, similarly to other patients with this type of SVT (orthodromic reciprocating tachycardia). SAN, sinoatrial node.

In WPW, the accessory connection conducts antegrade from the atria to the ventricles, much faster than the AV node, allowing a portion of the ventricle to depolarize early, thus creating the slurred delta wave and short PR interval.

When impulses conduct retrograde, from the ventricles to the atria via the accessory connection, SVT may occur by a mechanism identical with that in those patients whose concealed accessory connection only conducts one way.

> WPW patients have a manifest accessory connection only evident electrocardiographically during sinus rhythm; SVT appears the same for WPW patients as for those with concealed connections.

In rare patients with WPW, conduction via the accessory connection is so rapid – much faster than that which occurs via the AV node – that rapid atrial arrhythmias such as atrial flutter may result in very rapid atrial-to-ventricular conduction, ventricular fibrillation, and sudden death.

Patients with concealed accessory connections do not risk sudden death during primary atrial tachyarrhythmias because the only atrial-to-ventricular conduction is through the normal AV node, limiting the ventricular rate to 210 bpm or less.

Many cardiologists discourage the use of verapamil or digoxin in WPW patients, since these drugs may speed conduction through the accessory connection in rare WPW patients and thus increase the risk of life-threatening arrhythmia.

WPW syndrome may be present in patients without other cardiac anomalies and in patients with Ebstein's malformation or other structural malformations.

In the other rarer pre-excitation syndromes, the PR interval is short, but the QRS is of normal duration.

Prolonged atrioventricular conduction
Several forms of prolonged atrioventricular conduction have been described.

First-degree heart block
First-degree heart block (Figure 10.12) is represented by prolongation of the PR interval beyond the normal range; each P wave is also followed by a QRS complex. Digoxin, acute rheumatic fever, and acute infections can cause first-degree heart block. Certain neuromuscular diseases may also cause it, but it is also seen in a small number of otherwise normal individuals. It does not require treatment.

Second-degree heart block
In this form of heart block, each P wave is not followed by a QRS complex. A 2 : 1, 3 : 1, or greater block may exist between the atria and the ventricles.

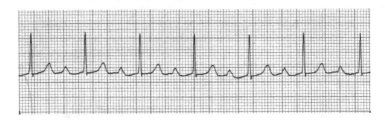

Figure 10.12 Electrocardiogram in first-degree heart block. Prolonged PR interval and 1 : 1 AV conduction.

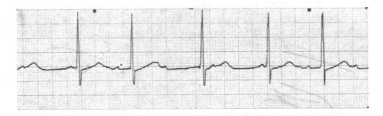

Figure 10.13 Electrocardiogram in second-degree heart block, Mobitz type I (Wenckebach). The PR interval lengthens each beat until conduction fails and a "beat is dropped." The QRS is typically "regularly irregular."

Two types occur, often named Mobitz types.

Mobitz type I (Wenckebach). This is characterized by a progressively lengthening PR interval until a P wave fails to conduct to the ventricles and a ventricular beat is "dropped" (absent) (Figure 10.13). Then the cycle resumes again. Type I second-degree block is usually benign and is often seen during drug therapy (especially digoxin) or minor metabolic derangements. It may occur in asymptomatic individuals with a structurally normal heart. Treatment is not indicated in asymptomatic patients.

Mobitz type II. This is characterized by sudden failure of AV node conduction without any sentinel abnormalities of the preceding beats (Figure 10.14). Type II second-degree AV block is often associated with serious AV node disease, and the propensity for progression to complete AV block is high. Patients often have syncopal episodes. A pacemaker is usually indicated.

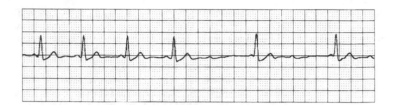

Figure 10.14 Electrocardiogram in second-degree heart block, Mobitz type II. The PR interval is normal and constant, until sudden failure of conduction from the atria to the ventricle occurs.

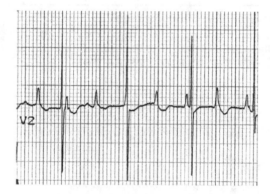

Figure 10.15 Electrocardiogram in complete heart block. P waves and QRS complexes are occurring independently and the ventricular rate is slow.

Third-degree heart block

This condition is complete AV block with dissociation between the atria and the ventricles, and the atrial impulse does not influence the ventricles (Figure 10.15). Since the ventricular rate is slow, ventricular stroke volume is increased, leading to a soft systolic ejection and a mid-diastolic murmur and cardiomegaly.

Third-degree heart block can occur from birth, often associated with maternal autoimmune disease (see Chapter 2). It has a good prognosis except in those cases with a family history of heart block from neuromuscular disease or myopathy or in neonates with major cardiac structural anomalies. It may also develop from digoxin toxicity or follow a cardiac operation. The prognosis for recovery from postoperative block is poor. Complete heart block may be associated with syncopal episodes (Stokes–Adams attacks) but is usually not tied to congestive cardiac failure, unless additional cardiac abnormalities exist, particularly those placing volume loads on the ventricles.

If the heart rate is persistently low (less than 40 bpm) or if syncopal episodes occur, a permanently implanted pacemaker is indicated. A pacemaker is usually indicated in children with postoperative heart block because of the high incidence of sudden death. Waiting for two weeks after operation, with careful monitoring, before implanting a permanent pacemaker is wise, as within that period sinus rhythm may return.

Acute management of bradyarrhythmia

Assess and manage ABC (Airway, Breathing, Circulation) *first*.

  Must differentiate *congenital complete AV block* (CCAVB, rare) versus *sinus bradycardia* from noncardiac causes (common).

IF

CCAVB *and*

Patient stable?

• Obtain 12-lead ECG and rhythm strip and call pediatric cardiologist.

OR
Patient unstable?

• Isoproterenol (Isuprel®) 0.1–0.5 μg/kg/min IV and/or
• Pace (transcutaneous/transvenous/transgastric).

See "Additional reading" for published pediatric and neonatal resuscitation guidelines.

GENERAL PRINCIPLES OF TACHYARRHYTHMIA DIAGNOSIS AND MANAGEMENT

Initial clinical assessment

Patients with tachycardia should be immediately assessed for hemodynamic stability. Stable infants and children may have no symptoms or minimal complaints, such as palpitations in a child old enough to articulate them. In a preverbal child, the parents may observe rapid forceful precordial activity.

Children showing hemodynamic compromise from their tachycardia have increased respiratory rate, resulting from pulmonary congestion and/or compensation of the metabolic acidosis that follows from inadequate cardiac output.

Inadequate cardiac output is reflected by poorly palpable pulses, decreased skin perfusion, agitation, listlessness, or unconsciousness.

A normal oxygen saturation by pulse oximeter is the rule and therefore is an unreliable means of assessing the hemodynamic effect of tachycardia, except in patients with a cyanotic cardiac malformation, such as unrepaired tetralogy of Fallot, or following a "fenestrated" Fontan or partial Fontan operation. In these cyanotic patients, oxygen saturation (and also cardiac output in the patients with a cavopulmonary anastomosis) falls dramatically during tachycardia.

Patients with significant reduction of cardiac output during tachyarrhythmia are obviously unstable; they die without immediate cardioversion (usually best accomplished by external DC shock) and other resuscitative and support measures.

Stable patients in tachycardia should be assessed using a 12-lead ECG (Table 10.1) to obtain valuable diagnostic and therapeutic information that cannot be gathered by a single-lead rhythm strip or by counting the heart rate during physical examination.

Differential diagnosis and management in stable patients

Most tachyarrhythmias in children are regular (each R–R interval varying by less than 10 ms). Stable regular tachycardia with wide QRS is either sinus rhythm with pre-existing bundle branch block, a variety of SVT with bundle branch block, or VT. The last should be suspected first, even in asymptomatic patients. The presence of AV dissociation (atria and ventricles contracting at different rates) during wide-QRS tachycardia is virtually pathognomonic of VT.

A regular narrow-QRS tachycardia is either sinus rhythm (but not at rates greater than about 210 bpm), a primary atrial tachyarrhythmia (e.g. atrial flutter), or, most commonly, one of the AV re-entrant tachyarrhythmias.

Sinus tachycardia varies in rate from minute to minute, whereas the last two tachyarrhythmias tend to have no rate variation, despite changes in the infant's activity level.

A 12-lead ECG allows better definition of P waves than a single lead recording. P waves are usually easily seen in sinus tachycardia, can appear, obvious or not, as a "sawtooth" pattern in atrial flutter, and are generally not well seen in AV tachycardias.

Table 10.1 Electrocardiographic differential diagnosis of the most common narrow-QRS (supraventricular) tachycardias in neonates, children, and adolescents.

Rhythm	P waves	Ventricular rate (bpm)	Minute-to-minute rate variation	Ventricular rhythm	Response to adequate adenosine dose or vagal stimulation
Sinus tachycardia	Distinct	≤230 neonates 210 infants and children 180–200 adolescents	Yes	Regular	*Gradual* slowing of atrial *and* ventricular rate ± transient second-degree AVB
AV re-entrant tachycardia					
ORT (any age)	Indistinct	240–280	No	Regular	*Sudden* conversion to sinus
AVNRT (≥4 years)	Indistinct	160–240	No	Regular	*Sudden* conversion to sinus
Primary atrial tachycardia					
Atrial flutter	Regular uniform flutter waves	120–280	No	Regular	Transient second-degree AVB, no change in atrial rate, atrial rate usually a multiple of ventricular rate
Atrial fibrillation	Irregular low voltage	120–280	±	Irregular	Transient ventricular slowing, no change in atrial rhythm
Automatic or "chaotic"	Irregular multiform	160–280	±	Irregular	Transient ventricular slowing, no change in atrial rhythm

AVB, atrioventricular nodal block; AVNRT, atrioventricular nodal re-entry tachycardia; ORT, orthodromic reciprocating tachycardia; bpm, beats per minute.

Adenosine or vagal maneuvers that slow AV node conduction can be used to differentiate these three main types of narrow-QRS tachycardia and can convert an AV tachycardia (Table 10.1). Adenosine is an endogenous purine that must be rapidly injected intravenously; its qualities include an ultrashort (seconds) duration of action, low risk, and effectiveness in patients when vagal stimulation fails.

The technique of adenosine administration is important to its effective use. Adequate doses, usually given in increasing increments until the desired effect is achieved, are essential. A central venous catheter is not necessary and peripheral intravenous sites are routinely used with success. The most rapid means of delivering a bolus to the central venous circulation, however, is by "chasing" the adenosine in rapid sequence with an injection of saline, to achieve effective concentrations at the AV node.

Contraindications include unpaced patients with sinus node dysfunction or second- or third-degree AV block and in patients with known hypersensitivity. Relative contraindications include use in wide-QRS tachycardias, particularly in WPW patients with a wide-QRS tachycardia, and in patients with asthma. Aminophylline and caffeine are adenosine receptor antagonists and greatly increase the dose of adenosine needed for effectiveness.

An ECG, preferably using at least three leads, must be recorded continuously during adenosine administration or the vagal maneuver, otherwise valuable information is lost.

(a) In sinus tachycardia, adenosine or a vagal maneuver transiently slows the sinus rate because of direct effects on the sinoatrial node (SAN). Transient second-degree AV block may be seen, yet the P-wave morphology remains unchanged.
(b) In atrial flutter or other primary atrial tachycardia, the AV node fails to conduct some atrial depolarizations (second-degree AV block), making the diagnosis obvious but not producing conversion. As soon as the adenosine or vagal effect subsides, the rapid ventricular rate resumes.
(c) In AV tachycardias, adenosine or vagal stimulation may produce a lasting conversion to sinus rhythm, or a transient conversion to sinus rhythm, followed by rapid reinitiation of tachycardia.

Failure to record an adequate ECG continuously during these interventions may lead to the erroneous conclusion that the maneuvers had no effect, as the brief decrease in ventricular rate may not be apparent by examination alone.

Acute management of tachyarrhythmia

Patient **unstable**?

- Cardiovert/defibrillate.

Patient **stable**?

- 12-lead ECG.
- *Run continuous rhythm strip (preferably a 3- or 12-lead) during conversion attempt.*
- Vagal maneuvers.
  Valsalva/gag/ice to face.

  (Avoid carotid and ocular massage and hypertension-producing drugs.)

- Adenosine (Adenocard®, 2 mL/vial × 3 mg/mL = 6 mg/vial) DRUG OF CHOICE.
- Start dose 100 µg/kg IV *push* (fastest bolus possible, follow immediately with saline flush).
- Increase by 100 µg/kg/dose to "maximum" 300 µg/kg/dose. (Some experts consider the currently recommended maximum of 300 µg/kg/dose to be lower than some patients may safely require for cardioversion; it is estimated that >90% of infant and pediatric patients will have successful cardioversion at the dose of 300 µg/kg/dose; consult specific drug literature or an expert; methylxanthines are adenosine receptor antagonists; patients so treated may not convert with a "maximum" adenosine dose.)
- *Verapamil is absolutely contraindicated* at age ≤12 months and relatively contraindicated at any age.
- *Digoxin and verapamil are contraindicated* in WPW.
- Obtain 12-lead ECG after conversion.

See "Additional reading" for published pediatric and neonatal resuscitation guidelines.

External DC shock

CARDIOVERSION – electrical termination of any arrhythmia other than ventricular fibrillation.
DEFIBRILLATION – electrical termination of one and only one arrhythmia: ventricular fibrillation.

- Use the *largest* paddles that will completely contact the skin over the entire surface.
- No dry contacts – electrolyte pad or paste must completely cover the contact area between paddles and skin. Do not use ultrasound gel.

Dose:

Cardioversion	SVT	1/4–1/2 J/kg
	Ventricular tachycardia	1–2 J/kg
Defibrillation	Ventricular fibrillation	2–4 J/kg

Biphasic defibrillators may allow for lower effective doses.
Avoid "pilot error:"

- *Never SYNC* (synchronize) for ventricular defibrillation.
- *Always SYNC* for cardioversion, even for atrial "fibrillation," whenever QRS is distinct.
- Connect 3- or 5-lead ECG *cable* for best sync during cardioversion.
- *Power on.*
- *Set dose.*
- *Charge.*
- Call *"Clear!!"* and observe that all personnel are not in contact with the patient.
- *Press hard* for good contact (minimal paddle-to-skin electrical resistance).
- Hold *both buttons* depressed for at least three seconds (sync takes time, particularly with relatively slow ventricular rates).
- Always record *rhythm strip* during procedure (some machines do this automatically).
- For subsequent cardioversion attempts, push *SYNC* again.

See "Additional reading" for published pediatric and neonatal resuscitation guidelines.

Long-term management

Treatment is influenced by the natural history. Following conversion to sinus rhythm, many infants and children do not have recurrent SVT and may not need prophylactic medication. The initial episode is converted by adenosine or vagal maneuvers and followed by administration of either digoxin (if there is no evidence of WPW) or a beta-blocker as needed for prophylaxis of recurrent SVT. Since in neonates and infants the tendency for tachycardia often resolves with age, generally, if there are no recurrences, the medication can be discontinued after one year. In older children with frequent episodes of tachycardia despite medications, often ablation is the treatment of choice.

The need for prophylactic antiarrhythmic medication is based on the hemodynamic severity of the tachycardia (or degree of symptoms in older children), the frequency of SVT episodes, the difficulty and/or risk of tachycardia conversion, and the possibility of whether or not the tachycardia poses other risks for the patient (e.g. the adolescent who has tachycardia-induced near-syncope and who wishes to drive a car).

Many patients require no prophylactic therapy as they can be easily converted with simple vagal maneuvers during infrequent mild episodes.

Patients with troublesome or potentially risky SVT, who fail drug therapy, or who have unacceptable side effects can essentially be cured using RF ablation at the time of electrophysiologic study (EPS) in the catheterization laboratory.

By probing using a catheter-mounted electrode, the location of an accessory connection is mapped by determining the site of earliest electrical activation during tachycardia. A burst of RF energy is delivered through the catheter to heat the accessory connection and destroy it. At some centers, cryoablation is used by way of a catheter to eliminate the aberrant pathway.

Unlikely complications include destruction of the AV node (complete AV block). Some patients with automatic foci can be cured by RF ablation.

In children with malignant forms of ventricular tachycardia who do not respond well to antiarrhythmic drugs, implantation of an implantable cardioverter-defibrillator (ICD) can be life-saving; however, such devices have important risks and limitations.

ADDITIONAL READING

de Caen, A.R., Berg, M.D., Chameides, L. et al. (2015). Part 12: pediatric advanced life support: 2015 American Heart Association guidelines update for cardiopulmonary resuscitation and emergency cardiovascular care. *Circulation* **132** (18 Suppl 2): S526–S542. https://doi.org/10.1161/CIR.0000000000000266. (Reprinted in Pediatrics 2015;**136** (Suppl 2):S176–S195. doi:10.1542/peds.2015-3373F.)

Van de Voorde, P., Turner, N.M., Djakow, J. et al. (2021). European Resuscitation Council Guidelines 2021: Paediatric Life Support. *Resuscitation* **161**: 327–387. https://doi.org/10.1016/j.resuscitation.2021.02.015.

Wren, C. (2011). *Concise Guide to Pediatric Arrhythmias*. Oxford: Wiley-Blackwell.

Chapter 11
Congestive heart failure in infants and children

Congestive cardiac failure is a frequent urgent medical problem in neonates and infants with a cardiac malformation and can occur in children with cardiac disease. It demands a level of care and attention similar to that for infants and children with an arrhythmia.

> Among children who develop cardiac failure, 80% do so in the first year of life, most commonly from congenital cardiac anomalies; of the 20% who develop cardiac failure after one year of age, in half it is related to congenital anomalies and in the other half to acquired conditions.

PATHOPHYSIOLOGY

Mechanisms

Two basic mechanisms are involved in the development of congestive cardiac failure. In each type, certain physiologic principles, such as the Laplace and

Moller's Essentials of Pediatric Cardiology, Fourth Edition.
Walter H. Johnson, Jr. and Camden L. Hebson.
© 2023 John Wiley & Sons Ltd. Published 2023 by John Wiley & Sons Ltd.

Starling relationships (see Chapter 4), describe the derangements that occur with ventricular dilation.

Increased cardiac work

Many neonates and infants experience heart failure from increased cardiac work (e.g. left-to-right shunts and valve regurgitation) despite normal or increased myocardial contractility. This type of heart failure is sometimes referred to as "high-output failure."

Reduced myocardial contraction

Myocardial contractility can be reduced as in dilated cardiomyopathy. Most adults and some children have failure of this type. Myocardial failure may result from myocarditis, chemotherapy, or familial cardiomyopathies.

In neonates and young infants, severe failure may result from an obstructive lesion including aortic stenosis, coarctation, or severe systemic hypertension. In these infants, myocardial function often improves following relief of obstruction or treatment of hypertension.

Patients with a morphologic right ventricle acting as the systemic pump (e.g. Norwood palliation of hypoplastic left heart syndrome, and the atrial switch repair of complete transposition) frequently develop systolic heart failure. Longstanding pulmonary regurgitation in a patient following tetralogy of Fallot repair may also lead to right ventricular failure, but since these patients have two functioning ventricles, the clinical manifestations are generally less acute.

Most therapy, either nonspecific or supportive, is designed to counteract the elevation of systemic and pulmonary vascular resistance that accompanies neuro-humoral abnormalities (including increased sympathetic tone and activation of the renin–angiotensin system) common to both types of failure.

Clinical features

> The clinical diagnosis of congestive cardiac failure rests upon the identification of the four cardinal signs: tachycardia, tachypnea, cardiomegaly, and hepatomegaly.

In addition, the patient often has a history of poor weight gain, fatigue upon eating (dyspnea on exercise), and excessive perspiration. Table 11.1 presents the most common clinical classifications of severity of cardiac failure, which are used to decide management and study outcomes of patients.

Table 11.1 Clinical classifications of heart failure.

Class	NYHA (Functional Class)[a]	Ross[b]
I	Adults and older children No limitation of physical activity; no symptoms with ordinary activity	Infants and children No limitations or symptoms
II	Slight limitation of physical activity; comfortable at rest; symptoms with ordinary activity	Mild tachypnea and/or diaphoresis with feedings; dyspnea on exertion in older children; no growth failure
III	Marked limitation of physical activity; comfortable at rest; symptoms with less than ordinary activity	Marked tachypnea and/or diaphoresis with feedings or exertion; prolonged feeding times with growth failure
IV	Inability to carry on any physical activity without discomfort; symptoms may be present at rest; symptoms increase withany activity	Symptomatic at rest with tachypnea, retractions, grunting, or diaphoresis

[a] New York Heart Association (NYHA) Functional Class. Adapted from American Heart Association Medical/Scientific Statement. 1994 revisions to classification of functional capacity and objective assessment of patients with diseases of the heart. *Circulation*, 1994, 90: 644–645. The Criteria Committee of the New York Heart Association. *Nomenclature and Criteria for Diagnosis of Diseases of the Heart and Great Vessels*, 9e, 253–256. Little, Brown; Boston, 1994.
[b] "Ross Classification" data from Ross, R.D., Daniels, S.R., Schwartz, D.C., et al. (1987). Plasma norepinephrine levels in infants and children with congestive heart failure. *Am. J. Cardiol.*, 59: 911–914.

MEDICAL MANAGEMENT

Once the diagnosis of cardiac failure has been made, treatment should be initiated with as many as four types of medication: an inotrope, a diuretic, an agent to reduce afterload, and a beta-blocker for chronic heart failure.

Inotropes

Inotropes include beta-receptor agonists (dopamine and dobutamine), inhibitors of myocardial phosphodiesterases (milrinone), and digoxin preparations (which inhibit cell-wall sodium–potassium pumps).

The common end effect of these inotropes is an increase in intracellular calcium ions available to the myocardial contractile proteins.

Inotropes, however, have limitations. A child with cardiac failure usually has maximum activation of compensatory mechanisms, including elevated catecholamines, and in chronic heart failure, beta-receptors and contractile elements show a blunted response to adrenergic stimulation. Administration of therapeutic inotropes in these children may have little added benefit.

Patients with certain types of heart failure, including ischemic cardiomyopathy, may actually do less well with inotropes and have a better long-term prognosis with beta-receptor blockers rather than beta-stimulants.

Other adverse effects of inotropes include increased heart rate and metabolic work with little increase in myocardial performance. High doses of some inotropic drugs, particularly digoxin or dopamine, may adversely increase systemic vascular resistance.

Intravenous inotropes

These include dobutamine (1–15 μg/kg/min) and dopamine (5–20 μg/kg/min). The inotropic effects of the two are similar, but dopamine may increase renal blood flow more than dobutamine. Dopamine doses in excess of 15 μg/kg/min stimulate alpha-receptors and may adversely increase systemic vascular resistance. Milrinone, inotropic by inhibition of the breakdown of phosphorylated "messenger" compounds within the cell, may exert their greatest beneficial effect by vasodilation (see the section "Afterload Reduction").

Oral therapy

Digoxin is the preferred and only oral introtropic drug for pediatric use, although oral phosphodiesterase inhibitors are under development.

Digoxin may exert its greatest beneficial effect through vagal stimulation and slowing of conduction and heart rate. Although it may be given orally, intramuscularly, or intravenously, digoxin is safest given orally. Digoxin can be initiated at the maintenance dose without a loading dose. This is a safer method of starting outpatient therapy but requires several days to reach full digitalization.

Digoxin loading dose

Great care must be exercised in the calculation of dosage and ordering the medication; dose errors have a potentially greater adverse effect than with many other drugs.

Recommended oral *total digitalizing doses* (TDD) per kilogram of body weight of digoxin:

- premature infants, 20 μg
- term neonates, 30–40 μg
- children up to two years of age, 40–60 μg
- children more than two years of age, 30–40 μg.

If given parenterally, these doses are reduced by 25%.

Usually, half of the TDD is given initially, one-fourth at six to eight hours after the first dose, and the final one-fourth at six to eight hours following the second dose.

If necessary, in emergency cases, three-fourths of the digitalizing dosage may be given initially.

Maintenance digoxin dose. Twenty-four hours after the initial dose of digoxin, maintenance therapy is started. The recommended maintenance dose is 25% of the TDD, in divided doses, with half of the maintenance dose given in the morning and the other half in the evening.

These recommendations are merely guidelines, and the dose may be altered according to the patient's response to therapy or the presence of digitalis toxicity.

Digoxin maintenance dosing

Except for premature infants and those with renal impairment, generally 10 µg/kg/day is given in two divided doses.

In children taking the elixir (50 µg/mL), a convenient dose is 0.1 mL × body weight in kilograms, twice daily. The authors round off the dose to the nearest (usually the lowermost) 0.1 mL. For example, a 4.4-kg infant may be given 0.4 mL b.i.d. A 2.8-kg infant can safely receive 0.3 mL b.i.d.

Toxicity. During digitalization, monitoring the patient clinically is important. If indicated, an electrocardiographic rhythm strip is used before the administration of each portion of the digitalizing dose to detect digitalis toxicity.

Slowing of the sinus rate and alterations in the ST segments are indications of digitalis effect but not of toxicity.

Digitalis toxicity is indicated by a prolonged PR interval or higher degrees of AV block and by cardiac arrhythmia, such as nodal or ventricular premature beats. Clinical signs of digitalis toxicity are nausea, vomiting, anorexia, and lethargy.

Digoxin should not be used in the presence of hypokalemia. Toxic effects, especially ventricular arrhythmias, are much more likely during hypokalemia, even with therapeutic digoxin levels.

Because digoxin is almost completely eliminated by the kidney, it should be used with caution and with appropriate dose modification in patients with renal impairment.

Diuretics

Diuretics are indicated in many patients with congestive cardiac failure. Although peripheral edema is uncommon in infants and children with cardiac failure, perhaps because they are supine much of the time, they do retain sodium and fluid. The major manifestations of tissue edema are tachypnea and dyspnea.

Furosemide (frusemide; Lasix®), the diuretic most commonly used in the acute treatment of cardiac failure, can be given parenterally, 1 mg/kg/dose. The oral dosage is 2–4 mg/kg/day. The effect of furosemide begins promptly.

> For infants who also commonly receive digoxin, parental stress is minimized by giving the same volume of furosemide suspension (10 mg/mL) as of digoxin at each dose, twice daily. For example, an infant weighing 3 kg can be given digoxin 0.3 mL and furosemide 0.3 mL orally twice per day.

With repeated use, serum sodium, chloride, and potassium levels become abnormal, and a contraction metabolic alkalosis may develop. Patients receiving chronic diuretic therapy may develop hypokalemia, and the low potassium enhances digitalis toxicity, even with normal digoxin blood levels.

Potassium supplementation should be given to such patients. Older children should be encouraged to eat potassium-rich foods, such as oranges, bananas, and raisins, as part of their regular diet.

With diuretics, the central fluid volume in some children may decrease, leading to higher renin (and angiotensin) levels than occur from heart failure alone. These adverse effects of chronic high-dose diuretic use may contribute to increased systemic vascular resistance and, paradoxically, worsen cardiac failure.

A variety of other diuretics, including hydrochlorothiazide or spironolactone, are used for chronic long-term management of congestive cardiac failure. Although they produce less electrolyte disturbance, their beneficial effect relative to that of furosemide has been questioned.

Furosemide and a potassium-sparing diuretic are often used in combination. Potassium-sparing diuretics must be used with caution if other aldosterone antagonists (angiotensin-converting enzyme [ACE] inhibitors) are used (see the next section, "Afterload reduction").

Afterload reduction

Natural mechanisms produce vasoconstriction and redistribution of organ blood flows in patients with hypotension. Although such events may be beneficial during acute hemorrhage, for example, vasoconstriction is disadvantageous in chronic heart failure.

Vasoconstriction increases the impedance to arterial blood flow that myocytes must overcome to propel blood from the heart. The mechanical load on the myocytes, known as afterload, is increased in heart failure.

Reducing the afterload on failing myocardial cells may improve their performance, lessen ongoing myocyte injury, and allow for recovery of injured myocytes, depending on the mechanism of the heart failure.

Afterload reduction is achieved by the administration of vasodilator drugs, which relax smooth muscle in systemic arterioles and decrease systemic vascular resistance.

These drugs may also partially redistribute blood flow toward more normal patterns. Increasing renal blood flow may lessen the overproduction of renin, a factor in elevated afterload.

Afterload reduction is titrated to prevent lowered blood pressure. According to the equation $P = Q_s \times R_s$, as systemic resistance (R_s) falls, myocyte performance is enhanced, cardiac output (Q_s) increases, and blood pressure (P) remains constant or rises.

In infants with a ventricular septal defect and a large left-to-right shunt, reduction of systemic vascular resistance (provided that the pulmonary vascular resistance does not fall to a similar extent) decreases the volume of blood shunted and relieves cardiac failure by lessening the left ventricular volume overload.

ACE inhibitors block the conversion of renin to its vasoconstrictor form, angiotensin, thereby producing afterload reduction. The prognosis for patients with chronic heart failure treated with ACE inhibitors appears better than for those treated with direct vasodilator agents, such as nitrates. Presumably, ACE inhibitors prevent maladaptive myocardial changes that occur as nonspecific responses to failure.

Two common ACE inhibitors used in infants and children are captopril and enalapril. If the liquid forms are not available, solutions have been made from tablets, but care must be taken in its preparation and storage, since captopril in particular degrades rapidly in solution. Oral enalapril can be used once daily in children able to take tablets. An intravenous form, enalaprilat, is also available.

Disadvantages of ACE inhibitors include an increase in bradykinins (also metabolized by ACE), which may both worsen pulmonary symptoms and cause renal injury. These drugs have an antialdosterone renal effect, so they are used with caution with potassium-sparing diuretics or potassium supplements.

Beta-receptor antagonists

Beta-receptor antagonists (beta-blockers) benefit some children with moderate chronic heart failure (class II–III; see Table 11.1), usually those with cardiomyopathy. Beta-blockers may reverse some neurohumoral derangements of chronic heart failure, especially the detrimental cardiac effect of high levels of endogenous catecholamines. Some beta-blockers (e.g. carvedilol) have both alpha-antagonist (promoting vasodilation and afterload reduction) and beta-antagonist properties.

Beta-blockers are for long-term use. Short-term treatment of heart failure may require an inotrope, including a beta-agonist (e.g. dopamine). Simultaneous use of beta-agonists and antagonists is irrational. Identifying patients who do not depend on high levels of catecholamines and will benefit from beta-blockers can be challenging.

These drugs are not useful for and may have adverse effects in children with high-output-type heart failure, as in a left-to-right shunt. These children are usually managed definitively with surgery.

In conclusion, one or more of the classes of drugs outlined in Table 11.2 are employed for the management of acute heart failure, and examples of commonly used agents are given. The specific drug literature should be consulted for precautions, contraindications, and details of use, including maximum doses.

Supportive measures

Other therapeutic measures may be useful in the treatment of children with congestive cardiac failure.

Oxygen

Oxygen should be administered initially. Long-term use of oxygen may be counterproductive, perhaps because of its effect as a systemic vasoconstrictor (thereby increasing afterload). Oxygen is administered using a rigid plastic hood in neonates and nasal cannulae in older children. The least aggravating method of delivery should be sought, since increased patient agitation in the presence of limited cardiac output will be counterproductive.

Mechanical ventilation

In the acute management of severe cardiac failure, endotracheal intubation and mechanical ventilation may be indicated. Children may present in extremis with respiratory failure due to fatigue of overworked ventilatory muscles. After intubation and mechanical ventilation, paralysis and deep sedation can reduce the patient's requirements for cardiac output, allowing time for more definitive management of their heart failure.

Table 11.2 Congestive heart failure – drug therapy.

Diuretics	Dose	Frequency	Route
Chlorothiazide (Diuril®)			
Age <6 months	2–8 mg/kg/day	b.i.d.	IV
	20–40 mg/kg/day	b.i.d.	PO
Age >6 months	4 mg/kg/day	q.d. or b.i.d.	IV
	20 mg/kg/day	b.i.d.	PO
Adult	100–500 mg/day	q.d. or b.i.d.	IV
	500 mg–2 g/day	q.d. or b.i.d.	PO
Furosemide (Lasix)	0.5–1 mg/kg/dose	q.d. or b.i.d.	IV
	1–4 mg/kg/day	q.d. or b.i.d.	PO
Spironolactone (Aldactone®)	1–3 mg/kg/day	q.d. or b.i.d.	PO
	Adult: 12.5–50 mg/ day	q.d. or b.i.d.	PO
Inotropes			
Digoxin (Lanoxin®)			
Load (TDD)	PO (avoid parenteral route)		
Premature	20 μg/kg		
Term neonates	30–40 μg/kg		
Infants to 2 years	40–60 μg/kg		
Children >2 years	30–40 μg/kg		
(Give ½ of TDD initially, ¼ of TDD in 6–8 hours, and last ¼ of TDD in 12–16 hours after first dose; reassess clinically before each increment of the TDD is given.)			
Maintenance			
25% of TDD/day b.i.d			PO
or			
10 μg/kg/day b.i.d			PO
Dobutamine (Dobutrex®)	1–15 μg/kg/min		IV
Dopamine (Intropin®)	5–20 μg/kg/min		IV
Epinephrine (adrenaline)	0.02–1.0 μg/kg/min		IV
Milrinone (Primacor®)			
bolus	50 μg/kg (over 15 min)		IV
infusion (± *bolus*)	0.25–1.0 μg/kg/min		IV
Afterload reducing agents			
Captopril (Capoten® tablets)	0.25–4 mg/kg/day t.i.d.		PO
	Adult: 12.5–25 mg/ dose t.i.d.		PO

(*continued*)

Table 11.2 (*continued*)

Diuretics	Dose	Frequency	Route
(No commercially available liquid dose form; captopril rapidly degrades in aqueous solution, mix fresh 1 mg/mL solution each dose, or compound according to *Am. J. Hosp. Pharm.* 1994, 51:95–96.)			
Enalapril (Vasotec® tablets; Epaned® 1 mg/mL)	0.1–0.5 mg/kg/day q.d. or b.i.d.		PO
	Adult: starting 5 mg/day, max 40 mg/day		PO
Enalaprilat (Vasotec)	Starting 5–10 μg/ kg/dose q6h–24h		IV
	Adult: 0.625– 1.25 mg/dose q6h		IV
Nitroglycerin	0.25–20 μg/kg/min		IV
Nitroprusside (Nitropress®)	0.25–10 μg/kg/min		IV

Morphine

Morphine (0.1 mg/kg) and other sedatives may be useful in treating a tachypneic, dyspneic, and dusky infant who has severe respiratory distress associated with congestive cardiac failure and pulmonary edema.

On the other hand, sedation may result in apnea in children who have impending respiratory failure from fatigue and in those with underlying pulmonary disease.

> Close monitoring and preparations for emergency intubation are warranted if sedatives are used.

Management of pulmonary consolidation. Conditions associated with increased pulmonary blood flow have an increased incidence of pneumonia. Atelectasis occurs more commonly in children because of bronchial compression from enlarged pulmonary arteries or cardiac chambers. Pneumonia, atelectasis, or other febrile illnesses can precipitate decompensation of a previously stable patient with congestive cardiac failure. Pulmonary consolidation should be sought in children with cardiac failure and treated appropriately if present.

Fever

Fever should be treated aggressively in children with heart failure if it results in decompensatory episodes. Fever increases cardiac output by 10–15% per degree Celsius.

Anemia management

Anemia often occurs in children with chronic cardiac failure. It is usually a mild normochromic anemia, not related to iron or nutrient deficiency, and may be similar to the "anemia of chronic disease." It may improve with heart failure treatment.

In patients with severe uncompensated heart failure, significant anemia imposes a cardiac volume overload proportional to the degree of anemia; the effects of compensatory changes in hemoglobin affinity for oxygen are negligible compared with the hemoglobin concentration.

> For example, if a child's hemoglobin concentration is 10 rather than 15 g/dL, cardiac output will be approximately one-third greater to deliver the same amount of oxygen to the tissues in the same amount of time.
>
> A dysfunctional left ventricle may lack the contractile reserve to compensate for anemia by increased cardiac output.

Transfusion is usually well tolerated if given slowly. Unfortunately, the small number of leukocytes that contaminate packed erythrocyte transfusions expose the patient to foreign antigens and may make tissue matching for subsequent cardiac transplantation problematic. Steps should be taken to filter the transfused erythrocytes.

DEFINITIVE DIAGNOSIS AND MANAGEMENT

Congestive cardiac failure is not a disease but a symptom complex caused by an underlying cardiac condition. After treatment of congestive cardiac failure, consideration must be given to the type of cardiac abnormality that produced the failure.

Operable lesions, such as coarctation of the aorta or patent ductus arteriosus, may cause the cardiac failure. Therefore, following the treatment of congestive failure in any infant, appropriate studies should be performed to establish the diagnosis.

Once a diagnosis has been made, either a palliative or a corrective procedure should be completed. For lesions with a favorable natural history (e.g. the infant with a moderate-sized ventricular septal defect that might close spontaneously, thereby avoiding operation) and if the infant gains weight and does well, a conservative approach may be appropriate.

Since in older children congestive cardiac failure often results from acquired cardiac conditions, cardiac catheterization may not be required because the etiology is frequently evident from history, physical examination, or laboratory findings. Catheterization may be indicated to determine pulmonary resistance in consideration for cardiac or cardiopulmonary transplantation.

If appropriate, specific treatment should be undertaken for the condition (e.g. fever from infection) triggering the failure.

Circulatory support and cardiac transplantation

Myocardial failure occurs from many causes (including myocarditis, primary cardiomyopathy, storage disease, and heart failure associated with congenital heart malformations), yet the exact mechanism of failure usually cannot be determined. Treatments are usually nonspecific. When the child does not respond to medical therapy and survival is threatened, circulatory support and/or transplantation may be indicated.

Circulatory support can be provided by extracorporeal membrane oxygenation (ECMO) or with other mechanical support devices. These are simply pumps connected to the patient's circulation that assume the entire work of the left heart, and sometimes of both ventricles. It is continued until the patient recovers their own intrinsic myocardial function (*bridge to recovery*) or is used as a *bridge to transplantation*. For some children transplantation may not be an option, and such devices are increasingly used as *destination therapy*. Cardiac transplantation remains the ultimate option for patients with severe myocardial dysfunction that is not expected to recover.

Limitations of transplantation include the need to identify an appropriate donor of compatible size and immunologic "match" in sufficient time to avoid end-organ damage (such as pulmonary hypertension or renal failure) that might preclude successful transplantation. Approximately one in four patients suffer a stroke, usually embolic, while being treated with mechanical circulatory support. More adult and pediatric patients die from their disease before coming to transplantation than are able to receive transplant. Currently, about 500 pediatric and adolescent cardiac transplantations occur annually in the United States.

Survival to the point of transplant is limited primarily by patient-related factors (e.g. end-organ damage such as renal failure and pulmonary hypertension) and donor organ availability.

The surgical procedure for transplantation is relatively straightforward. Either the donor atria are anastomosed to the recipient atria (leaving the recipient's native venoatrial connections unaltered, except in those children with heterotaxy), called a *biatrial* technique, or the vena cavae are individually anastomosed, the *bicaval* technique. The latter is generally preferred as it preserves the recipient right atrium, resulting in less dilation and tricuspid valve dysfunction, and reduces arrhythmia and the need for postoperative pacing. The donor and recipient great arteries are anastomosed. Surgical survival is usually very good.

Long term prognosis refers to survival of both the patient and the transplanted heart. The most common threat to long-term survival is loss of graft (heart function) due to rejection, and coronary artery microvascular disease. The latter can lead to sudden death and is an indication for a second transplant in children affected by it. Periodic cardiac catheterization is routinely used (i) to obtain biopsy specimens of the right ventricular myocardium, looking for histologic signs of rejection, and in (ii) coronary arteriography to screen for luminal disease.

Long-term quality of life is affected by a balance of medications designed to combat rejection against the toxicity and adverse effects of these drugs (Table 11.3).

Table 11.3 Typical therapeutic scheme for pediatric cardiac transplant patients.

Antirejection therapy	Duration
Calcineurin inhibitors (e.g. cyclosporine, tacrolimus)	Lifelong
Antiproliferatives (e.g. mycophenolate, azathioprine)	Lifelong
Steroids	For first year, and subsequently as needed during rejection episodes
Anti-infective therapy	
Antivirals (e.g. ganciclovir)	For first year
Antibacterials (e.g. trimethoprim/sulfamethoxazole)	For first year
Endocarditis prophylaxis, if valvulopathy, according to AHA guidelines (see Table 12.10)	Lifelong
Immunizations (influenza vaccine; avoid live virus such as MMR, varicella, and some polio vaccines)	Influenza vaccine annually
Antihypertensive therapy	
Generally, calcium channel antagonists over other antihypertensives	Lifelong, as indicated
Antihyperlipidemia therapy	
Therapy of secondary causes (diabetes) and drug therapy (statins, etc.)	Lifelong, as indicated
Diabetes therapy	
Oral hypoglycemics and/or insulin; diet; discontinue steroids if possible; transition from tacrolimus if possible	Lifelong, as indicated
Antineoplastic therapy	
Reduction of antirejection agents when possible, and/or active treatment of neoplasia	Lifelong

AHA, American Heart Association.

Some patients after transplantation have relatively few episodes of clinical rejection (with symptoms). Others have only subclinical rejection that may only be detected using biopsy, but which can nevertheless damage the transplanted heart. Still others have multiple severe episodes of rejection that must be aggressively treated to maintain survival.

Long-term survival and quality of life can be excellent, however, and extend for decades beyond transplantation. Some patients can eventually arrive at a point where medical therapy and its potential adverse effects are minimal (Table 11.3).

ADDITIONAL READING

Chatfield, K., Nakano, S., J., and Everitt, M., D. (2019). General pediatric care for a patient after heart transplant: what the practitioner needs to know. *Curr. Opin. Pediatr.* **31** (5): 592–597. https://doi.org/10.1097/MOP.0000000000000803.

Kirk, R., Dipchand, A., I., Rosenthal, D., N. et al. (2014). The International Society for Heart and Lung Transplantation guidelines for the management of pediatric heart failure: executive summary [corrected]. *J. Heart Lung Transplant.* **33** (9): 888–909. http://doi.org/10.1016/j.healun.2014.06.002. Epub 2014 Jun 17. [Erratum appears in *J. Heart Lung Transplant.* 42(5):1104.] www.ishlt.org (accessed 5 January 2022).

Kleinman, K., McDaniel, L., and Molloy, M. (ed.) (2021). *The Harriet Lane Handbook. A Handbook for Pediatric House Officers*, 22e. Philadelphia, PA: Elsevier.

Law, Y., M., Lal, A., K., Chen, S. et al. (2021). Diagnosis and management of myocarditis in children: a scientific statement from the American Heart Association [published correction appears in *Circulation* 144 (6):e149]. *Circulation* **144** (6): e123–e135. https://doi.org/10.1161/CIR.0000000000001001.

Lorts, A., Conway, J., Schweiger, M. et al. (2021). ISHLT consensus statement for the selection and management of pediatric and congenital heart disease patients on ventricular assist devices. Endorsed by the American Heart Association. *J. Heart Lung Transplant.* **40** (8): 709–732. http://dx.doi.org/10.1016/j.healun.2021.04.015, www.ishlt.org. (accessed 5 January 2022).

Masarone, D., Valente, F., Rubino, M. et al. (2017). Pediatric heart failure: a practical guide to diagnosis and management. *Pediatr. Neonatol.* **58** (4): 303–312. https://doi.org/10.1016/j.pedneo.2017.01.001.

McDonagh, T., A., Metra, M., Adamo, M. et al. (2021). ESC guidelines for the diagnosis and treatment of acute and chronic heart failure [published correction appears in *Eur. Heart J.* Oct 14]. *Eur. Heart J.* **42** (36): 3599–3726. https://doi.org/10.1093/eurheartj/ehab368.

Taketomo, C. (ed.) (2021). *Pediatric and Neonatal Drug Dosage Handbook*, 28e. Hudson, OH: Lexicomp.

US National Library of Medicine (2022). *Drug Information* (with links to International Drug Information sites). http://druginfo.nlm.nih.gov (accessed 6 March 2022).

Chapter 12
A healthy lifestyle and preventing heart disease in children

In this chapter, we discuss the prevention of cardiac disease both for patients with cardiac malformations and cardiac disease acquired during childhood and for children and adolescents with a normal heart who may be at risk for the development of atherosclerotic heart disease in adulthood. We discuss the environmental and genetic factors that influence cardiac disease in these two groups of patients.

PREVENTION FOR CHILDREN WITH A NORMAL HEART

Risk factors for adult-manifest cardiovascular disease

Many risk factors have been identified for the development of atherosclerotic disease of coronary, cerebral, and other arteries. Some factors are more important and/or prevalent in childhood than others, and their impact in adulthood begins with exposure in childhood and adolescence. We discuss factors that are generally regarded to have the greatest preventive benefit if effective modification can be

Moller's Essentials of Pediatric Cardiology, Fourth Edition.
Walter H. Johnson, Jr. and Camden L. Hebson.
© 2023 John Wiley & Sons Ltd. Published 2023 by John Wiley & Sons Ltd.

achieved early in life. Several factors are strongly interrelated (e.g. obesity and abnormal lipid and glucose metabolism).

Tobacco

Tobacco use is the single most important independent risk factor for the development of atherosclerotic cardiovascular disease that is purely environmental, and thereby potentially modifiable. Adults who smoke have a two- to fourfold increased risk of myocardial infarction.

Smoking and tobacco use

The mechanism of adverse cardiovascular effect is related to multiple factors:

(1) Endothelial cell dysfunction and injury from various toxins and oxygen free radicals.
(2) Hypercoagulable effects and platelet activation.
(3) Induced hyperlipidemia.
(4) Increased myocardial work, caused by nicotine.
(5) Decreased oxygen delivery, caused by carbon monoxide.

Because of the poor rate of recovery from tobacco addiction, prevention of first use of smoking and other tobacco products among children and adolescents is the single most important means of avoiding adverse health effects in adulthood. The long-term abstinence rate among adults without physician-based intervention is less than 5% and yet with intervention it is only about 40%.

Passive smoking is risky for children, so family members and household contacts should be counseled not to smoke. The cardiovascular risk is related to both dose and duration, and a safe lower limit of passive exposure has not been determined.

Factors in tobacco addiction

Nicotine is highly addictive and shares features common to other addictive substances:

(1) Psychoactive properties – substance use causes pleasurable central nervous system response.
(2) Tolerance – (tachyphylaxis) occurs by multiple physiologic mechanisms, including receptor downregulation, and is overcome by increased dose.

---

(3) Physiologic dependency – results in physiological reaction and adverse withdrawal symptoms upon cessation of use.

Other factors have been observed regarding tobacco addiction:

(1) Genotype. Certain individuals may be biologically predisposed to addiction; a familial tendency has been demonstrated.
(2) Age of introduction. Patients who begin smoking as children or adolescents are more likely to continue smoking as adults. Prevention of addiction must begin in childhood.
(3) Chemical dependency. Chemical dependency on other substances is associated with increased rates of tobacco addiction.
(4) Depression, other mental illness, and high emotional stress are associated with increased rates of tobacco addiction.
(5) Other smokers in the household.
(6) Lack of access to smoking-cessation resources.

Cessation management

The risk of cardiovascular disease declines after cessation and, after a number of years, may approach the risk level of those who have never smoked.

The reported long-term abstinence rate of counseling, psychotherapy, and/or nicotine replacement (chewing gum, transdermal patches, nasal spray, etc.) is 20% or less (for adolescents, it is less than 5%).

The addition of antidepressants, such as bupropion (a dopamine reuptake inhibitor), increases success rates to just over 20%.

The use of drugs (e.g. varenicline) that act on the nicotine receptor increases success rates to more than 40%. Such drugs are partial nicotine receptor agonists (which serve to blunt withdrawal and craving) and receptor blockers (which prevent nicotine binding, eliminating the positive reinforcement from tobacco use).

Hypercholesterolemia

Coronary atherosclerosis is a highly prevalent problem in developed societies and less common in other cultures, suggesting that diet, lifestyle, and other environmental factors are important. A strong genetic component also influences the metabolism of lipids, which has an important effect on individual disease.

Mechanism of cardiovascular effect. Atheroma, the basic lesion of coronary and other arteriosclerosis, is an erosion of the arterial endothelium capped by a lipid-laden plaque. These plaques may slowly narrow the coronary arterial lumen, leading to intermittent insufficiency of arterial blood flow (creating myocardial ischemia and symptoms of angina). They can also rupture, lead to acute thrombosis and occlusion of the artery, and result in myocardial infarction and/or sudden cardiac death. The exact role of lipids in the initial endothelial injury is unclear. Atheromas are known to begin in childhood; therefore, prevention of adult cardiovascular disease should also begin in childhood.

Heart-diet theory

Coronary atherosclerosis is strongly associated with high blood levels of certain lipids. Dietary fats influence the concentration of circulating lipids, which are transported by lipoproteins:

(1) Low-density lipoprotein cholesterol (LDL-C), the "bad cholesterol," promotes atheroma formation, transports cholesterol to tissues such as the endothelium, binds to the low-density lipoprotein (LDL) receptor on cells, and thereby allows the cholesterol to enter the cell.

   LDL receptors on liver cells can be modified by drugs (statins) to reduce circulating LDL-C.

   LDL-C can be measured but is often estimated using the Friedewald equation:

$$LDL - C = TC - (HDL - C + triglycerides / 5),$$

   where *TC* is total cholesterol and *HDL-C* is high-density lipoprotein cholesterol. This equation is invalid if the patient is nonfasting, if abnormal lipoprotein is present (type III; see under "Screening and intervention"), and when triglycerides (TGs) exceed 400 mg/dL. Current estimates in adults suggest that calculated LDL-C levels vary from measured levels by as much as 25%. Other formulas have been developed in an attempt to overcome this, but all only approximate directly measured lipids.

(2) HDL-C, the "good cholesterol," may inhibit atheroma formation by transporting cholesterol away from tissues such as the endothelium and into the liver for excretion as bile acids. It can be measured in nonfasting children. HDL-C levels may be congenitally low, but more commonly they fall with smoking, obesity, or lack of exercise and, conversely, rise with intervention for these factors.

(3) Other lipids, including TGs, transported by very low-density lipoproteins (VLDLs), and chylomicrons, are less strongly associated with cardiovascular risk, and blood levels are more subject to dramatic postprandial shifts. Interventions targeting LDL-C, HDL-C, and TC generally improve levels of these lipids also.

(4) TC is a collective measure of LDL-C, HDL-C, and VLDL.

Measurement of LDL-C, HDL-C, VLDLs, and TGs has traditionally been performed after a 12-hour fast (nothing to eat or drink except water), yet fasting is a problem when screening patients. Currently, nonfasting studies are recommended, unless there are additional risk factors or a strong family history.

Because TC is less affected by postprandial change, it can be drawn in fasting and nonfasting patients. Therefore, TC (or TC and non-HDL-C) is the value most often used for screening.

(5) Non-HDL-C is a way of expressing all of the atherogenic components of a lipid profile. It is simply the HDL-C subtracted from the TC value. Some have suggested that it correlates as well or better than LDL-C with adult disease. It has the advantage of being less affected by nonfasting and has been recommended, along with TC, as a screening test.

(6) Apolipoproteins (e.g. ApoB, ApoA-1) are the proteins that allow transport within the bloodstream of otherwise insoluble lipids when the two combine to form lipoproteins. Apolipoproteins also function with enzymes and receptors in the regulation of lipid metabolism. Many genetic polymorphisms have been described and this may account for some of the wide clinical variations in disease that lipid concentrations alone fail to explain. ApoB is the main protein component of atherogenic LDL-C, and ApoA-1 is the protein component of anti-atherogenic HDL-C. They are not typically used in screening tests.

In adults with myocardial infarction, 25% have LDL-C ≤130 mg/dL (corresponding to TC ≤200 mg/dL), yet myocardial infarction is rare in adults with LDL-C ≤100 mg/dL (TC ≤150 mg/dL).

Screening and intervention. The goals of screening include identification of children with familial dyslipidemia (1–2% of patients), secondary causes of hyperlipidemia (1%), and those at highest risk for adult-manifest cardiovascular disease (10–25% of all children).

Screening of blood lipid levels in children has been controversial because of lack of consensus about which children to screen, the age of screening, and the lipid level limits (cut points) at which to consider a patient for further testing or intervention.

One approach has been to risk-stratify children for screening (targeted screening); another is to screen all children (universal screening).

However, risk-stratification is part of both screening strategies. Children and adolescents are evaluated according to their body mass index (BMI), blood pressure, family history, and the presence of conditions associated with increased risk of coronary artery disease, such as diabetes, familial hypercholesterolemia (FH), renal disease, Kawasaki disease, and chronic inflammatory disease such as lupus. Note that those with a high risk (Tier I) have lower values for cut points. For Tier II patients, the cut points are higher (Figure 12.1). Depending on the individual child's level of risk, differing cut points for lipids, blood pressure, and so on are then targeted for intervention.

Controversy also exists concerning the most appropriate intervention to offer when an affected child is identified. The safety and efficacy of dietary restriction of essential fatty acids on growth and central nervous system development are unknown. The advisability and safety of drug therapy are uncertain. Some guidelines have been criticized for placing increased emphasis on drug therapy in children and adolescents. Also, in general, guidelines have proved to be complicated and unwieldy in clinical use, and with low adherence by medical providers and parents. Recommendations continue to evolve as more data become available.

The 1992 National Cholesterol Education Program (NCEP) and the 2012 National Heart, Lung, and Blood Institute (NHLBI) guidelines adopt similar approaches.

With regard to lipids, these guidelines emphasize:

(1) Lower lipid levels in all persons through population-wide education and changes in diet and lifestyle.
(2) Identification and treatment of children at the highest risk for adult-manifest heart disease by:

- identification of an individual child's risk factors;
- family history;
- lipid measurement;
- diet and exercise to achieve acceptable lipid levels;
- drug therapy when indicated;
- referral to a lipid specialist when indicated.

Specific and detailed recommendations are available from National Heart, Lung, and Blood Institute (2012) *The Expert Panel on Integrated Guidelines for Cardiovascular Health and Risk Reduction in Children and Adolescents. Full Report*, NIH Publication No. 12-7486, National Institutes of Health, Bethesda, MD; www.nhlbi.nih.gov.

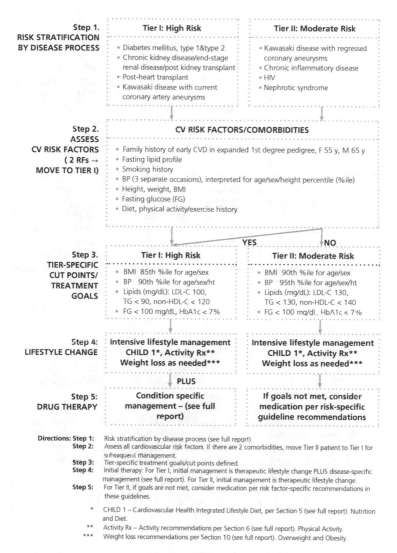

Step 1. **RISK STRATIFICATION BY DISEASE PROCESS**	**Tier I: High Risk**	**Tier II: Moderate Risk**

	• Diabetes mellitus, type 1&type 2
	• Chronic kidney disease/end-stage
	  renal disease/post kidney transplant
	• Post-heart transplant
	• Kawasaki disease with current
	  coronary artery aneurysms
		• Kawasaki disease with regressed
		  coronary aneurysms
		• Chronic inflammatory disease
		• HIV
		• Nephrotic syndrome

Step 2.
**ASSESS
CV RISK FACTORS
(2 RFs →
MOVE TO TIER I)**

CV RISK FACTORS/COMORBIDITIES

• Family history of early CVD in expanded 1st degree pedigree, F 55 y, M 65 y
• Fasting lipid profile
• Smoking history
• BP (3 separate occasions), interpreted for age/sex/height percentile (%ile)
• Height, weight, BMI
• Fasting glucose (FG)
• Diet, physical activity/exercise history

YES   NO

Step 3. **TIER-SPECIFIC CUT POINTS/ TREATMENT GOALS**	**Tier I: High Risk**	**Tier II: Moderate Risk**

	• BMI 85th %ile for age/sex
	• BP 90th %ile for age/sex/ht
	• Lipids (mg/dL): LDL-C 100,
	  TG < 90, non-HDL-C < 120
	• FG < 100 mg/dL, HbA1c < 7%
		• BMI 90th %ile for age/sex
		• BP 95th %ile for age/sex/ht
		• Lipids (mg/dL): LDL-C 130,
		  TG < 130, non-HDL-C < 140
		• FG < 100 mg/dl , HbA1c < 7%

Step 4: **LIFESTYLE CHANGE**	**Intensive lifestyle management CHILD 1*, Activity Rx** Weight loss as needed***	**Intensive lifestyle management CHILD 1*, Activity Rx** Weight loss as needed***

PLUS

Step 5: **DRUG THERAPY**	**Condition specific management – (see full report)**	**If goals not met, consider medication per risk-specific guideline recommendations**

Directions:	**Step 1:**	Risk stratification by disease process (see full report)
	Step 2:	Assess all cardiovascular risk factors. If there are 2 comorbidities, move Tier II patient to Tier I for subsequent management.
	Step 3:	Tier-specific treatment goals/cut points defined.
	Step 4:	Initial therapy: For Tier I, initial management is therapeutic lifestyle change PLUS disease-specific management (see full report). For Tier II, initial management is therapeutic lifestyle change.
	Step 5:	For Tier II, if goals are not met, consider medication per risk factor-specific recommendations in these guidelines.

*   CHILD 1 – Cardiovascular Health Integrated Lifestyle Diet, per Section 5 (see full report). Nutrition and Diet.
**   Activity Rx – Activity recommendations per Section 6 (see full report). Physical Activity.
*** Weight loss recommendations per Section 10 (see full report). Overweight and Obesity.

Figure 12.1 Risk stratification and management for children with conditions predisposing to accelerated atherosclerosis and early cardiovascular disease. BP, blood pressure; CV, cardiovascular; CVD, cardiovascular disease; F, female; ht, height; M, male; RFs, risk factors; Rx, recommendations; y, years. Source: National Heart, Lung, and Blood Institute, National Institutes of Health, US Department of Health and Human Services. See full guidelines and references in National Heart, Lung, and Blood Institute (2012) *The Expert Panel on Integrated Guidelines for Cardiovascular Health and Risk Reduction in Children and Adolescents. Full Report*, NIH Publication No. 12-7486, National Institutes of Health, Bethesda, MD; www.nhlbi.nih.gov.

Guidelines have been criticized for fixed lipid cutoff values, which, depending on the age of the child at screening, identify not just the top quartile, but up to 75% of children as being at risk. Concerns have been expressed about the number of blood samples required and the potential for a large number of children to experience "medicalization" of a preventive health issue that will not be manifest for decades.

One screening strategy has been to advise universal screening but to restrict it to children 9–12 years old, an age at which childhood lipid levels may best correlate with their adult values; postpubertal lipid levels tend to be lower, before rising again to adult levels in late adolescence. It is hoped that those at greatest risk, such as those with FH, can be identified.

Adults in the upper quartile for lipid concentration are at the highest risk for cardiovascular disease. Most of these adults and their children do not have a specific lipid metabolism disorder. Their children tend to be those with lipid levels in the highest quartile and who "track" along similar percentiles into their adult years. Screening and preventive measures are designed to identify and improve risk for these 25% of children also.

Fredrickson classification (types I–V)

This system describes five major phenotypes of hyperlipidemia, but more than one genotype (or acquired condition, such as diabetes) can be associated with a particular phenotype. Cardiovascular risk tends to correlate better with genotype.

Strictly applied, all patients in the top quartile for TC and LDL-C can be classified as type II, but traditionally, the Fredrickson classification is used only for those with lipid levels more than the 98th percentile. It is not useful for most children screened in a general practice, but may be helpful in the management and referral of the patient with a recognized primary lipid disorder. It requires a fasting blood sample.

Type I (high chylomicrons),

Type III (high abnormal VLDL), and type V (high VLDL and chylomicrons) are rare (less than 1 in 1 million children).

Type II (high TC, high LDL-C, ± high TGs) and

Type IV (normal TC, high TGs)

are more common (1 in 200 to 1 in 100), but type II patients (which include the two most common diagnoses encountered in general practice, familial hyperlipidemia and familial combined hyperlipidemia) have significantly increased risk of cardiovascular disease.

Familial combined hyperlipidemia (FCHL)

This group of disorders may be caused by one of many various mutations in apolipoproteins and yet display a similar phenotype. FCHL is relatively common, with as many as 1 in 100–200 children affected. However, the term "combined hyperlipidemia" can also refer to acquired forms with a similar lipid profile. Both forms are likely to be seen with obesity.

Familial hypercholesterolemia (FH)

Some patients showing a type II pattern have FH caused by an LDL receptor defect; they may be heterozygotes (TC 250–500 mg/dL) or, more rarely, homozygotes (TC 500–1200 mg/dL).

Although homozygous FH patients are rare (1 in 1 million children), heterozygotes are not (1 in every 500 children), and early detection and intervention are important since the risk of early-onset cardiovascular disease can be greatly reduced.

Children can present with xanthomas (nodular deposits of lipid in skin or tendons), arcus juvenilis (and other ocular deposits of lipids), and diffuse atherosclerosis, which may manifest at a very young age.

These children (including heterozygotes) need referral to a specialist experienced in the management of dyslipidemias, as diet and many drugs often prove inadequate. Effective therapy requires careful monitoring and balancing of the potential long-term benefit against the risks.

Primary versus secondary hyperlipidemia

Secondary causes of hyperlipidemia that must be ruled out include the following:

(1) Nonfasting sample.
(2) Metabolic: renal failure, nephrotic syndrome, anorexia nervosa, inborn errors of metabolism.
(3) Hepatic disorders: biliary atresia, hepatitis.
(4) Drugs: corticosteroids, hormone contraceptives, retinoic acid, anticonvulsants.
(5) Endocrine disorders: diabetes mellitus, thyroid disease, pregnancy.

Blood lipid levels vary by age, gender, and, to some extent, ethnicity. Ethnicity may involve environmental factors (diet and lifestyle may vary between cultures) and also genetic factors.

In general, lipid levels in the late teenage years best predict adult levels, but for younger children, the lipid percentile level correlates better with the adult percentile rank. Values by age and gender are presented in Table 12.1. Acceptable lipid

Table 12.1 Blood lipid levels in a sample of US children.

Lipid	Age (years)	Males (percentiles)					Females (percentiles)				
		5	25	50	75	95	5	25	50	75	95
TC	0–4	114	137	151	171	203	112	139	156	172	200
	5–9	121	143	159	175	203	126	146	163	179	205
	10–14	119	140	155	173	202	124	144	158	174	201
	15–19	113	132	146	165	197	120	139	154	171	200
	20–24	124	146	165	186	218	122	143	160	182	216
LDL-C	0–4										
	5–9	63	80	90	103	129	68	88	98	115	140
	10–14	64	81	94	109	132	68	81	94	110	136
	15–19	62	80	93	109	130	60	78	93	110	135
	20–24	66	85	101	118	147	–	80	98	113	–
HDL-C	0–4										
	5–9	38	49	54	63	74	36	47	52	61	73
	10–14	37	46	55	61	74	37	45	52	58	70
	15–19	30	39	46	52	63	35	43	51	61	73
	20–24	30	38	45	51	63	–	43	50	60	–
TGs	0–4	29	40	51	67	99	34	45	59	77	112
	5–9	30	40	51	65	101	32	44	55	71	105
	10–14	32	45	59	78	125	37	54	70	90	131
	15–19	37	54	69	91	148	39	52	66	84	124
	20–24	44	63	86	119	201	36	51	64	84	131

TC, total cholesterol; LDL-C, low-density lipoprotein cholesterol; HDL-C, high-density lipoprotein cholesterol; TGs, triglycerides.
Plasma lipid values are expressed as mg/dL and are based on a sample of White males and females (not taking hormone contraceptives). Values for black males and females (not shown) were based on a smaller sample size, but tended to be up to 5% higher for TC in the 0–9 years age group.
For TC, LDL-C, and HDL-C, to convert from mg/dL to mmol/L multiply mg/dL by 0.0259.
For TG, to convert from mg/dL to mmol/L multiply mg/dL by 0.0113. Source: Data from National Heart, Lung, and Blood Institute. (1980). *The Lipid Research Clinics Population Studies Data Book*, Vol. I, NIH Publication 80-1527, National Institutes of Health, Bethesda, MD.

values have been presented in 2012 NHLBI guidelines (Tables 12.2 and 12.3). Lipid levels alone do not perfectly predict future coronary artery disease.

For a child identified with a lipid abnormality, three levels of care may be advisable: primary care, referral, and/or comanagement with a lipid specialist.

In general, healthy children with a family history of coronary artery disease and/ or LDL-C values in the top quartile should be counseled and followed by their primary care provider.

Children with secondary causes of hyperlipidemia (e.g. diabetes, nephrotic syndrome) may be followed jointly by other subspecialists (e.g. pediatric endocrinologist, nephrologist) and usually do not require further evaluation by a specialist in dyslipidemia.

Table 12.2 Acceptable, borderline-high, and high plasma lipid, lipoprotein, and apolipoprotein concentrations (mg/dL) for children and adolescents[a].

Category	Acceptable	Borderline-high	High[b]
LDL-C	<110	110–129	≥130
LDL-C	<110	110–129	≥130
Non-HDL-C	<120	120–144	≥145
ApoB	<90	90–109	≥110
TGs:			
0–9 years	<75	75–99	100
10–19 years	<90	90–129	130

Category	Acceptable	Borderline-low	Low[b]
HDL-C	>45	40–45	<40
ApoA-1	>120	115–120	<115

Values given are in mg/dL. To convert to SI units, divide the results for TC, LDL-C, HDL-C, and non-HDL-C by 38.6; for TGs, divide by 88.6.

[a] Values for plasma lipid and lipoprotein levels are from the NCEP Expert Panel on Cholesterol Levels in Children. Non-HDL-C values from the Bogalusa Heart Study are equivalent to the NCEP Pediatric Panel cut points for LDL-C. Values for plasma ApoB and ApoA-1 are from the National Health and Nutrition Examination Survey III.

[b] The cut points for high and borderline-high represent approximately the 95th and 75th percentiles, respectively. Low cut points for HDL-C and ApoA-1 represent approximately the 10th percentile.Source: National Heart, Lung, and Blood Institute, National Institutes of Health, US Department of Health and Human Services. Full references are available in National Heart, Lung, and Blood Institute. (2012). *The Expert Panel on Integrated Guidelines for Cardiovascular Health and Risk Reduction in Children and Adolescents. Full Report*, NIH Publication No. 12-7486, National Institutes of Health, Bethesda, MD; www.nhlbi.nih.gov.

Table 12.3 Recommended cut points for lipid and lipoprotein levels (mg/dL) in young adults[a].

Category	Acceptable	Borderline-high	High
TC	<190	190–224	≥225
LDL-C	<120	120–159	≥160
Non-HDL-C	<150	150–189	≥190
TGs	<115	115–149	≥150

Category	Acceptable	Borderline-low	Low
HDL-C	>45	40–44	<40

Values given are in mg/dL. To convert to SI units, divide the results for TC, LDL-C, HDL-C, and non-HDL-C by 38.6; for TGs, divide by 88.6.
[a] Values provided are from the Lipid Research Clinics Prevalence Study. The cut points for TC, LDL-C, and non-HDL-C represent the 95th percentile for subjects aged 20–24 years and are not identical with the cut points used in the most recent NCEP Adult Treatment Panel III, which are derived from combined data on adults of all ages. The age-specific cut points given here are provided for pediatric care providers to use in managing this young adult age group. For TC, LDL-C, and non-HDL-C, borderline-high values are between the 75th and 94th percentiles, whereas acceptable values are less than the 75th percentile. The high TG cut point represents approximately the 90th percentile, with borderline-high between the 75th and 89th percentiles; acceptable is less than the 75th percentile; the low HDL-C cut point represents roughly the 25th percentile, with borderline-low between the 26th and 50th percentiles; acceptable is more than the 50th percentile.
Source: National Heart, Lung, and Blood Institute, National Institutes of Health, US Department of Health and Human Services. Full references are available in National Heart, Lung, and Blood Institute. (2012). *The Expert Panel on Integrated Guidelines for Cardiovascular Health and Risk Reduction in Children and Adolescents. Full Report*, NIH Publication No. 12-7486, National Institutes of Health, Bethesda, MD; www.nhlbi.nih.gov.

Children with heterozygous FH can be managed jointly. The rare child with homozygous FH or another rare lipid disorder requires intensive therapy by a lipid specialist who works with dietitians specializing in the treatment of primary hyperlipidemia. The mainstays of therapy are diet and, for selected children, drug therapy.

Diet
Diet, although simple in concept, remains difficult to execute, requires a high level of motivation and cooperation from the family and child, and usually represents a considerable commitment in counseling. A professional dietitian is helpful but is a resource not usually available to a primary care provider.

Various diets have been advocated as interventions for children with primary hyperlipidemia, and they have common characteristics, most importantly the proportion of daily calories from fat (Table 12.4).

The Cardiovascular Health Integrated Lifestyle Diet (CHILD 1) is used for children whose LDL-C is borderline or high, with the goal of reducing LDL-C to the acceptable range.

As a next step, two different CHILD 2 diets can be used that are similar to the CHILD 1 diet, except that the levels of saturated fat and cholesterol are less, and for targeting of elevated TGs, with replacement of simple sugars with complex carbohydrates (Table 12.4).

A detailed assessment by a trained specialist, such as a dietitian, is required; the diet must be carefully monitored to ensure adequate nutrient intake.

Medication

Drug therapy is inappropriate for most children with hyperlipidemia, as most respond to diet and exercise. When drugs are indicated, they are most effective in combination with diet therapy.

Table 12.4 Cardiovascular Health Integrated Lifestyle Diet (CHILD).

CHILD 1 (for children with elevated LDL-C)

- Total fat 25–30% of daily kcal/EER
- Saturated fat 8–10% of daily kcal/EER
- Avoid *trans* fat
- Monounsaturated and polyunsaturated fat up to 20% of daily kcal/EER
- Cholesterol <300 mg/day

CHILD 2-LDL (for children with elevated LDL-C additional risk factors or unresponsive to CHILD 1)

- Saturated fat <7% of daily kcal/EER
- Cholesterol <200 mg/day

CHILD 2-TG (for children with elevated TG)

- Same as CHILD 2 but replaces simple sugars with complex carbohydrates

EER, estimated (daily) energy requirement.
Many characteristics are similar to the American Heart Association Step 1 and Step 2 diets and to the NCEP Pediatric Panel diets.
Specifics of CHILD 1 and 2 diets and detailed information regarding their indications and use are available from National Heart, Lung, and Blood Institute. (2012). *The Expert Panel on Integrated Guidelines for Cardiovascular Health and Risk Reduction in Children and Adolescents. Full Report*, NIH Publication No. 12-7486, National Institutes of Health, Bethesda, MD; www.nhlbi.nih.gov.

(1) Bile binding agents like cholestyramine prevent enterohepatic recycling of bile acids, thus leading to increased conversion of blood and hepatic cholesterol to bile acids.

Although relatively safe with few side effects, they are usually not necessary if dietary compliance can be achieved. They are useful in children with FH and in the management of some secondary hyperlipidemias. Side effects include gastrointestinal symptoms.

(2) Nicotinic acid (niacin) lowers lipid levels by an unknown mechanism. It has unpleasant side effects, including vasodilation, hepatic toxicity, and hyperuricemia, and is usually reserved for children with homozygous FH.

(3) 3-Hydroxy-3-methylglutaryl-coenzyme A (HMG-CoA) reductase inhibitors ("statins") result in lower hepatocyte cholesterol levels. This decrease causes an increase in the LDL receptors on liver cells and leads to increased uptake of LDL-C by the liver. Blood levels of TC, LDL-C, and TGs decrease; HDL-C increases.

Although statins have become first-line drugs for adults, their recommended use in children (except in those with disorders such as FH, in consultation with a lipid specialist) remains controversial. Side effects include skeletal muscle, hepatic, and gastrointestinal toxicity.

Other drugs commonly used in adults have had increasing use in children, usually in those with severe forms of hyperlipidemia. These drugs include fibrates, which lower TG (by accelerating enzymatic clearance of TG-rich particles) and raise HDL, and ezetimibe, a molecular inhibitor of cholesterol absorption in the small bowel. Evolocumab is an antibody which inhibits PCSK9, an enzyme that clears LDL receptors; by increasing the number of LDL receptors, LDL clearance improves and plasma LDL-C levels decrease.

Nonpharmacologic treatments have included stem cell (bone marrow) transplantation for rare children with metabolic errors, such as homozygous FH.

Obesity

Mechanism of cardiovascular effect and definitions of obesity. Obesity is strongly associated with cardiovascular disease. It is multifactorial: 30% of cases are estimated to be genetic and 70% are from environmental factors that are modifiable. These factors may act through multiple interrelated mechanisms, including hyperlipidemia, hypertension, increased left ventricular mass, diabetes and insulin resistance, and obstructive sleep apnea (OSA), which may cause increased pulmonary resistance and right heart abnormalities.

Obesity is the presence of excess body fat, usually expressed as a proportion of total body mass. Like hyperlipidemia, the definition of obesity is somewhat arbitrary and depends on population "normals." Although controversial, a commonly used definition of the term overweight in children is a proportion of body fat greater than the 85th percentile; the term obesity is reserved for those above the 95th percentile.

Comparing children in the 1990s with children studied in the 1960s, the number of "obese" children doubled.

Techniques for assessing obesity include indices of weight or mass compared with some reference, such as height, and also various measures of the proportion of body mass that is comprised of fat. Indices such as BMI, although rapid and simple to determine, do not reliably express adiposity, especially in children with lean body mass who are at the highest percentiles for age.

BMI (or Quetelet Index) is most often used in adults. Normal values are published for children.

$$BMI = \text{weight in kilograms} / (\text{height in meters})^2$$

or

$$BMI = \text{weight in pounds} \times 705 / (\text{height in inches})^2$$

For adults, overweight is defined as BMI $\geq 25\,kg/m^2$ and obesity as BMI $\geq 30\,kg/m^2$.

Note that in this index, the denominator *does not* represent body surface area.

Ideal weight for height

This can be calculated from a standard growth chart showing both height and weight for age.

Ignoring the child's true age, plot the child's true height along the 50th percentile line, then find the "ideal weight" along the 50th percentile for the age corresponding to the plotted height (draw a perpendicular line from the height to the weight curve to find the "ideal weight").

Overweight is defined as weight $\geq$ ideal body weight $\times 1.2$ (which corresponds to approximately the 85th percentile for BMI) and obesity as weight $\geq$ ideal body weight $\times 1.3$.

Various measures of the proportion of body mass consisting of fat can be determined. Varying with age and gender, it may be as much as 25% in normal infants. Measurements of triceps skin-fold thickness and bioelectric impedance are commonly used methods; they are more difficult to perform, require special equipment and/or training, and have limited reproducibility.

Clinical observation of a patient's body fat and habitus is also important in interpreting measures of obesity.

Management. Management of overweight and obese children has become an important priority in preventive medicine because of the rising prevalence of obesity in developed societies. Effective intervention remains challenging, partly because of the difficulty in changing the strong societal factors that influence overweight and obesity in individual patients.

Although the definitions of overweight and obese are to some extent arbitrary, one should avoid classifying as obese any large-for-age child with high lean body mass who appears nonobese.

Rare hormonal and genetic causes (e.g. Klinefelter syndrome, hypothyroidism) should be ruled out. This can be done clinically, as most such affected children will be short (height ≤ 5th percentile) and have other physical clues to the diagnosis.

Increased physical activity rather than direct dietary intervention is the primary therapy for simple obesity. This is most effective when the patient has prescribed time for unstructured outdoor play, with less screen-time and other sedentary pursuits. It may work by (i) increasing energy expenditure, (ii) decreasing total caloric intake (presumably because the child is spending less time near food), and (iii) altering the type of food ingested (e.g. lower percentage of fat calories) by an unknown mechanism.

Morbidly obese children or those who are refractory to simple management techniques benefit from an intensive team approach and require referral to a specialist in pediatric obesity.

Nutrition

Nutrition is an independent risk factor for cardiovascular disease through multiple mechanisms, most of which are interrelated to other risk factors, such as hyperlipidemia and obesity.

In general, the risk increases with a diet high in total calories, total fat, saturated fat, and salt and low in fiber, complex carbohydrates, antioxidants, and certain vitamins.

Commonsense guidelines for improving diet include eating a wide variety of foods, increasing the proportion of whole grains, fruits, and vegetables, and reducing overall fat intake, saturated fat, simple sugars, and salt.

Some specific nutrients have been associated with increased risk of cardiovascular disease, notably increased dietary consumption of *trans*-fatty acids. These fatty acids are chemically different to *cis*-fatty acids, leading to straighter and stiffer molecules when they are incorporated into cellular structures such as membranes.

Exercise

Even moderate-intensity exercise, if performed regularly, exerts a beneficial protective effect against adult-manifest cardiovascular disease. Its effect is mediated through lower blood pressure, less risk of obesity and diabetes, and more favorable lipid profile (particularly increased HDL-C). Exercise may confer a direct benefit to the endothelium, a tissue responsive to mechanical changes, such as increased blood flow and pressure. Children who pursue regular physical activity are more likely to remain active as adults.

Light and moderately intense exercise has low risk. The risks of more intense physical activity, particularly participation in competitive sports, have been studied in relation to sudden death in young athletes, which is estimated to occur at a rate of 1 in 300 000 to 1 in 100 000 each year. Approximately half of deaths of athletes result from trauma, infection, or heat illness, and the other half of this group have pre-existing medical conditions, such as asthma or unrecognized heart disease.

Sports preparticipation evaluation

This examination is designed to identify young athletes who may be at risk for death with intense exercise. Various screening guidelines have been proposed. Heart disorders causing sudden death include hypertrophic cardiomyopathy and coronary artery anomalies, which together account for more than 50% of cases. Other rare causes (e.g. myocarditis and arrhythmogenic right ventricular dysplasia) are difficult to diagnose. Unfortunately, not all patients at risk can be identified by screening tests. US and European recommendations include the screening elements outlined in Table 12.5.

Table 12.5 Preparticipation screening of competitive athletes.

Item	AHA (2007)	ESC (2005) and IOC (2009)
History	Chest pain, exertional	Chest pain, exertional
	Syncope, exertional	Syncope, exertional
	Dyspnea/fatigue, exertional	Dyspnea/fatigue, exertional
	Murmur	Murmur

(continued)

Table 12.5 (*continued*)

Item	AHA (2007)	ESC (2005) and IOC (2009)
	Elevated blood pressure	High blood pressure
		Seizure
		Epilepsy
		Asthma (five questions)
		High cholesterol
		Ever told to give up sports
		Racing heart/skipped beats
		Arrhythmia
		Dizziness, exertional
		Any other history of heart problems
		Severe recent viral infection
		Allergies
		Medications (current and last two years)
Family history	Premature death at age <50 years	Anyone <50 years old:
	Cardiac disability at age <50 years	• sudden unexpected death
		• recurrent fainting
		• unexplained seizure
		• unexplained drowning
		• unexplained car accident
		• heart transplantation
		• pacemaker or defibrillator
		• treated for irregular heart beat
		• heart surgery
	Specific heritable disorders	Marfan syndrome
		SIDS, crib death, cot death
Physical examination	Murmur	Murmur (≥2/6 systolic or any diastolic)
		Systolic click
		Abnormal S_2
		Rate and rhythm
	Femoral pulses (coarct)	Radial and femoral pulses
	Marfan stigmata	Marfan stigmata
	Arm blood pressure	Blood pressure

Table 12.5 (continued)

Item	AHA (2007)	ESC (2005) and IOC (2009)
Laboratory examination	–	Electrocardiogram (abnormal T-wave inversion, ST-segment depression, pathologic Q waves, left atrial enlargement, QRS axis deviation, right ventricular hypertrophy, complete bundle branch block, long or short QT, Brugada findings, or ventricular arrhythmia)

AHA, American Heart Association; ESC, European Society of Cardiology; IOC, International Olympic Committee; SIDS, sudden infant death syndrome. Items refer to screening only; following a positive screening evaluation, additional laboratory studies (e.g. echocardiogram, exercise testing) may be indicated under both sets of recommendations.

Sources: AHA (2007): Maron, B.J., Thompson, P.D., Ackerman, M.J., et al. (2007) Recommendations and considerations related to preparticipation screening for cardiovascular abnormalities in competitive athletes: 2007 update. A scientific statement from the American Heart Association Council on Nutrition, Physical Activity, and Metabolism. endorsed by the American College of Cardiology Foundation. *Circulation*, 115 (12): 1643–1655; www.heart.org. ESC (2005): Corrado, D., Pelliccia, A., Bjørnstad, H.H., et al. (2005). Cardiovascular preparticipation screening of young competitive athletes for prevention of sudden death: proposal for a common European protocol. Consensus Statement of the Study Group of Sport Cardiology of the Working Group of Cardiac Rehabilitation and Exercise Physiology and the Working Group of Myocardial and Pericardial Diseases of the European Society of Cardiology. *Eur. Heart J.*, 26 (5): 516–524. IOC (2009): International Olympic Committee. (2009). *The International Olympic Committee (IOC) Consensus Statement on Periodic Health Evaluation of Elite Athletes*, http://www.olympic.org/documents/reports/en/en_report_1448.pdf.

Laboratory studies have not been accepted as universal screening tools, but the 12-lead electrocardiogram (ECG) has been proposed, as 95% of hypertrophic cardiomyopathy patients will have an abnormal ECG. The ECG is often abnormal in coronary artery anomalies, and it is the most effective means of screening for long QT syndrome (LQTS) and Wolff–Parkinson–White syndrome. Because ECG is not very specific and requires age-appropriate interpretation, many normal children could face unnecessary referral for "borderline" ECGs.

Other risk factors for acquired atherosclerotic disease

Family history and gender. Genetics determines an individual child's future risk for adult-manifest cardiovascular disease in an important but variable fashion. Even when familial risk factors (such as hyperlipidemia) cannot be identified, family history remains an independent risk factor that cannot be modified. With greater understanding of lipid metabolism and endothelial function, many of these patients may become candidates for therapy to lessen their risk. Premenopausal women are relatively protected from atherosclerotic disease when all other risk factors are equal.

Diabetes. Juvenile and adult-onset diabetes are major independent risk factors for cardiovascular disease in adults, as they damage the endothelium by hyperglycemia and glycosylation and, less directly, via hyperlipidemia, hypertension, and autonomic neuropathy, which may worsen microvascular dysfunction.

Insulin resistance is a spectrum of metabolic derangements (type 2 diabetes is at one end), including hyperinsulinemia, that are related to obesity, inactivity, and advancing age and are associated with a greater risk of coronary artery atherosclerosis.

Rarely, young adults and adolescents may have angina and other symptoms of coronary arterial insufficiency but without narrowed proximal coronary arteries – the so-called syndrome X. This condition may represent an abnormality of the coronary microvascular bed and has been associated with insulin resistance.

Systemic hypertension. This is a risk factor for adult-manifest cardiovascular disease, and children with a strong family history of essential hypertension tend to "track" into adulthood with the highest blood pressures relative to their same-age peers. Some other risk factors, such as obesity and dyslipidemia, usually associate with essential hypertension, leading to speculation that a group of abnormal genes is responsible.

Renal disease. Chronic and end-stage kidney disease is associated with early-onset coronary artery disease, likely due to multiple mechanisms, including systemic hypertension, abnormal lipid and calcium metabolism, elevated homocysteine, and the effects of inflammation and uremia on endothelial function. Calcification of soft tissues, including coronary arteries, can develop in children with chronic renal disease, especially those on dialysis.

Homocysteine and hypercoagulable states. High blood levels of the amino acid homocysteine are associated with atherosclerosis and a hypercoagulable state. The observation was first made in homocystinuric children, rare individuals with an inborn metabolic error. For most individuals, adequate dietary intake of folate and other vitamins can decrease homocysteine levels.

Heart transplantation. A diffuse form of coronary artery narrowing occurs in most children and adults following transplantation and may be due primarily to low-grade chronic rejection. In at least one-third of children it is a major factor in death or need for retransplantation. Although the pathology of transplant vasculopathy differs from that of atheroma, modifying traditional risk factors such as systemic hypertension and lipids has been proposed as a means to improve the outcome for these patients.

Substance abuse. In addition to tobacco, excessive alcohol consumption may adversely affect other risk factors, such as lipids, but it also has a direct toxic effect on the myocardium, which can result in a dilated cardiomyopathy. Cocaine and similar illicit drugs are associated with acute myocardial ischemia and sudden death. Anabolic steroids may result in systemic hypertension and dyslipidemia.

Dental disease and bacterial infection. These are speculative factors in the genesis of atheromas, presumably by direct (infection) or indirect (toxin or inflammatory) injury to the endothelium.

ISSUES FOR CHILDREN AND YOUNG ADULTS WITH HEART DISEASE

General considerations

Almost all of the preventive health issues discussed earlier also apply to children and young adults with congenital or acquired heart disease, and in some, such as children with coronary artery abnormalities from Kawasaki disease, these preventive issues become even more important.

Optimum care of the child with congenital cardiac disease entails attention to the effect of the disease on the behavioral, psychological, and intellectual growth of the child and on the family. Other considerations include the proper definition of the disease and medical and surgical management. In the current age of sophisticated diagnostic and surgical procedures, the common psychological factors of chronic disease are frequently overlooked.

Some patients undergo expensive and extensive operative procedures to correct their cardiac malformations but suffer from the "crippling" effect of the severe emotional problems common to many children with chronic disease. Because of a murmur or cardiac disease, many potential problems can develop in the family. The physician must make the recognition of these problems of the utmost importance. On the initial visit, following review of the clinical and laboratory findings with the parents, the parents should be given ample opportunity to express their feelings and to ask questions. Listening to them and reassuring them are wise. A feeling of guilt, although seldom expressed, is often present. Many parents are helped by the practitioner who, when explaining cardiac anomalies, points out that, except for rare cases, the medical community knows little of the etiology of the condition. Parents should be told that their child's malformation was not the result of something they did wrong or did not do right.

Many parents, because of feelings of guilt or sympathy, assume an overprotective and solicitous attitude toward the child with cardiac abnormalities; in part, this can be fostered by the physician's attitudes. Unless there are contraindications, the child should be treated in the same way as his or her siblings or peers in chores, responsibilities, and discipline. He or she should partake as fully as possible in family activities. Family life should not center on the cardiac patient. Stressing the emotional needs of other children in the family is also important. Whenever possible, the affected child should attend regular school. Grandparents in particular must be cautioned of the dangers of an overly sympathetic or solicitous approach.

In summary, the child must be treated like other children to the greatest possible extent.

Family counseling

This involves consideration of the type and severity of maternal heart disease, the risk to the mother and fetus, and the recurrence risk in offspring.

Both maternal and fetal risk largely depends on the type of cardiac disorder. In general, for women with well-repaired congenital malformations with normal or near-normal hemodynamics, the risk of pregnancy is similar to that in unaffected women.

Disorders conferring the highest risk of maternal and fetal death include Marfan syndrome, severe dilated cardiomyopathy, pulmonary vascular obstructive disease (PVOD) or primary pulmonary hypertension, and severe unrepaired malformations (e.g. severe left ventricular outflow tract obstruction), especially those with severe cyanosis and polycythemia.

Maternal cardiovascular medications (e.g. certain antiarrhythmics and antithrombotic therapy) may confer high risk to the fetus.

Reproductive issues and pregnancy

Reproductive issues, including pregnancy, recurrence risk, and contraception, are issues of concern to young persons with congenital or acquired heart disease. An adolescent patient who presents with an unplanned and unintended pregnancy can be challenging, particularly if they have not had regular medical visits and is discovered with worsening heart condition independent of the pregnancy. Such adverse cardiac changes that would ordinarily need catheter intervention or an operation may present a problem during pregnancy, or such treatments may be impossible until after delivery.

Maternal risks. Pregnancy may increase risk for both mother and fetus, with the risk depending on the type of cardiac condition and the functional status of the patient. In general, the highest risk of maternal mortality during (and just following) pregnancy is associated with maternal pulmonary hypertension and/or Eisenmenger physiology. The pulmonary hypertension may increase during pregnancy, but, perhaps more importantly, systemic vascular resistance falls during pregnancy. If a shunt is present then the degree of right-to-left shunt may increase, cyanosis deepens, and the mother's clinical status may worsen, or sudden death may occur. Other physiologic changes during pregnancy include increased cardiac output. In patients with limited cardiac output reserve, such as with cardiomyopathy, pulmonary hypertension, or severe (usually left heart) obstructive lesions, the demand for increased cardiac output accompanying pregnancy may outstrip available supply. Maternal risk is also high in Marfan syndrome when the aorta is >40 mm in diameter, or in a patient with Turner syndrome who has achieved a pregnancy through oocyte donation, hormonal support, and other reproductive technologies.

Intermediate levels of maternal risk accompany pregnancies in which the mother has unrepaired cyanotic congenital heart disease (CHD), palliated single ventricle lesions (after Fontan or total cavopulmonary anastomoses), moderately severe left heart obstructive lesions, systemic hypertension related to coarctation, significant arrhythmia, or the need for anticoagulation.

The lowest maternal risk exists in young women with successful repair of a left-to-right shunt or who have a small hemodynamically insignificant shunt, a mild obstructive lesion, and following repair of cyanotic heart disease. These mothers have essentially the same medical risk as women without CHD.

However, the recurrence risk for congenital cardiac malformation or other cardiac disease to occur in the offspring may still be higher and is discussed in other chapters and with regard to specific cardiac malformations and conditions such as Marfan syndrome. In general, there are relatively few cardiac lesions that alter the medical management of a pregnancy. Certain lesions may alter the conduct of delivery or mandate that delivery be planned at a center able to provide timely congenital heart surgery or intervention rather than transferring the newborn from the delivering hospital. Fetal echocardiography offers promise for an expectant parent with CHD; although it lacks perfect sensitivity and specificity, it can be useful in the prenatal diagnosis of cardiac conditions and allow appropriate staging of resources for neonatal care.

Fetal risks. The highest levels of risk for fetal death or very premature delivery occur in pregnancies of mothers needing anticoagulation (such as for prosthetic valves), with unrepaired cyanotic heart malformations, or with poor functional class (including women with cardiomyopathy or pulmonary hypertension).

Obviously, the risk of fetal death goes hand-in-hand with the maternal death risk during early and mid-gestation.

Contraception and pregnancy planning. Contraception can be considered from two perspectives: reversible and irreversible. For common types of reversible forms, such as hormonal contraception, the primary risk is the potential increase in thrombogenicity with estrogen-containing preparations. Low-estrogen or estrogen-free options are available. For women with the highest risk cardiac conditions, when the risk of pregnancy is much higher than for contraceptive surgery, the primary concern is the chance of becoming pregnant while using contraception. In these circumstances, irreversible contraception methods are usually advised. These may include surgical versus laparoscopic fallopian tube ligation or alternative methods such as endoscopic tubal ablation.

A young woman presenting with an unintended pregnancy and a high-risk maternal cardiac problem is very challenging and management must be individualized. Although pregnancy termination is often advised, there is considerable risk, particularly in the second or third trimester. When pregnancy termination is an option, its risks must be weighed against those of continuing the pregnancy.

For young adults contemplating a planned pregnancy, a reasonable approach involves a preconception cardiac re-evaluation to plan maternal cardiac intervention, if indicated. The potential recurrence risk of CHD, evaluation by fetal echocardiography, and maternal management by high-risk pregnancy specialists are discussed.

Recurrence risk

This varies with lesion and even with which parent is affected. In general, maternal CHD is more likely than paternal CHD to recur in offspring. Some lesions, such as ventricular septal defect (VSD) and atrial septal defect (ASD), have a relatively low recurrence risk, except in families where multiple members are affected despite the absence of a recognizable syndrome. Left heart obstructive lesions, such as aortic stenosis, have a relatively high recurrence risk (estimated at 10–15%). A parent affected by DiGeorge or Noonan syndrome has a 50% risk of recurrence.

Following the discovery of CHD in one of their children, parents become concerned with the risks of having a second child who would be similarly affected. If, in the proband, the cardiac malformation is not part of a recognized syndrome (including microdeletions of chromosome 22 or translocation-type trisomies) and no previous family history of cardiac anomalies exists, the risk of a second child being affected is probably twice that of the first. The incidence of CHD in the population is 0.7%, reflecting an incidence of 1 in 135. If a second child in a family is affected, the form of cardiac anomaly will be concordant in half. Some families have several members of one generation who show the same form of cardiac malformation. Interestingly, one exception seems to be complete transposition of the great vessels, where the occurrence of multiple, or even two, instances in a family is rare. If a second child does have a cardiac anomaly, the risk of a subsequent child also having a cardiac anomaly is even higher.

If the child shows one of the recognizable syndromes associated with cardiac malformations, specific genetic counseling should be given. The physician's responsibility is not to instruct parents about whether they should or should not attempt to have more children, but they should be advised of the available information so that they can reach an appropriate decision.

Exercise limitations

These have been based on limited evidence and much speculation. Wide differences exist in the advice given to parents regarding exercise.

General exercise. Most children with a cardiac anomaly can be allowed a normal range of physical activity; however, they should realize that the anomaly may limit their ability to exercise. The child may be permitted to participate in physical education in school, but teachers must understand that the child may have to stop and rest sooner than the other children. The child should not be pushed to extremes of physical activity or to perform in unfavorable situations, such as extreme heat or cold, and dehydration should be avoided. More severe exercise restrictions are indicated for children with disorders such as severe aortic stenosis, hypertrophic cardiomyopathy, and Marfan syndrome, as exertion can be fatal in these children.

Sports. Some pediatric cardiologists advise avoidance of any competitive sports activity for all unrepaired and some repaired patients (such as those with tetralogy of Fallot); these patients may participate in fun physical activities provided that they are in charge of when they cease activity, but presumably they are at greater risk if they are "pushed" to more intense exertion, such as during a competitive sports situation. The 26th Bethesda Conference in 1994, and revised as the 36th Conference in 2005, with additional revisions in 2015, sought to determine eligibility for athletic competition based on the type and severity of the cardiac abnormality and the type and intensity of the sport (Tables 12.6 and 12.7).

Inappropriate restriction. Children with cardiac abnormalities may be inappropriately restricted by school authorities, even when the school has been informed that no need for exercise restriction exists. This reflects an unrealistic fear that teachers sometimes have about children with cardiac disease, which arises from ignorance of cardiac anomalies and from the association of all cardiac disease with heart attacks and sudden death. In any correspondence regarding a child with a cardiac abnormality, whether to a referring physician or to a school, the recommended level of exercise should be clearly defined.

Table 12.6 Classification of Sports – 36th Bethesda Conference.

		A. Low (<40% Max O_2)	B. Moderate (40–70% Max O_2)	C. High (>70% Max O_2)
Increasing Static Component	**III. High (>50% MVC)**	Bobsledding/Luge[a,b], Field events (throwing), Gymnastics[a,b], Martial arts[a], Sailing, Sport climbing, Water skiing[a,b], Weight lifting[a,b], Windsurfing[a] (1)	Body building[a,b], Downhill skiing[a,b], Skateboarding[a,b], Snowboarding[a,b], Wrestling[a] (2)	Boxing[a], Canoeing/Kayaking, Cycling[a,b], Decathlon, Rowing, Speed-skating[a,b], Triathlon[a,b] (3)
	II. Moderate (20–50% MVC)	Archery, Auto racing[a,b], Driving[a,b], Equestrian[a,b], Motorcycling[a,b] (4)	American football[a], Field events (jumping), Figure skating[a], Rodeoing[a,b], Rugby[a], Running (sprint), Surfing[a,b], Synchronized swimming (5)	Basketball[a], Ice hockey[a], Cross-country skiing (skating technique), Lacrosse[a], Running (middle distance), Swimming, Team handball (6)
	I. Low (<20% MVC)	Billiards, Bowling, Cricket, Curling, Golf, Riflery (7)	Baseball/Softball[a], Fencing, Table tennis, Volleyball (8)	Badminton, Cross-country skiing (classic technique), Field hockey[a], Orienteering, Race walking, Racquetball/Squash, Running (long distance), Soccer[a], Tennis (9)

Increasing Dynamic Component ⟶

This classification is based on peak static and dynamic components achieved during competition. It should be noted, however, that higher values may be reached during training. The increasing dynamic component is defined in terms of the estimated percentage of maximum oxygen uptake (Max O_2) achieved and results in an increasing cardiac output. The increasing static component is related to the estimated percentage of maximum voluntary contraction (MVC) reached and results in an increasing blood pressure load. The lowest total cardiovascular demands (cardiac output and blood pressure) are shown in cell (7) and the highest in cell (3). Cells (4) and (8) show low–moderate, cells (1), (5), and (9) show moderate, and cells (2) and (6) show high–moderate total cardiovascular demands.

[a] Danger of bodily collision.

[b] Increased risk if syncope occurs.

Source: Reprinted from Mitchell, J.H., Haskell, W., Snell, P., and Van Camp, S.P. Task Force 8: Classification of Sports. *J. Am. Coll. Cardiol.* 45: 1364–1367, Copyright © 2005 American College of Cardiology Foundation, with permission from Elsevier.

Table 12.7 Sports recommendations for athletes with cardiovascular abnormalities.

Condition	Sport
ASD, untreated	
Small defects, nl RV volume, no PA htn	All
Large ASD, nl PA pressure	All
ASD, mild PA htn	IA
ASD, PVOD, cyanosis, R-to-L shunt	None vs IA
ASD, closed at operation or catheterization	
After 3–6 months, if no PA htn, arrhythmia, AVB, or myocardial dysfxn	All
Or, if residual abnormalities	Individualize; consider IA
VSD, untreated	
VSD, nl PA pressure	All
VSD, large, with R_p allowing repair	Repair first
VSD, large, with PA htn	IA
VSD, closed at operation or catheterization	
After 3–6 months, if no sxs, no or small residual defect, no PA htn, no arrhythmia, and no myocardial dysfxn	All
Symptomatic arrhythmias, AVB, PA htn, myocardial dysfxn	Individualize
PDA, untreated	
Small PDA, nl LV size	All
Moderate or large PDA with LV enlargement	Repair first
Moderate or large PDA, severe PA htn, cyanosis	IA
PDA, closed at operation or catheterization	
After recovery, if no PA htn	All
With residual PA htn	None vs IA
PS, untreated	
≤40 mmHg peak systolic gradient, nl RV fxn, no sxs; reeval annually	All
>40 mmHg peak systolic gradient	IA, IB; prior to gradient relief
PS, treated by operation or balloon valvuloplasty	
No or mild (≤40 mmHg gradient by Doppler) residual PS	All
Mod or severe (>40 mmHg gradient) residual PS and/or severe PI with RV enlargement	IA, IB
AS, untreated (reeval annually)	
Mild (mean Doppler gradient <25 mmHg or peak instantaneous Doppler gradient <40 mmHg), no sxs, nl ECG, no exercise intolerance, no arrhythmia	All

(continued)

Table 12.7 (*continued*)

Condition	Sport
Moderate (mean Doppler gradient 25–40 mmHg or peak instantaneous Doppler gradient 40–70 mmHg), no sxs, mild or no LVE by echo, nl ECG, nl exercise test	IA, IB, IIA
Severe (mean Doppler gradient >40 mmHg or peak instantaneous Doppler gradient >70 mmHg)	None vs IA
AS, treated by operation or balloon valvuloplasty (reeval annually)	
Mild, moderate, or severe residual AS	See untreated AS
Moderate to severe AI	See AI
AI (reeval annually)	
Mild to moderate AI, no sxs, nl EF, no, mild, or moderate LV dilation, nl exercise tolerance on GXT	All
Severe AI, no sxs, nl EF, no change in AI or LV size, nl exercise tolerance on GXT	All
Severe AI, sxs, EF <50%, LVE, or progressive LV dilation	None
Bicuspid aortic valve	
No aortic root dilation (>40 mm, or z-score >+2), no significant AS or AI	All
Dilated aortic root 40–45 mm (adult)	IA, IB, IIA, IIB (+ no collision)
Dilated aortic root >45 mm (adult)	None[a]
Coarctation, untreated	
Mild, no large collaterals, ascending aortic z-score ≤+3.0, resting gradient ≤20 mmHg, nl exercise test and max exercise peak systolic BP ≤95th percentile predicted	All
Resting gradient >20 mmHg, or exercise-induced htn (>95th percentile predicted), or ascending aortic z-score ≤+3.0	IA, until treated
Coarctation, treated by surgery or balloon/stent	
At least 3 months after treatment, no sxs, resting gradient ≤20 mmHg, nl resting and exercise systolic BP	Avoid IIIA, IIIB, IIIC and collision
Significant aortic dilation, site aneurysm, or associated valve disease	IA, IB
Elevated pulmonary resistance with CHD[b]	
PA mean ≤25 mmHg	All
PA mean ≥25 mmHg	None vs IA; perform full evaluation and individualize

Table 12.7 (*continued*)

Condition	Sport
Ventricular dysfunction after cardiac surgery (reeval periodically)	
Normal or near-normal function (EF ≥50%)	All
Mild depression of function (EF 40–50%)	IA, IB, IIA, IIB
Moderate to severe depression of function (EF <40%)	None vs IA
Cyanotic CHD	
Unrepaired, clinically stable, and no heart failure sxs, after full evaluation including exercise testing	IA
Tetralogy of Fallot[b]	
EF >50%, no arrhythmia, outflow tract obstruction, or arrhythmia or other adverse findings on exercise test	II and III
EF <40%, severe outflow tract obstruction, or recurrent or uncontrolled atrial or ventricular arrhythmia	None vs IA
d-TGV, repaired[b] (evaluation should include exercise testing)	
Atrial switch, if no cardiac symptoms, nl ventricular fxn, no tachyarrhythmia, nl exercise test	All
Atrial switch, with normal exercise test but more than mild hemodynamic abn or ventricular dysfunction	IA, IB, IC, IIA
Arterial switch, with ischemia by exercise test	None vs IA
l-TGV ("corrected" transposition) (reeval periodically)	
Asymptomatic and no abnormalities on clinical eval	II, IIIB, IIIC
No clinically significant arrhythmias, ventricular dysfunction, exercise intolerance, or exercise-induced ischemia	IA, IB
Severe clinical systemic RV dysfunction, severe RV outflow tract obstruction, or recurrent or uncontrolled atrial or ventricular arrhythmias	None vs IA
Fontan (evaluation should include exercise testing)	IA; individualize
Ebstein's	
Mild; no cyanosis, nl RV size, no arrhythmia	All
Severe TR, no significant arrhythmia on ambulatory ECG	IA

(*continued*)

Table 12.7 (*continued*)

Condition	Sport
Congenital coronary artery anomalies	
Anomalous origin from PA, unoperated	IA
Anomalous origin from PA, operated; based on infarct and fxn	Individualize
Wrong sinus origin	
Right coronary from left sinus of Valsalva, unoperated; no sxs, nl GXT	Individualize and consider uncertainty in risk determination
Right coronary from left sinus of Valsalva, unoperated; sxs, arrhythmia, or abn GXT	IA
Left coronary from right sinus, especially if intramural course, unoperated	None vs IA
>3 months after repair of wrong sinus origin, if no sxs, and no ischemia or arrhythmia on exercise testing	All
Systemic hypertension	
Prehypertension (120/80 mmHg up to 139/89 mmHg)	All
Stage 1 htn (140–159 mmHg/90-99 mmHg) without target organ damage including LVH or concomitant heart disease	All (monitor BP)
Stage 2 htn (≥160/100 mmHg)	Avoid IIIA-C until BP controlled
Kawasaki disease	
Normal coronary arteries, if no exercise-induced ischemia or arrhythmia, beginning 8 weeks after resolution of illness	All
Transient aneurysm, if no exercise-induced ischemia or arrhythmia, beginning 8 weeks after resolution of illness; reassess every 3–5 years	All
Aneurysms, no exercise-induced ischemia or arrhythmia; reassess periodically	IA, IB, IIA, IIB[c]
After MI or revascularization, after ≥3 months, LV >50%, no symptoms, no inducible ischemia or electrical instability	All[c]
Patients on antithrombotic therapy	Avoid collision sports
Myocarditis	
Full recovery = nl LV fxn, wall motion, and cardiac dimensions; nl ECG; no significant arrhythmia on ambulatory ECG and GXT; serum markers of inflammation and heart failure normalized	None until full recovery (3–6 months)

Table 12.7 (*continued*)

Condition	Sport
Pericarditis	
Acute phase	None
Full recovery (no evidence of active disease, no effusion by echo, and serum markers of inflammation normal)	All
With myocarditis	See myocarditis
Constrictive	None
Inherited arrhythmia syndromes (long QT syndrome, short QT syndrome, Brugada syndrome, catecholaminergic polymorphic ventricular tachycardia [CPVT], early repolarization syndrome, idiopathic ventricular fibrillation)	
Asymptomatic, genotype-positive, phenotype-negative	All, with appropriate precautionary measures (see reference)
Previously symptomatic or electrocardiographically evident (except CPVT)	All, with disease-specific treatments and appropriate precautionary measures if asymptomatic >3 months (see reference, including additional considerations for treatment with pacing/ICD)
CPVT	None vs IA
Cardiomyopathy	
Hypertrophic cardiomyopathy	None vs IA
Arrhythmogenic right ventricular cardiomyopathy (ARVC)	None vs IA
Dilated cardiomyopathy	None vs IA
Noncompaction of LV myocardium	None vs IA
Marfan syndrome[b]	
No more than one of the following: aortic root dilation (>40 mm, or z-score >+2), moderate–severe MR; EF<40%; family hx dissection at aortic diameter <50 mm	IA, IIA
Ehlers–Danlos syndrome (vascular form); if no aortic dissection or dilation (Ao <+2 z), < moderate MR, and no extracardiac organ involvement increasing risk	IA

(*continued*)

Table 12.7 (*continued*)

Condition	Sport
Loeys–Dietz syndrome; if no aortic dissection or dilation (Ao < +2 z), < moderate MR, and no extracardiac organ involvement increasing risk	IA
Other genetic aortopathies, and aortic dilation in isolation	See reference

abn, abnormality; AI, aortic insufficiency; AS, aortic stenosis; ASD, atrial septal defect; AVB, atrioventricular nodal block; BD, balloon dilation; BP, blood pressure; CV, cardiovascular; dTGV, d-transposition of the great vessels; dysfxn, dysfunction; EF, ejection fraction; Elev, elevated; fxn, function; GXT, graded exercise test; htn, hypertension; hx, history; l-TGV, l-transposition of the great vessels; LV, left ventricle or left ventricular; LVE, left ventricular enlargement; LVEDD, left ventricular end-diastolic diameter (echo); LVH, left ventricular hypertrophy; mmHg, millimeters of mercury; MI, myocardial infarct; MR, mitral regurgitation; MVP, mitral valve prolapse; nl, normal; p, pressure; PA, pulmonary artery; PDA, patent ductus arteriosus; PI, pulmonary insufficiency; PS, pulmonary stenosis; pts., patients; PVOD, pulmonary vascular obstructive disease; reeval, re-evaluate/re-evaluation; R_p, pulmonary vascular resistance; RV, right ventricle or right ventricular; sat, oxygen saturation; sxs, symptoms; TR, tricuspid regurgitation; VO$_2$ max, maximum oxygen consumption (exercise); VSD, ventricular septal defect.
[a] Author's note: this and other recommendations regarding aortic dilation remain controversial.
[b] Author's note: many conditions, including repaired tetralogy of Fallot, d-TGV, single ventricle, and pulmonary vascular obstructive disease, are associated with a risk of sudden death at rest and during exertion.
[c] Author's note: the recommendation for post-MI or revascularization patients is less restrictive than for patients with aneurysm and a similar clinical picture otherwise, and appears paradoxical.
Source: Adapted from (2005) 36th Bethesda Conference: Eligibility Recommendations for Competitive Athletes with Cardiovascular Abnormalities. *J. Am. Coll. Cardiol.* 2005, 45: 1312–1375; and (2015) Eligibility and Disqualification Recommendations for Competitive Athletes With Cardiovascular Abnormalities: A Scientific Statement From the American Heart Association and American College of Cardiology. *J. Am. Coll. Cardiol.* 2015;66(21): 2343–2450, and *Circulation.* 2015;132(22): e256–e349.

Postoperative. Following pediatric cardiac operations, the level of exercise can be gradually increased to full participation four to six weeks postoperatively, if no major complication (e.g. congestive cardiac failure or pericardial effusion) is present. After recovery from operation, the child should be permitted normal activity as tolerated and dictated by the postoperative hemodynamics.

Modified bedrest. This has very limited indications. In the presence of an active inflammatory disease involving the myocardium, such as acute rheumatic carditis or myocarditis, it may be advisable. Complete bedrest is difficult to achieve because of a child's natural activeness; it may even have adverse consequences compared with modified bedrest. As an alternative, children can spend most of their time sitting or lying on the couch and can be allowed up to the bathroom and dinner table.

Sports classification is shown in Table 12.6. Recently, other expert organizations including the European Society of Cardiology have taken a different approach, avoiding lesion-specific recommendations, and focusing on functional and pathophysiologic groupings based on ventricular function, pulmonary hypertension, aortic dilation, arrhythmia, and systemic arterial oxygen saturation.

Nutrition

Diet. Most children with cardiac anomalies do not require a special diet, except for those with cardiac failure, in whom a high-caloric-density diet and perhaps a low-sodium diet may be indicated. In older children, salt restriction varies from recommendations of no added salt and avoidance of foods with high salt content, such as potato chips and pizza, to a modified diet limiting sodium. Sodium restriction has less impact on symptoms and prognosis than once thought; it is less important (and more difficult to achieve) than avoiding excess sodium intake.

Infants with congestive heart failure (CHF). Nutrition is most critical for infants with CHF because of large left-to-right shunts, such as VSD. These infants may feed poorly because of dyspnea and tachypnea and may have emesis and/or gastroesophageal reflux because of intestinal edema, thoracic hyperinflation, and esophageal compression from left atrial enlargement. They have greater energy expenditure because of cardiac and respiratory overwork and often require 30–40% more calories than normal infants to achieve minimally acceptable weight gain. If timely surgery is not feasible, alternative feeding methods, such as continuous gastric or transpyloric tube feedings of hypercaloric formula, may be indicated.

Growth and small stature. Children with a cardiac anomaly may be small in stature because of the effect of the condition upon the circulation or because of problems coexisting with the cardiac anomaly (e.g. DiGeorge syndrome). In most children, the latter applies, as evidenced by the observation that growth rates and stature for age often remain unchanged after successful cardiac repair.

Between the ages of one and four years, the appetite of many children is considered poor by their parents. The parents of healthy children in this age range often complain about their child's eating habits. The rate of weight gain compared with the first year of life decreases markedly at about one year of age. However, many small-statured children with a cardiac problem have a normal rate of growth. Comparison with published "normal" growth curves may help to allay parental anxiety. Each of these factors leads to concern for many parents, and these concerns are increased in the parents of children with a cardiac anomaly who are small statured. They believe that stature would become normal if the child would only eat. This leads to turmoil, unpleasant meal experiences, and frustration. These problems can be reduced by using anticipatory guidance to discuss with the parents what they should expect as their child grows older.

Follow-up medical care

Most children with cardiac anomalies require periodic evaluation. The reasons for the evaluation and the type of information sought depend in large part upon the natural history of the cardiac condition. For instance, in a patient with a large VSD, evidence of the development of pulmonary hypertension or congestive cardiac failure would be sought, whereas in aortic stenosis, evidence of increasing gradient, left ventricular strain, and/or important aortic insufficiency would be looked for. Hence the frequency of return visits and the type of diagnostic studies performed on the patient's return are dictated by the symptoms and the natural history of the defect.

Usually infants are evaluated more frequently than older children because changes in circulation take place more rapidly during the first year of life.

Children with cardiac anomalies also require routine pediatric care. In infants with cardiac failure or other major symptoms, physicians can easily overlook or fail to administer routine immunizations, but these are an important component of the child's health care.

Most children with repaired cardiac malformations and many with acquired heart disease are at risk for late complications, such as dysrhythmia, endocarditis, and progressive obstruction of previously relieved stenosis. Some patients are at long-term risk for sudden life-threatening events.

Many children with repaired patent ductus arteriosus (PDA), ASD, or VSD are not at great risk for complications and may not require frequent follow-up care by a pediatric cardiologist after they have fully recovered from their cardiac intervention.

Many centers for adults with CHD have established follow-up programs, which usually include the expertise of pediatric cardiologists.

Insurability and occupational issues

For the young adult with heart disease, insurability and occupational issues remain difficult problems for many patients, especially for those with important physical limitations (e.g. CHF, PVOD, or Marfan syndrome) that severely limit their available employment options to sedentary or light-activity jobs (Table 12.8), particularly in countries where health insurance is closely tied to employment and where health

Table 12.8 Occupational guidelines for adults with CHD.

Work→	Sedentary	Light	Medium	Heavy	Very heavy
Peak lift→	≤10lb	≤20lb	≤50lb	≤100lb	>100lb
Frequent carry→	small objects	≤10lb	≤25lb	≤50lb	≥50lb
Peak load→	≤2.5cal/min	2.6–4.9cal/min	5.0–7.5cal/min		≥7.6cal/min
↓ Condition					
AI	–	Severe	Moderate	Mild	–
AS	–	Severe[a]	Moderate	Mild	–
ASD	–	Mod–severe PVOD[a]	Mild–mod PVOD	–	No PVOD
Cardiomyopathy[a]	Dilated	Hypertrophic	–	–	–
COA	–	–	± op; htn	–	Repaired, nl BP rest and exercise
Hypertension	–	–	–	Mild	–
MR	Severe (CM and/or AFib)	Mod–severe	Moderate (mild–mod CM)	Mild (no CM)	–
MS	Severe	Moderate	Mild	–	–
MVP	–	–	–	–	Mild, no sxs
PDA	–	Mod–severe PVOD[a]	Mild–mod PVOD	–	No PVOD
PS	–	Severe	Moderate	–	Mild
PA hypertension (primary)[a]	PA_p ≥0.5 systemic	PA_p ≤0.5 systemic	–	–	–
TOF, post op[a]	–	–	RV_p >50mmHg	RV_p <50mmHg	–
VSD	–	Mod–severe PVOD[a]	Milc–mod PVOD	–	No PVOD
Other major defects[a]	–	Unop or palliated only	Postop	–	–

(continued)

Table 12.8 (*continued*)

Work→	Sedentary	Light	Medium	Heavy	Very heavy
Peak lift→	≤10lb	≤20lb	≤50lb	≤100lb	>100lb
Frequent carry→	small objects	≤10lb	≤25lb	≤50lb	≥50lb
Peak load→	≤2.5cal/min	2.6–4.9cal/min	5.0–7.5cal/min		≥7.6cal/min
Arrhythmia	–	VT[a]	PVC with CHD	AVB; pacemaker[b,c]; SVT; VT (nl otherwise)	PAC; PVC (nl heart); WPW[a]

AI, aortic insufficiency; AS, aortic stenosis; ASD, atrial septal defect; AVB, atrioventricular block; cal/min, calories/minute; CHD, congenital heart disease; CM, cardiomegaly; COA, coarctation; GXT, graded exercise test; htn, hypertension; lb, pound; mmHg, millimeters of mercury; mod, moderate; MR, mitral regurgitation; MS, mitral stenosis; MVP, mitral valve prolapse; nl, normal; op, operation; PA, pulmonary artery; PAp, pulmonary artery pressure; PDA, patent ductus arteriosus; postop, postoperative; PS, pulmonary stenosis; PVC, premature ventricular contraction; PVOD, pulmonary vascular obstructive disease; RVp, right ventricular pressure; SVT, supraventricular tachycardia; TOF, tetralogy of Fallot; TR, tricuspid regurgitation; unop, unoperated; VSD, ventricular septal defect; VT, ventricular tachycardia.

Wide variation exists among patients with similar diagnoses (Diller et al., 2005); recommendations must be individualized. Exercise testing may be advisable for many patients.

Diller, G.-P., Dimopoulos, K., Okonko, D., et al. (2005). Exercise intolerance in adult congenital heart disease: comparative severity, correlates, and prognostic implication. *Circulation*, 112(6): 828–835.

[a] Some conditions may be associated with sudden death, even in patients at rest.

[b] Use of certain equipment (e.g. arc welding) or repetitive shoulder motion may damage pacing system.

Source: Data adapted from Gutgesell, H.P., Gessner, I.H., Vetter, V.L., Yabek, S.M., and Norton, J.B. (1986). Recreational and occupational recommendations for young patients with heart disease. A statement for physicians by the Committee on Congenital Cardiac Defects of the Council on Cardiovascular Disease in the Young, American Heart Association. *Circulation* 74(5): 1195A–1198A.

care is not universal and independent of insurance. Worldwide, however, many children with CHD do not survive to adulthood due to lack of adequate local medical resources to treat their conditions.

Altitude and air travel

Both residence at higher altitudes and travel by air may affect children and adults with heart disease. Patients with unrepaired cyanotic congenital heart malformations or cavopulmonary anastomoses may be at particular risk because of the adverse effect on pulmonary vascular resistance of lower oxygen tension at high altitudes. Patients with pulmonary hypertension also may be at risk.

Air travel obviously presents a much shorter duration of exposure than does residing at relatively high altitude. Commercial flights in pressurized airliners do not achieve a pressure equal to sea level; rather, the cabin pressure equals an elevation of 8000 ft (~2400 m). This results in a partial pressure of oxygen of about 75% of that at sea level and an arterial hemoglobin saturation of ~90–93% for persons with normal physiology. Supplemental oxygen, which for an adult can be 2 L/min when administered by nasal cannula, essentially restores the pulmonary venous oxygen tension to that of sea level, but has the disadvantages of inconvenience, cost, and limited availability, as not all airlines will accept passengers who need to use it. Observational studies of adults with CHD traveling by commercial airline suggest that very few adverse events occur in those not using supplemental oxygen. Patients with chronic cyanosis may have a rightward shift in their oxyhemoglobin dissociation curve, which may attenuate the effect of hypoxia by resulting in higher saturations at any given arterial oxygen pressure (PaO_2). Although the theoretical risks vary with the patient's age, their cardiac lesion, and their pathophysiology, and with factors not directly related to hypoxia, such as dehydration, prophylactic oxygen use is often individualized. No clear consensus regarding the use of supplemental oxygen for air travel has emerged.

Altitude may also affect the prevalence of certain types of CHD; for instance, PDA tends to occur with greater frequency and in infants without other risk factors, such as prematurity, in locations at relatively high altitude.

Infective endocarditis prophylaxis

Endocarditis is a serious, life-threatening condition that requires lengthy medical treatment and in some patients surgical treatment. Therefore, prevention is a worthy goal. Many patients who develop endocarditis, however, have received recommended antibiotic prevention prior to an appropriate procedure, so the efficacy of antibiotics appears limited.

These issues are addressed in the most recent guidelines from the American Heart Association and approved by the American Dental Association, published in 2007 (Figure 12.2). They are similar to 2008 British and 2009 European assessments

PREVENTION OF INFECTIVE (BACTERIAL) ENDOCARDITIS
Wallet Card

This wallet card is to be given to patients (or parents) by their physician. Healthcare professionals: Please see back of card for reference to the complete statement.

Name: _____
needs protection from
INFECTIVE (BACTERIAL) ENDOCARDITIS
because of an existing heart condition.

Diagnosis: _____
Prescribed by: _____
Date: _____

You received this wallet card because you are at increased risk for developing adverse outcomes from infective endocarditis (IE), also known as bacterial endocarditis (BE). The guidelines for prevention of IE shown in this card are substantially different from previously published guidelines. This card replaces the previous card that was based on guidelines published in 1997.

The American Heart Association's Endocarditis Committee together with national and international experts on IE extensively reviewed published studies in order to determine whether dental, gastrointestinal (GI), or genitourinary (GU) tract procedures are possible causes of IE. These experts determined that there is no conclusive evidence that links dental, GI, or GU tract procedures with the development of IE.

The current practice of giving patients antibiotics prior to a dental procedure is no longer recommended **EXCEPT** for patients with the highest risk of adverse outcomes resulting from IE (see below on this card). The Committee cannot exclude the possibility that an exceedingly small number of cases, if any, of IE may be prevented by antibiotic prophylaxis prior to a dental procedure. If such benefit from prophylaxis exists, it should be reserved **ONLY** for those patients listed below. The Committee recognizes the importance of good oral and dental health and regular visits to the dentist for patients at risk of IE.

The Committee no longer recommends administering antibiotics solely to prevent IE in patients who undergo a GI or GU tract procedure.

Changes in these guidelines do not change the fact that your cardiac condition puts you at increased risk for developing endocarditis. If you develop signs or symptoms of endocarditis—such as unexplained fever —see your doctor right away. If blood cultures are necessary (to determine if endocarditis is present), it is important for your doctor to obtain these cultures and other relevant tests **BEFORE** antibiotics are started.

Antibiotic prophylaxis with dental procedures is reasonable only for patients with cardiac conditions associated with the highest risk of adverse outcomes from endocarditis, including:

- Prosthetic cardiac valve or prosthetic material used in valve repair
- Previous endocarditis
- Congenital heart disease only in the following categories:

    –Unrepaired cyanotic congenital heart disease, including those with palliative shunts and conduits

    –Completely repaired congenital heart disease with prosthetic material or device, whether placed by surgery or catheter intervention, during the first six months after the procedure*

    –Repaired congenital heart disease with residual defects at the site or adjacent to the site of a prosthetic patch or prosthetic device (which inhibit endothelialization)

- Cardiac transplantation recipients with cardiac valvular disease

*Prophylaxis is reasonable because endothelialization of prosthetic material occurs within six months after the procedure.

Dental procedures for which prophylaxis is reasonable in patients with cardiac conditions listed above.

Figure 12.2 Prevention of infective endocarditis wallet card. Source: Reprinted with permission, www.heart.org, © 2008 American Heart Association.

All dental procedures that involve manipulation of gingival tissue or the periapical region of teeth, or perforation of the oral mucosa*

*Antibiotic prophylaxis is NOT recommended for the following dental procedures or events: routine anesthetic injections through noninfected tissue; taking dental radiographs; placement of removable prosthodontic or orthodontic appliances; adjustment of orthodontic appliances; placement of orthodontic brackets; and shedding of deciduous teeth and bleeding from trauma to the lips or oral mucosa.

Antibiotic Prophylactic Regimens for Dental Procedures

Situation	Agent	Regimen—Single Dose 30-60 minutes before procedure	
		Adults	Children
Oral	Amoxicillin	2 g	50 mg/kg
Unable to take oral medication	Ampicillin OR	2 g IM or IV*	50 mg/kg IM or IV
	Cefazolin or ceftriaxone	1 g IM or IV	50 mg/kg IM or IV
Allergic to penicillins or ampicillin— Oral regimen	Cephalexin**†	2 g	50 mg/kg
	OR		
	Clindamycin	600 mg	20 mg/kg
	OR		
	Azithromycin or clarithromycin	500 mg	15 mg/kg
Allergic to penicillins or ampicillin and unable to take oral medication	Cefazolin or ceftriaxone†	1 g IM or IV	50 mg/kg IM or IV
	OR Clindamycin	600 mg IM or IV	20 mg/kg IM or IV

*IM—intramuscular; IV—intravenous
**Or other first or second generation oral cephalosporin in equivalent adult or pediatric dosage.
† Cephalosporins should not be used in an individual with a history of anaphylaxis, angioedema or urticaria with penicillins or ampicillin.

Gastrointestinal/Genitourinary Procedures: Antibiotic prophylaxis solely to prevent IE is no longer recommended for patients who undergo a GI or GU tract procedure, including patients with the highest risk of adverse outcomes due to IE.

Other Procedures: Procedures involving the respiratory tract or infected skin, tissues just under the skin, or musculoskeletal tissue for which prophylaxis is reasonable are discussed in the updated document (reference below).

Adapted from *Prevention of Infective Endocarditis: Guidelines From the American Heart Association,* by the Committee on Rheumatic Fever, Endocarditis, and Kawasaki Disease. *Circulation,* 2007; 116: 1736-1754. Accessible at http://circ.ahajournals.org/cgi/reprint/CIRCULATIONAHA.106.183095.

Healthcare Professionals—Please refer to these recommendations for more complete information as to which patients and which procedures need prophylaxis.

American Heart Association® | American Stroke Association®
Learn and Live.

National Center
7272 Greenville Avenue
Dallas, Texas 75231-4596
americanheart.org

50-1605 0805

Figure 12.2 (*continued*)

of endocarditis risk and the limited effectiveness of antibiotics in prevention (Table 12.9). With their assessment, the British guidelines no longer advise antibiotic prophylaxis (Table 12.10) for any circumstance. It is interesting that the guidelines from three organizations are not identical, despite the fact that they reviewed essentially the same evidence. The authors of the guidelines acknowledge that the scientific basis for many of the recommendations is lacking and much still rests solely on expert opinion. The current recommendations represent a considerable departure from those of the previous decades, and substantially reduce the number of patients, and the types of conditions, for which endocarditis prophylaxis is recommended prior to dental or other procedures.

Children with most forms of congenital cardiac anomalies and those with acquired valvar anomalies are at some risk of developing infective endocarditis, but for many lesions this risk is low or similar to that in unaffected patients.

Endocarditis is very rare in repaired and unrepaired ASD, repaired VSD and PDA (after six months and with no residual abnormality), and mitral valve prolapse without regurgitation. Children with functional murmurs and those with a normal heart following Kawasaki disease or rheumatic fever also are not at risk.

Table 12.9 Reasons cited for revision of endocarditis prophylaxis guidelines (AHA, Wilson et al. 2007; NICE 2008; ESC, Habib et al. 2009).

Epidemiology	Majority of endocarditis cases cannot be linked to a causative dental or medical procedure
Procedural	Bacteremia more likely to result from daily activities (brushing, flossing, chewing) than from dental, genitourinary, or gastrointestinal procedures
Benefit	Lack of scientific evidence that preprocedural antibiotics prevent endocarditis or that only a very small number of cases may be prevented by antibiotics
Risk	Antibiotic adverse effects (non-life-threatening events, anaphylaxis[a], or increased microbial resistance) may exceed the small, if any, benefit
Alternatives	Dental hygiene and regular dental care may be important for prevention

[a] The risk of fatal anaphylaxis with antibiotic doses employed for prophylaxis is unknown, and estimates have varied widely, yet the 2007 AHA guidelines state: "For 50 years, the AHA has recommended a penicillin as the preferred choice for dental prophylaxis for IE. During these 50 years, the Committee is unaware of any cases reported to the AHA of fatal anaphylaxis resulting from the administration of a penicillin recommended in the AHA guidelines for IE prophylaxis."

Table 12.10 Comparison of recent infective endocarditis (IE) prophylaxis guidelines; highest risk patients for which preprocedure antibiotics may be reasonable.

		AHA, USA 2007[a,b]	NICE, UK 2008[b]	ESC, Europe 2009[b]
High-risk patients	Prosthetic valve or prosthetic material valve repair	Yes	Yes	Yes
	Previous IE	Yes	Yes	Yes
	Cyanotic CHD, unrepaired or palliated	Yes	Yes	Yes
	Repaired CHD within 6 months of repair	Yes	Yes	Yes
	Repaired CHD with residual defects	Yes	Yes	Yes
	Cardiac transplant with valve disease	Yes	–	No
	Hypertrophic cardiomyopathy	–	Yes	–
Procedures	Dental	Some	No	Some
	Respiratory	Some		No
	Gastrointestinal	No		No
	Genitourinary	No		No
	Infected skin/musculoskeletal	Some		No
	Cosmetic tattooing	No		No
	Cosmetic piercing	No		No

AHA, American Heart Association; CHD, congenital heart disease; ESC, European Society of Cardiology; NICE, National Institute for Health and Clinical Excellence; –, not addressed.
[a] See Figure 12.2
[b] See reference citations in Table 12.9 and in "Additional reading and references."

Children considered at high risk are those with:

(1) a prosthetic valve;
(2) an unrepaired cyanotic lesion;
(3) a surgically created systemic-to-pulmonary artery shunt;
(4) a conduit;
(5) a past history of endocarditis;
(6) a patient within six months of a repair (surgical or catheter based);
(7) a patient after repair who has a residual shunt adjacent to the site of prosthetic material impairing neoendothelialization.

The risk of an adverse outcome from endocarditis varies with the type of cardiac lesion and with the type of repair or palliation. Therefore, antibiotic prophylaxis is no longer based on the individual patient's lifetime risk of acquiring endocarditis but rather on the risk associated with developing endocarditis, and is advised only for those with the highest risk if endocarditis is acquired.

Antibiotic prophylaxis (Figure 12.2) is given within the hour before a procedure and not sooner. Antibiotic administration in this time interval assures a high antibiotic blood level at the time of greatest bacteremia. Beginning antibiotics a day or two before the procedure is unwise as it promotes the development of antibiotic-resistant organisms. Dental work is the predominant procedure for which endocarditis prophylaxis is indicated.

In patients receiving continuous antibiotics for prophylaxis of asplenia, rheumatic fever, or urinary tract infection and in patients receiving antibiotics for other acute indications, relatively resistant flora appear in the oropharynx and gut after only a few days of treatment, so an antibiotic of a different class from that currently being taken is indicated for endocarditis prevention.

Although endocarditis is rare, timely recognition of the possibility (such as with persistent unexplained fever) is important so that appropriate blood cultures may be obtained, ideally before any antibiotics are administered (Figure 12.2).

ADDITIONAL READING AND REFERENCES
General
National Heart, Lung, and Blood Institute (2012). *The Expert Panel on Integrated Guidelines for Cardiovascular Health and Risk Reduction in Children and Adolescents. Full Report*. NIH Publication No. 12-7486. National Institutes of Health, Bethesda, MD. www.nhlbi.nih.gov (accessed 12 March 2022).

Diet
Gidding, S.S., Dennison, B.A., Birch, L.L. et al. (2006). Dietary recommendations for children and adolescents a guide for practitioners [erratum appears in *Pediatrics* 118 (3):1323; *Circulation* 113 (23):e857]. *Pediatrics* 117 (2): 544–559.

Hyperlipidemia
American Academy of Pediatrics, National Cholesterol Education Program (1992). Report of the expert panel on blood cholesterol levels in children and adolescents. *Pediatrics* 89 (3 Pt 2): 525–584.

Magnussen, C.G., Raitakari, O.T., Thomson, R. et al. (2008). Utility of currently recommended pediatric dyslipidemia classifications in predicting dyslipidemia in adulthood: evidence from the Childhood Determinants of Adult Health (CDAH) study, Cardiovascular Risk in Young Finns Study, and Bogalusa Heart Study. *Circulation* 117 (1): 32–42.

National Cholesterol Education Program (2002). Third report of the National Cholesterol Education Program (NCEP) expert panel on detection, evaluation, and treatment of high blood cholesterol in adults (adult treatment panel III) final report. *Circulation* 106 (25): 3143–3421.

Nordestgaard, B.G., Chapman, M.J., Humphries, S.E. et al. (2013). Familial hypercholesterolaemia is underdiagnosed and undertreated in the general population: guidance for clinicians to prevent coronary heart disease: consensus statement of the European Atherosclerosis Society [published correction appears in *Eur. Heart J.* 2020;41 (47):4517]. *Eur. Heart J.* **34** (45): 3478–3490a. https://doi.org/10.1093/eurheartj/eht273.

US Preventive Services Task Force, Bibbins-Domingo, K., Grossman, D.C. et al. (2016). Screening for lipid disorders in children and adolescents: US Preventive Services task force recommendation statement [published correction appears in *JAMA* **316** (10):1116]. *JAMA* **316** (6): 625–633. http://dx.doi.org/10.1001/jama.2016.9852. www.uspreventiveservicestaskforce. org. (accessed 12 March 2022).

Obesity

Barlow, S.E. and Expert Committee (2007). Expert Committee recommendations regarding the prevention, assessment, and treatment of child and adolescent overweight and obesity: summary report. *Pediatrics* **120** (Suppl. 4): S164–S192.

Centers for Disease Control and Prevention (2022). *Body Mass Index-for-Age* (including CDC and WHO pediatric growth charts). http://www.cdc.gov/growthcharts (accessed 12 March 2022).

Jebeile, H., Kelly, A.S., O'Malley, G., and Baur, L.A. (2022). Obesity in children and adolescents: epidemiology, causes, assessment, and management. *Lancet Diabetes Endocrinol.* **10** (5): 351–365. https://doi.org/10.1016/S2213-8587(22)00047-X.

US Preventive Services Task Force, Grossman, D.C., Bibbins-Domingo, K. et al. (2017). Screening for obesity in children and adolescents: US Preventive Services task force recommendation statement. *JAMA* **317** (23): 2417–2426. http://dx.doi.org/10.1001/jama.2017.6803, www.uspreventiveservicestaskforce.org. (accessed 12 March 2022).

Tobacco

Fiore, M.C., Bailey, W.C., Cohen, S.J., et al. (2008). *Treating Tobacco Use and Dependence: 2008 Update. Clinical Practice Guideline.* US Department of Health and Human Services, Public Health Service, Rockville, MD. www.surgeongeneral.gov (accessed 12 March 2022).

US Department of Health and Human Services (2012). *Preventing Tobacco Use Among Youth and Young Adults. A Report of the Surgeon General.* US Department of Health and Human Services, Centers for Disease Control and Prevention, National Center for Chronic Disease Prevention and Health Promotion, Office on Smoking and Health, Atlanta, GA. www.surgeongeneral.gov (accessed 12 March 2022).

US Department of Health and Human Services (2016). *E-Cigarette Use Among Youth and Young Adults. A Report of the Surgeon General.* US Department of Health and Human Services, Centers for Disease Control and Prevention, National Center for Chronic Disease Prevention and Health Promotion, Office on Smoking and Health, Atlanta, GA. www.surgeongeneral.gov (accessed 12 March 2022).

Sports and heart conditions

Budts, W., Pieles, G.E., Roos-Hesselink, J.W. et al. (2020). Recommendations for participation in competitive sport in adolescent and adult athletes with congenital heart disease (CHD): position statement of the Sports Cardiology & Exercise Section of the European Association of Preventive Cardiology (EAPC), the European Society of Cardiology (ESC) Working Group on Adult Congenital Heart Disease and the Sports Cardiology, Physical Activity and Prevention Working Group of the Association for European Paediatric and Congenital Cardiology (AEPC). *Eur. Heart J.* **41** (43): 4191–4199. https://doi.org/10.1093/eurheartj/ehaa501.

Maron, B.J., Thompson, P.D., Ackerman, M.J. et al. (2007). Recommendations and considerations related to preparticipation screening for cardiovascular abnormalities in competitive athletes: 2007 update. A scientific statement from the American Heart Association Council on Nutrition, Physical Activity, and Metabolism: endorsed by the American College of Cardiology Foundation. *Circulation* **115** (12): 1643–1655.

Maron, B.J., Udelson, J.E., Bonow, R.O. et al. (2015). Eligibility and disqualification recommendations for competitive athletes with cardiovascular abnormalities: a scientific statement from the American Heart Association and American College of Cardiology. *J. Am. Coll. Cardiol.* **66** (21): 2343–2450; and *Circulation* **132** (22):e256–e349.

Mont, L., Pelliccia, A., Sharma, S. et al. (2017). Pre-participation cardiovascular evaluation for athletic participants to prevent sudden death: position paper from the EHRA and the EACPR, branches of the ESC. Endorsed by APHRS, HRS, and SOLAECE. *Eur. J. Prev. Cardiol.* **24** (1): 41–69. https://doi.org/10.1177/2047487316676042.

Oswald, D., Dvorak, J., Corrado, D. et al. (2004). *Sudden Cardiovascular Death in Sport Lausanne Recommendations: Preparticipation Cardiovascular Screening.* Lausanne: International Olympic Committee.

Pelliccia, A., Sharma, S., Gati, S. et al. (2021). 2020 ESC guidelines on sports cardiology and exercise in patients with cardiovascular disease [published correction appears in *Eur Heart J.* **42** (5):548–549]. *Eur. Heart J.* **42** (1): 17–96. https://doi.org/10.1093/eurheartj/ehaa605.

Altitude and air travel

Luks, A.M. and Hackett, P.H. (2022). Medical conditions and high-altitude travel. *N. Engl. J. Med.* **386**: 364–373. https://doi.org/10.1056/NEJMra2104829.

Smith, D., Toff, W., Joy, M. et al. (2010). Fitness to fly for passengers with cardiovascular disease. *Heart* **96** (Suppl. 2): ii1–ii16.

Endocarditis prevention

Habib, G., Hoen, B., Tornos, P. et al. (2009). Guidelines on the prevention, diagnosis, and treatment of infective endocarditis (new version 2009): the task force on the prevention, diagnosis, and treatment of infective endocarditis of the European Society of Cardiology (ESC). Endorsed by the European Society of Clinical Microbiology and Infectious Diseases (ESCMID) and the International Society of Chemotherapy (ISC) for infection and cancer. *Eur. Heart J.* **30** (19): 2369–2413.

NICE (2008). *Prophylaxis Against Infective Endocarditis.* NICE Clinical Guideline No. 64. National Institute for Health and Clinical Excellence, London. http://www.nice.org.uk/cg064.

Wilson, W., Taubert, K.A., Gewitz, M. et al. (2007). Prevention of infective endocarditis: guidelines from the American Heart Association. A guideline from the American Heart Association Rheumatic Fever, Endocarditis and Kawasaki Disease Committee, Council on Cardiovascular Disease in the Young, and the Council on Clinical Cardiology, Council on

Cardiovascular Surgery and Anesthesia, and the Quality of Care and Outcomes Research Interdisciplinary Working Group [published erratum appears in *Circulation* 116 (15):e376–e377]. *Circulation* 116 (15): 1736–1754.

Adults with congenital heart disease

Baumgartner, H., De Backer, J., Babu-Narayan, S.V. et al. (2021). 2020 ESC guidelines for the management of adult congenital heart disease. *Eur. Heart J.* 42 (6): 563–645. https://doi.org/10.1093/eurheartj/ehaa554. PMID: 32860028.

Gatzoulis, M.A., Swan, L., Therrien, J., and Pantely, G.A. (2005). *Adult Congenital Heart Disease: A Practical Guide*. Oxford: Wiley Blackwell.

John, A.S., Jackson, J.L., Moons, P. et al. (2022). Advances in managing transition to adulthood for adolescents with congenital heart disease: a practical approach to transition program design: a scientific statement from the American Heart Association. *J. Am. Heart Assoc.* 2022: e025278. https://doi.org/10.1161/JAHA.122.025278.

Sable, C., Foster, E., Uzark, K. et al. (2011). Best practices in managing transition to adulthood for adolescents with congenital heart disease: the transition process and medical and psychosocial issues: a scientific statement from the American Heart Association. *Circulation* 123 (13): 1454–1485. https://doi.org/10.1161/CIR.0b013e3182107c56.

Stout, K.K., Daniels, C.J., Aboulhosn, I.A. et al. (2019). AHA/ACC guideline for the management of adults with congenital heart disease: a report of the American College of Cardiology/American Heart Association task force on clinical practice guidelines [published correction appears in *Circulation* 139 (14):e833–e834]. *Circulation* 139 (14): e698–e800. https://doi.org/10.1161/CIR.0000000000000603.

Additional reading

The following are encyclopedic reference works covering all aspects of pediatric cardiology:

Moller, J.H. and Hoffman, J.I.E. (ed.) (2012). *Pediatric Cardiovascular Medicine*, 2e. Oxford: Wiley Blackwell www.mollerandhoffmantext.com (accessed 23 March 2022).

Shaddy, R.E., Penny, D.J., Feltes, T.F. et al. (ed.) (2021). *Moss and Adams' Heart Disease in Infants, Children, and Adolescents Including the Fetus and Young Adult*, 10e. Philadelphia, PA: Lippincott Williams and Wilkins.

Wernovsky, G., Anderson, R.H., Kumar, K. et al. (ed.) (2020). *Anderson's Paediatric Cardiology*, 4e. Philadelphia, PA: Elsevier.

Index